YOGA

FOR THE

HEART

AND CIRCULATION

YOGA
FOR THE
HEART
AND CIRCULATION

Shashi K. Agarwal, MD

First Edition

Disclaimer

This book presents research information on the role of yoga in heart and vascular health and illness. Readers should be aware that knowledge of medicine is constantly evolving. This book is not intended as a substitute for the medical advice of your physicians or other trained health care professional.

Do not disregard professional medical advice or delay seeking it because of something you have read in this book. Do not stop taking any medicines. Do not embark on any lifestyle change without seeking your health care provider's advice. It is clinicians' responsibility, relying on their experience and knowledge of their patients, to determine the best plan of care, including lifestyle change advice.

Reviewing or following information contained on this book, does not constitute a physician-patient relationship. The authors, editors, and publisher accept no liability for any injury arising out of the use of material contained herein, and make no warranty, express or implied, with respect to the contents of this publication.

Copyright © 2019 Shashi K. Agarwal, MD
All rights reserved.
ISBN - 9781095383179

CONTENTS

Introduction	7
What is Yoga?	9
The Heart and the Vascular System	14
Prophylactic and Therapeutic Benefits of Yoga on the Heart and the Vascular System	20

1. Alcohol — 21
2. Alcoholism/Alcohol Abuse — 24
3. Anti-oxidants — 25
4. Atherosclerosis — 26
5. Autonomic Nervous System — 28
6. Biochemicals — 31
7. Blood Pressure/Hypertension — 40
8. Blood Sugar/Diabetes — 44
9. Cardiac Arrythmias — 49
10. Cardiac Output — 50
11. Cardiac Rehabilitation — 51
12. Congestive Heart Failure — 52
13. Coronary Artery Disease — 54
14. Diet — 57
15. Drug Abuse/Addiction — 62
16. Erectile Dysfunction — 63
17. Exercise — 65
18. Heart Rate — 68
19. Heart Rate Variability — 70
20. Lipids — 72
21. Lymphedema — 77
22. Metabolic Syndrome — 78
23. Negative Emotions — 80
24. Obesity — 85
25. Peripheral Artery Disease — 89
26. Positivity/Happiness/Laughter — 90
27. Sedentary Behavior/Excessive Sitting — 92
28. Sleep — 94
29. Smoking/Tobacco Use — 97
30. Social Isolation/Loneliness — 101
31. Spirituality — 103
32. Stroke — 104
33. Stroke Rehabilitation — 105
34. Vascular Dementia — 107
35. Vascular Elasticity — 108

36. Vascular Inflammation	110
37. Venous Diseases	112
38. Other Cardio-vasculo-protective Lifestyles	116

Yoga program for the Heart and Vascular System — 124

1. Opening Prayer — 125
2. Loosening Exercises — 126
3. *Asanas* — 129
4. *Pranayama* — 158
5. *Dhyana* — 161
6. Yoga *Nidra* — 164
7. Closing Prayer — 167

Yogic Lifestyle — 168

Yoga and Safety — 171

Closing Remarks — 176

Appendix — 178

Glossary — 191

References — 198

Resources — 333

INTRODUCTION

Cardiovascular disease is the number one killer worldwide. The data shows that globally (in 2013), 31 percent of all deaths were due to cardio-vascular diseases, with 80 percent of these deaths occurring in low- and middle-income countries. Stroke (a neuro-vascular disease) accounted for 11.8 percent of these deaths. Other vascular diseases that commonly affect humans are peripheral artery disease, venous diseases of the legs, lymphedema and erectile dysfunction.

USA has a large population with vascular disease. According to data released by the American Heart Association, in 2016, nearly half of all adults in the United States in 2016 — 48% or 121.5 million — had some form of heart, cardiovascular or neurovascular disease - these include coronary artery disease, heart failure, and stroke.

Cardiovascular disease (and stroke) is also a major killer in the USA. Coronary heart disease (43.8%) is the leading cause of deaths attributable to cardiovascular disease (CVD) in the US, followed by stroke (16.8%), high blood pressure (9.4%), heart failure (9.0%), and other CVDs (17.9%).[1]

Life style appears to play an important role in vascular health and disease. According to the World Health Organization (WHO), 60% of related factors to individual health and quality of life are related to lifestyle.[2] Estimates suggest that 9 out of 10 Americans lead a poor lifestyle.

Healthy lifestyles not only help prevent non-fatal heart attacks and strokes, but also decrease fatal cardiovascular events. In a recent study involving 58,319 women in the Nurses' Health Study (1984-2010) and 29,854 men in the Health Professionals' Follow-up Study (1986-2010), nine unhealthy lifestyles resulted in an increase of death from cardiovascular diseases by 2.85 times, death due to coronary heart disease by 3,37 times and death due to stroke by 1.75 times.

Healthy lifestyles also prolong life. In a recent study, researchers from Harvard T.H. Chan School of Public Health looked at 34 years of data from 78,865 women in the Nurses' Health Study and 27 years of data from 44,354 men in the Health Professionals Follow-up Study and found that women with five healthy lifestyles gained, on average, 14 years of life, and men, 12 years of life, when compared with those with unhealthy lifestyles.

Yoga has demonstrated beneficial effects not only for general health, but also in several disease processes. Yoga also encourages a healthy lifestyle.

This book presents scientific studies that have demonstrated benefits of yoga practice in the prevention and adjunct management of diseases of the heart and circulation.

This book also presents a simple, illustrated one-hour yoga practice, which along with a healthy 'yogic' life-style, will positively impact your 'heart and circulation' health. Incorporating the yoga practice and lifestyle changes gradually, you will not only live a healthier and better life but also a longer life – your lifespan should increase by several years.

Shashi K. Agarwal, MD

WHAT IS YOGA?

"Yoga chitta vritti nirodha"
Yoga is the cessation of the fluctuations of the mind

Several millennia ago, astute human ancestors recognized the health benefits of engaging the body in several physical postures – as an exercise. These series of poses were devised by watching living things, especially animals, and many poses are therefore named after them. This knowledge was transferred from generation to generation verbally and via physical illustration. These practices, along with breathing exercises and meditation, would, after several thousand years, become united under the term 'yoga'. The term "yoga," is found in ancient India's earliest known scripts — the Vedas.

"Yujyate anena iti yogah"
That which joins is Yoga

These writings (the Vedas) date from the Vedic period, which began in 1500 BCE. They are composed in Vedic Sanskrit and are the oldest writings of Hinduism and Sanskrit literature. The word 'yoga' means 'to join' or 'to yoke' or 'to unite' and is derived from the Sanskrit root '*yuj*'. According to the sages, yoga unites the human consciousness with that of the Universal Consciousness. This leads to a perfect harmony between the mind and body, and the humans and nature.

Several ancient Indian scriptures allude to various aspects of yoga practice – these include the Bhagvad Gita, Upanishads, Yoga Vasishta, Hatha Yoga Pradeepika, Gheranda Samhita, Siva Samhita and the Puranas. Some notable sayings from these:

Bhagvad Gita*: "Yogah Karmasu Kaushalam"* = yoga is dexterity in action.

Kathopanisad (Upnishad): *"Tam yogamiti manyante sthiramindriyadharanam"* = yoga allows the *indriyas* (or the senses) to be held steadily.

Yoga Vasishta: *"Manah prashamana Upaya yoga ityabhidhiyate"* = yoga skillfully calms the mind.

Hath Yoga Pradeepika: *"kuryāttad āsanaṃ sthairyam ārogyaṃ ca aṅga lāghavan"* = *asana* practice brings steadiness, reduced illness and a lightness of limb.

Gheranda Samhita: *"Abhya satkardi varnana, yatha shasvani bodhyet, tatha yoga samasadh tatvagyan cha labhyate"* = just as one learns the alphabet to read and understand the scriptural teachings, so can one learn about the ultimate reality by practicing yoga.

Siva Samhita: *'Ek gyan nitya madhant shunya, nanat kichdwate te vastu satyam, yandosmi trindriyopadhina vaye gyanasya bhaste nanyathev"* = *jnana* (gnosis) is the only thing eternal and is without beginning and without an end. There is no other substance except sense related illusions.

Puranas: "*aham mamabhimanotthaih, kama-lobhadibhir malaih, vitam yada manah suddham, aduhkham asukham samam*"= When one is completely cleansed of the impurities of lust and greed produced from the false identification of the body as "I" and bodily possessions as "mine," one's mind becomes purified. In that pure state he transcends the stage of so-called material happiness and distress.

Patanjali, often considered the father of yoga, systematically organized (approximately 1700 years ago) this ancient knowledge into aphorisms, collectively known as the' Yoga-Sûtras' (*sutra* = a rule or aphorism).

> *"The five points of yama, together with the five points of niyama, remind us of the Ten Commandments of the Christian and Jewish faiths, as well as of the ten virtues of Buddhism. In fact, there is no religion without these moral or ethical codes. All spiritual life should be based on these things. They are the foundation stones without which we can never build anything lasting."*

Swami Satchidananda, The Yoga Sutras

This compilation of yoga in Sanskrit contains 196 sutras. These sutras lay out an 8-limb path of yoga, with details of how to practice, ways to treat oneself, ways to treat others and guidance to remain on the path of spirituality. These limbs are *yama* (morality), *niyama* (personal observances) *asanas* (postures), *pranayama* (breathing exercises), *dharna* (concentration), *dhyana* (meditation) and *samadhi* (union with the divine) – these are described in more detail in the chapter on yogic philosophy.

Modern yoga is based on these sutras. Yoga was introduced to the West in the late 1800s and early 1900s by yogic '*gurus*' from India. Swami Vivekananda in the late 19th and early 20th century made an important contribution towards this. Swami Vivekananda and Sri Aurobindo clarified the concept of yoga philosophy, and its benefit to the human life. Swami Sivananda, an Indian yogi, commercialized yoga in the West through his English-language publications and Divine Life Society in the 1930s.[1]

The real popularity of yoga in the US started after Indra Devi (a Russian yoga teacher) opened her yoga studio in Hollywood in 1947. In the early 1950s, yoga studios started opening across the USA. Theos Bernard's 'Hatha Yoga: The Report of a Personal Experience', became a 'major sourcebook' for yoga practitioners in the 1950s.[2] Charismatic Indian gurus, started teaching yoga devoid of a religious connection. In 1961, Richard Hittleman brought 'non-religious yoga...with an emphasis on its physical benefits' into America's living rooms via the TV.[3] Yoga gradually became mainstream in the USA.[4]

Today, yoga is a popular system of physical exercise across the Western world.

As practiced in the West, 'multimodal yoga' usually is done in classes and incorporates three processes: postures, breathing exercises and meditation. Most yoga sessions last about an hour and despite the workout, are relaxing and invigorating. They are often practiced with soft background yoga music, and with the room filled with a pleasant aroma. Yoga retreats are also very popular – they take the practitioners away from the hustle and bustle of daily life, usually immerse them in nature, and are even more beneficial to the health than attending intermittent sessions in a city class. Schmidt and colleagues[5] evaluated cardiovascular risk factors in subjects who stayed in a yoga training center. The participants had only vegetarian nutrition. Following 3 months of stay in yoga retreat, there was a significant reduction in body mass index, total- and LDL-cholesterol, fibrinogen and blood pressure, especially in those with elevated levels.

The number of adult yoga practitioners in the US exceeds 13 million.[6] It is a popular CAM (Complementary and Alternative Medicine) modality among lay population.[7] The medical community all over the world has also recognized that yoga practice is associated with a plethora of health benefits. Noting its blossoming popularity, and validation of its evidence-based health benefits, the United Nations General Assembly proclaimed every June 21 as the International Yoga Day.

Yoga is a low-impact, low-intensity exercise.[8] It is simple and easy to do.[9] It is non-competitive. It can be practiced in a non-secular way.[10] It can be done by all communities, irrespective of the race or income.[11-13] Its practice is feasible in both physically disabled[14] and mentally challenged people.[15] It can also be done by those with low vision or blind people.[16] It is non-pharmacological and non-surgical. It does not require any special equipment – except maybe a mat. It can however be done without a mat – on a carpet, the grass or even the sand.[17] It can be individually tailored, especially for the seniors.[18] It is inexpensive and is a potential attractive cost-effective adjunct to many traditional medical therapies. (compared to pharmaceutical or surgical interventions). Serious complications are rare.[19] It can be done at any time, including during working hours.[20] Its practice is possible in all age groups.[21-24] Adherence is good[25] with only a few drop outs. One study in adults reported an attrition rate of only 16%.[26] This compares to an attrition rate of 30% in a study which involved walking and balance exercises.[27] Increasing scientific evidence, also confirms its therapeutic feasibility in many medical conditions.[28]

Yoga has no known interactions with prescription medications.[29] It can be practiced anywhere – home, club, airport, hotel, office – and even in prison.[30,31] Healthy yoga practitioners also tend to practice healthy lifestyles: levels of obesity (4.9%), smoking (2%), and fruit and vegetable consumption are favorable in yoga practitioners when compared to national norms.[32] Yoga practitioners report that the more yoga they do, the healthier they feel.[32] Length of lifetime yoga practice is significantly associated with better physical health, suggesting yoga has a potential cumulative benefit over time.[33] As mentioned earlier, emerging scientific data strongly indicates that healthier lifestyles have the potential to increase the human life span by as much as 12 years(*and probably more*).[34]

Common types of yoga practiced in the West

In the West, several 'forms' of yoga are advertised, and this can be confusing[30]. Basic explanation of some of these types is as follows:

Anusara yoga: Established by American-born yoga teacher John Friend in 1997 – it involves basic hatha yoga postures and emphasizes attitude, alignment, and action.

Ashtanga yoga: Founded by K. Pattabhi Jois, ashtanga yoga is a dynamic, physically demanding practice (will make you sweat) – it synchronizes breath and movement. The series of postures help build core muscles and tone the entire body.

Bikram Yoga: Consists of a series of 26 postures and two breathing exercises performed in a room heated to 35–42 °C (95–108 °F) with a humidity of 40%.

Hatha yoga: The most common form of yoga – it incorporates postures, regulated breathing, and meditation.

Iyengar yoga: This form of hath yoga focuses on the precise structural alignment of postures.

Jivamukti yoga: Physically challenging postures combining other ethical principles of yoga: *shastra* (scripture), *bhakti* (devotion), *ahimsā* (nonviolence, non-harming), *nāda* (music), and *dhyana* (meditation).

Kundalini yoga: It primarily focuses on awakening the *kundalini* energy via a practice of meditation, *pranayama*, chanting mantra and yoga *asanas*.

Kripalu yoga: It stresses willful practice, willful surrender, willful meditation and willful relaxation.

Sivananda yoga: This yoga practice consists of *Kapalbhati* and *Anuloma-Viloma* breathing, followed by Surya namaskar and 12 basic yoga postures. It also emphasizes proper relaxation, proper diet and positive thinking and proper meditation.

Yin yoga: In Yin yoga, the poses are held for held for longer periods of time - from 45 seconds to two minutes. It is a slow-paced practice.

Multi-modal yoga

Irrespective of the style, most yoga centers and retreats in the West practice 'multi-modal' yoga:

Opening prayers
Loosening exercises
Asanas (fast and slow poses)

Pranayamas (breathing exercises
Dhyana (meditation)
Yoga *Nidra* (relaxation)
Closing prayers

There may also be lectures on yogic philosophy and yogic lifestyle. Some centers may also incorporate group meditative chanting or music/singing classes.

The above modalities are usually done together – hence the entire practice is often called 'multi-modal' yoga. The increasing health benefits of multi-modal yoga are numerous and are seen in healthy individuals as well as those suffering from disease. The health benefits of individual yoga modalities and multi-modal yoga are enumerated in the appendix.

Throughout this book, health benefits will usually be limited to those derived from the practice of multi-modal yoga and involving the vascular systems – cardiovascular, neurovascular and peripheral vascular.

"Yoga is a benevolent friend that is always there to greet you with a smile."

David Swenson

THE HEART AND THE VASCULAR SYSTEM

CARDIOVASCULAR

Heart is the size of two fists if you are an adult. It weighs about eight ounces in women and about ten ounces in men. Circulates the blood around the body via the arteries and veins, delivering fresh oxygen and nutrients to organs and tissues and carrying away carbon dioxide and other waste products away. It also equalizes temperature in the body.

The heart has four chambers – the right and left atria and the right and left ventricles. The right atrium receives blood from the veins and pumps it to the right ventricle. The right ventricle receives blood from the right atrium and pumps it to the lungs, where it is loaded with oxygen. The left atrium receives oxygenated blood from the lungs and pumps it to the left ventricle. The left ventricle (the strongest chamber) pumps oxygen-rich blood to the rest of the body (and the heart tissues), via the aorta.

If you use an average of 80 beats per minute, your heart beats about 4,800 times per hour. The adult heart pumps five quarts of blood each minute throughout the body – adding up to approximately 2,000 gallons of blood each day.

Heart muscle:

The muscle of the heart (myocardium) is an involuntary striated (striped – under the microscope the appearance is dark (A-bands) and light (I-bands) bands) muscle which contracts to pump blood to the rest of the body. It is covered on the outside by the epicardium and on the inside by the endocardium. Cardiac muscle cells (cardiomyocytes) are typically unicellular (110 μm in length and 15 μm in width) and from sheets - an arrangement that enables the cardiac muscle to contract quickly, repeatedly, and non-stop, throughout our life. The heart muscle works as a unit (functional syncytium - millions of cells working together), getting its orders from a natural pacemaker in the right atrium, called the SA node (sinoatrial node).

The electrical system of the heart:

The SA node cells demonstrate auto-rhythmicity (normal heart beat generated is at a rate of 60-100 per minute), but also respond to signals from the autonomic nervous system (ANS) and various hormones – this makes them speed up or slow down the heart rate.

Each electrical impulse generated by the SA node spreads throughout the atria through specialized internodal pathways (anterior, middle, and posterior) and the AV node (atrioventricular node), in approximately 50 milliseconds. The electrical impulse can only pass to the ventricles via the atrio-ventricular node (AV node) (the cardiac skeleton prevents the impulse from spreading directly to the ventricles without passing through the AV node), which takes about 100 milliseconds. From here the impulse enters the atrioventricular bundle, or bundle of His. This specialized conducting tissue divides into two branches, appropriately called the left and right bundle branches and transmits the electrical impulse to the ventricles via the Purkinje fibers. It takes about 0.03–0.04 seconds for the impulse to travel from the bundle of His to the ventricular muscle (total time for the electrical impulse to travel from the SA node to the ventricles is approximately 225 ms) The left ventricle contracts an instant before the right ventricle. The contraction of the ventricles squeezes the blood out. The blood not only travels to the lungs from the right ventricle and to the rest of the body from the left ventricle – but also to the coronary arteries which nourish the heart structures, especially the heart muscle. Following this contraction, the walls of the ventricles relax and wait for the next electrical signal from the SA node. Each contraction of the ventricles represents one heartbeat.

The normal heart beat varies according to age:

0-3 months of age - 99-149 per minute

3-6 months of age – 89-119 per minute

6-12 months of age – 79-119 per minute

1-10 years of age - 69-129 per minute

10-adulthood – 60-100 per minute

The heart rate varies in response to the needs of the body's cells for oxygen and nutrients under varying conditions. It is controlled by the autonomic nervous system. The sympathetic system (fight and flight system) releases the hormones (epinephrine and norepinephrine) to accelerate the heart rate while the parasympathetic system (rest and digest system) releases the hormone acetylcholine to slow the heart rate. The sympathetic system is activated to increase the heart rate during exercise, emotional excitement, or under various pathological conditions (e.g., infections, heart failure). The parasympathetic system dominates during rest, sleep, or emotional tranquility, and helps keep the resting heart rate around 60-75 bpm. At any given time, the heart rate is determined by net balance between the opposing actions of the sympathetic and parasympathetic systems.

Cardiac Output:

Cardiac output is the amount of blood the heart pumps in 1 minute, and it is dependent on the heart rate, contractility and several peripheral regulatory mechanisms. It is expressed in liters/minute. For a healthy person weighing 154 lbs, the cardiac output at rest averages about 5 Liters/min - assuming a heart rate of 70 beats/min. The normal range for cardiac output is about 4 to 8 L/min, but it can vary depending on the body's metabolic needs. During exercise, cardiac output and oxygen consumption increase linearly with work rate.

The amount of blood pumped by each ventricle per beat is the stroke volume. Cardiac output is therefore equal to the product of the stroke volume and the number of beats per minute (heart rate). The average stroke volume for a 154 lbs (70kg) person is 70 ml per beat (between 60 and 130 mL/beat in healthy individuals).

Ejection fraction reflects the proportion of blood ejected with each heartbeat relative to total ventricular volume (measured in percent). The left ventricle pumps oxygenated blood to the rest of the body - ejection fraction is usually measured only in the left ventricle (LV). An LV ejection fraction of 55 percent or higher is considered normal.

An adequate cardiac output is necessary for adequate tissue perfusion and adequate oxygenation.

Heart Circulation:

The coronary arteries arise from the aorta (the main artery into which the blood is pumped by the left ventricle) and run along the surface of the heart and provide oxygen and nutrients to the heart muscle.

Right Coronary Artery (RCA): The RCA branches off the right aortic sinus (a dilation on the right just above the aortic valve) and travels down the groove between the right atrium and right ventricle. It supplies the AV Node, most of the right atrium and right ventricle, and the posterior third of the inter-ventricular septum. In about 50% of individuals, the SA node is also supplied by a branch from the RCA.

Left Coronary Artery (LCA): The LCA arises from the left aortic sinus (a dilation on the left just above the aortic valve) and travels down the groove between the left atrium and left ventricle. Its major branches are the anterior descending artery and the left circumflex artery. The LCA supplies the anterior two-thirds of the inter-ventricular septum, the left atrium, and most of the left ventricle.

The aorta also has a non-coronary sinus – a posterior dilation just above the aortic valve with no coronary arising from it. Together, these are called the sinuses of Valsalva.

Coronary Sinus: The coronary venous system drains the myocardium of oxygen-depleted blood via two systems of veins – the greater cardiac venous system uses the coronary sinus to drain into the right atrium while the smaller cardiac venous system, also known as the Thebesian vessels, drain directly into the respective chambers.

NEUROVASCULAR

In an adult, the brain is nourished by about 750 milliliters per minute of blood or 15% of the cardiac output. Arterial blood supply to the human brain is provided by two pairs of large arteries, the right and left internal carotid and the right and left vertebral arteries. The internal carotid arteries supply the anterior brain. The two vertebral arteries combine to form the basilar artery and together they supply the posterior brain – occipital lobes, cerebellum and the brain stem. The basilar artery joins the two internal carotid arteries to form a complete anastomotic ring at the base of the brain known as the circle of Willis. This circle gives rise to three pairs of main arteries, the anterior, middle, and posterior cerebral arteries, providing nourishment to the cerebrum. The middle cerebral artery supplies a large territory of the cerebral cortex. These arteries give rise to pial arteries and arterioles that run on the surface of the brain – they form a heavily interconnected network and give rise to penetrating arterioles which enter the substance of the brain, and to the brain's capillary network, which feeds into the venous system. Venous outflow from the cerebrum is via the superficial cortical veins and the deep or central veins, which eventually drain into the sigmoid sinuses. These go on to form the two jugular veins, which drain blood into the superior vena cava – and back to the right atrium.

PERIPHERAL VASCULAR

The heart generates the tremendous pressures necessary to actuate the flow of blood throughout the entire circulation. From the heart, blood enters arteries which progressively branch and become narrower. This branching pattern is true of both the systemic and pulmonary circulations.

Arteries

The arteries are designed to rapidly conduct pressurized blood downstream within the circulation without significant loss of blood pressure.

Arterioles

Arterioles are the final and smallest branches of the arterial system and are the primary regulators of blood flow to downstream capillaries. When arterioles are dilated, the downstream capillary bed can receive large amounts of blood flow. However, if arterioles are constricted, blood flow through the downstream capillaries can be tremendously limited.

Capillaries

Capillaries are the primary location in which exchange of nutrients, metabolites, and waste products occurs between the blood and the tissues. Capillaries are very thin, approximately 5 micrometers in diameter, and are composed of only two layers of cells; an inner layer of endothelial cells and an outer layer of epithelial cells. They are so small that red blood cells need to flow through them in a single file. If all the capillaries in the human body were lined up in single file, the line would stretch over 100,000 miles. It's been estimated that there are 40 billion capillaries in the average human body. Surrounding the outer layer of cells is something called the basement membrane, a layer of protein surrounding the capillary. The capillaries are responsible for facilitating the transport and exchange of gases, fluids, and nutrients in the body. While the arteries and arterioles act to transport these products to the capillaries, it is at the level of capillaries where the exchange takes place.

Venules

Capillary converge on one another and form venules which drain the blood from capillary beds and conduct the blood to larger veins.

Veins

Veins are designed to conduct blood at low pressures back to the heart for oxygenation (via the lungs), re-pressurization and recirculation. Veins also act as important reservoirs for spare blood volume which can be rapidly called upon to meet physiological demands. Veins bring oxygen-depleted blood from the organs and tissues to the heart and lungs, where it is re-oxygenated. Blood return to the heart tends to be passive and is enabled by muscle contraction in the arms and legs. The venous system is a low pressure one.

The system of blood vessels – arteries, veins and capillaries – is over 60,000 miles long. That's long enough to go around the world more than twice! In one day, the blood travels a total of 12,000 miles – which is roughly four times the distance across the U.S. from coast to coast.

Lymphatics

Lymphatic vessels serve as conduits for return of protein and particle-laden interstitial fluid back to the circulation. These vessels direct this fluid through a series of lymph nodes and in doing so play an important anatomical role in the physiological immune function.

The architecture of lymphatic vessels allows for unidirectional entry of fluid along with high molecular weight proteins and particulates (especially nutrients from the intestinal tract) that would normally not be able to cross blood vessels. This is a result of the loose connections between certain lymphatic endothelial cells that result in the creation of large inter-cellular flaps. Fluid and particles can enter the lymphatic vessel through the flaps but cannot exit, thus creating a one-way valve.

Lymph fluid flows from the ends of lymphatic capillaries into progressively larger lymphatic vessels that ultimately combine to form the thoracic duct. The phenomenon which appears to actuate lymphatic flow from the interstitium back to the vasculature appears to be intermittent squeezing of lymphatic capillaries by surrounding muscles. Because lymphatic vessels possess intra-vascular unidirectional valves, like those found in veins, squeezing of the lymphatic vessel tends to cause directional flow toward the vasculature. Lymph vessels also remove excess fluid and waste from tissues and transport it back to the circulation. Lymph capillaries are like a cobweb in the skin - they drain to lymphatic vessels in the subcutaneous plane and ultimately to the deeper system and finally the thoracic duct. The thoracic duct is the main lymphatic channel for the return of chyle (the milky fluid containing emulsified fat and other products of digestion, to the left subclavian vein. It drains lymph from both lower limbs, abdomen (except the convex area of the liver), left hemithorax, left upper limb and left face and neck. The right lymphatic duct drains the right side of the thorax, right upper extremity, and right side of the neck and head. It usually empties into the right subclavian vein, the internal jugular vein, or the union of the two. The lymph nodes in our body drain into these lymphatic ducts. Maturation of immune cells takes place in the lymphatic system – this system is thus a major and critical defense mechanism in the human body.

Erectile Circulation

Erectile function is dependent on three physiologic mechanisms - neurogenic, arteriogenic, and venogenic. The neurogenic stimulus for erection either comes via the supraspinal centers (central nervous system) or stimulation of the dorsal nerve (peripheral nervous system).

The descending aorta divides into left and right common iliac arteries which in turn give rise to the internal iliac artery. A branch of this artery, the internal pudendal artery, gives rise to a penile artery. Since there are two internal iliac arteries, the penile arteries are paired. The penile artery has four terminal branches: the cavernous, dorsal, bulbar, and urethral arteries. When stimulated, there are several biochemicals released, the most important one being nitric oxide. This induces the production of the second messenger cyclic guanosine monophosphate, and there is a relaxation of the smooth muscle of the arteries. Blood moves in to the corpora cavernosa, raising the intra-cavernous pressure up to three to four times - leading to penile erection.

Venous outflow results from post cavernous venules, which form emissary veins and drain into the cavernous, the deep dorsal, and the superficial dorsal veins. These drain into the corresponding superficial external pudendal vein, a tributary of the great saphenous vein. Efficient veno-occlusion helps hold the blood in the penile corpora cavernosa during penile erection.

PROPHYLACTIC AND THERAPEUTIC BENEFITS OF YOGA ON THE HEART AND THE VASCULAR SYSTEM

The scientific literature on the effects of yoga practice on the heart and the circulatory system has exploded in the past decade or so. It is virtually impossible to refer to every published study on this topic – so I have elected to list only some illustrative studies that accomplish the aim – to provide evidence based data supporting the beneficial effects of yoga practice on these organs, both during healthy states as well during disease states. Since the heart muscle is the main pump responsible for the circulation, heart muscle disease affected by yoga, such as heart failure, and irregular heart function due to electrical abnormalities such as cardiac arrhythmias, are also included.

I frequently refer to the kind of study in providing evidence-based support to the vascular benefits of yoga – a brief definition of commonly used studies:

Meta-analysis: This provides a formal statistical analysis that integrates the quantitative results of several independent studies – providing a true 'evidence based' result.[1]

Review article: A systematic review article is a very detailed and comprehensive literature surveying on the selected topic.[2]

Randomized controlled trial: Randomized controlled clinical trials (RCTs) are the gold standard for ascertaining the efficacy and safety of a treatment – and can demonstrate the superiority of a new treatment over an existing standard treatment or a placebo.[3] Subjects are allocated randomly into a control group and or an intervention group.

Observational studies: Reports of observations without any intervention. These include cohort studies, case-control studies and cross-sectional studies.[4]

The scientific data keeps changing as more studies come in, so some tweaking may be needed. In general, the associations and trends do not change significantly over time.

1. Alcohol

Drinking an alcoholic beverage in a common social practice in many parts of the world. Drinking alcohol in mild to moderate quantities has been associated with some health benefits.[1]

Frequent alcohol intake is related to a lower prevalence of common cold episodes.[2,3] Alcohol intake reduces the risk of gall bladder stones.[4,5] Drinking alcohol in moderation also helps improve insulin resistance[6,7] and reduce diabetes mellitus.[8,9] In a meta-analysis (15 original prospective cohort studies) a 30% reduced risk of type 2 diabetes was found with moderate drinking (0.5-4 drinks a day) in 369,862 participants followed for an average of 12 years.[8] Recent meta-analytic studies have confirmed the protective effects of alcohol on the insulin and glycemic profile.[9]

Besides the effects of alcohol on lowering diabetes, alcohol intake also reduces several other risk factors for atherosclerotic vascular disease. These include raising the protective high-density lipoprotein cholesterol (the 'good cholesterol')[10,11] and decreasing the harmful oxidation of the low-density lipoprotein cholesterol (the 'bad' cholesterol).[12] It also decreases the levels of fibrinogen, thereby protecting against blood clots. There is decreased tendency for platelets to aggregate and there is an increased blood flow to the heart.[13,14] Alcohol also increases insulin sensitivity (as mentioned above) and this mechanism may be active in the suppression of atherosclerosis by alcohol drinking.[15] Alcohol also exerts several other protective effects on the vasculature, and these include increased nitric oxide bioavailability,[16] increase in circulating bone marrow-derived endothelial progenitor cells which reduce atherosclerosis,[17,18] improved prooxidant/antioxidant balance,[19] and reduced levels of inflammation.[20]

Moderate drinking - up to 1 drink per day for women and up to 2 drinks per day for men, is associated with a decreased risk of heart disease, stroke, diabetes mellitus – and death.[21-25] A standard drink in the US is considered to be approximately a 12-US-fluid-ounce (350 ml) glass of beer, 8-9 oz. of malt liquor, a 5-US-fluid-ounce (150 ml) glass of wine, 3-4 oz. of fortified wine, 2-3 oz. of a cordial, a 1.5-US-fluid-ounce (44 ml) glass of a 80 US proof spirit or a 1 oz. of 100-proof spirits. It has 0.6 ounces (18ml) of alcohol.[26]

Researchers from the University of Calgary, University of Texas Health Science Center, and Harvard Medical School identified 4,235 studies dealing with the effects of alcohol on the cardiovascular system. These studies included more than two million men and women who were followed for an average of 11 years. They concluded that when compared with no alcohol use, moderate alcohol use reduced the risk of a new diagnosis of coronary artery disease by 29%.[27] In this study mortality was also reduced – moderate alcohol used reduced the risk of dying from any cardiovascular disease by 25%, reduced the risk of dying from a heart attack or coronary artery disease by 25% and reduced the risk of dying from any cause by 13%. A subsequent meta-analysis suggests that women with moderate (to heavy) alcohol intake may have a higher risk of total mortality compared with men.[28]

Alcohol intake in moderate amounts also appears to be beneficial in reducing heart failure.[29-32] The incidence of stroke is also affected - ischemic stroke is reduced by 8% - however, hemorrhagic (bleeding) stroke incidence increases by 14%.[27]

A recent study has illustrated that the benefits of moderate drinking are not universal. Alcohol intake even in small amounts (especially in those with low socio-demographic index) is associated with an increased occurrence of tuberculosis, road accidents, self-harm, cancers, alcohol-attributable deaths and disability-adjusted life-years, in low socio-demographic index countries. (socio-demographic index is a summary measure of overall development, based on educational attainment, fertility, and income per capita within a location).[33] The benefits from moderate alcohol intake (for example in ischemic heart disease) in societies with high socio-demographic index, were however, confirmed.[33]

Alcohol intake is associated with a J or U-shaped curve as far as vascular system is concerned – moderate drinkers exhibit less risk for adverse events (heart attack/stroke) and less overall mortality than abstainers, while heavy drinkers demonstrate an increased risk.[34] Exceeding the recommended limits of alcohol intake may cause serious vascular health problems, including high blood pressure,[35] coronary heart disease[36] and heart failure.[37] Heavy drinking can also lead to an increased risk of all kinds of strokes.[38] Other serious cardiovascular conditions that excessive alcohol intake can cause include cardiomyopathy,[39] cardiac arrhythmias[40] and sudden cardiac death.[41]

Vascular dementia

Dementia (including vascular) is reduced with reliable benefits within the moderate range of alcohol intake.[42,43] This may be related to the atherosclerotic reducing effects of alcohol,[44] although many other factors may also be playing a role. However, alcohol is damaging to the brain in excess. The neurotoxicity of alcohol was recognized by Sabia and group, who reported increased levels of dementia with excessive alcohol consumption - moderate alcohol consumption was associated with a lower risk of dementia compared to those abstaining from drinking.[45]

Peripheral arterial disease

Alcohol also helps prevent peripheral artery disease - the risk is lower in light-to-moderate drinkers than in abstainers.[46-49]

A recent study (14,082 participants enrolled in the Atherosclerosis Risk in Communities Study - mean follow-up of 19.9 years) indicated that compared with those who drank no alcohol, those who had 1–6 drinks/week had a lower risk of developing incident peripheral artery disease.[50] Moreover, drinkers with PAD reportedly showed lower mortality than did nondrinkers with PAD. On the other hand, heavy drinking has been reported to be positively associated with the risk of PAD.[51]

Erectile dysfunction

Alcohol abuse is a leading cause of impotence and other sexual disturbances.[52-54] Alcohol is known to affect virtually all aspects of the human sexual response, especially sexual desire and erection.[55] Vijayasenan[56] found that of 97 male inpatients admitted for the treatment of alcoholism, 71% suffered from sexual dysfunction for a period of more than 12 months prior to admission to a hospital. The disturbances noted in this study included diminished sexual desire (58%), ejaculatory incompetence (22%), erectile impotence (16%) and premature ejaculation (4%).

Varicose veins

Ahti and group reported an increase in the incidence of new varicose veins in 2,202 individuals with regular alcohol intake.[57] However, there is a beneficial connection with deep vein thrombosis – low to moderate alcohol consumption is associated with a decreased risk of DVT. [58-60]

Yoga and alcohol

Alcohol may be frowned upon by Yoga - Chapter 1, verse 59 of the Hatha Yoga Pradipika, lists alcohol as one of the foods to be avoided by the yogi.

However, it appears that the evidence based medical data is persuasive, and most yoga practitioners continue to drink moderate amounts of alcohol, especially in the West, where data is available.

In a study of 4,307 randomly selected individuals from 15 US Iyengar yoga studios (n = 18,160), representing 41 states; 1,087 individuals responded, with 1045 (24.3%) surveys completed.[61] In the respondents, 69.7% of the yoga practitioners claimed that they drank alcohol, compared to 64.5% of the US national average. Almost one half of the respondents said that yoga practice did not affect their alcohol intake.

2. Alcoholism/Alcohol Abuse

Alcohol intake when in excess or associated with craving, inability to stop drinking, physical dependence characterized by withdrawal symptoms and gradual development of tolerance (the need to drink more and more to feel the same effect) – represents alcohol abuse disorder. Almost 6% of American adults (15.1 million) have alcohol use disorder.[1]

Alcohol abuse is related to more than 100 pathological conditions. The liver is especially susceptible – alcoholism results in conditions such as fatty liver,[2] alcoholic hepatitis,[3] and liver cirrhosis.[4-6] Other conditions often related to alcohol abuse include malnutrition,[7] esophagitis,[8] gastritis,[9] enterocolitis,[10] pancreatitis,[11] liver[12] and other cancers,[13] pulmonary infections,[14,15] polyneuritis, myelitis, encephalitis, delirium tremens,[16,17] and some blood disorders.[18]

Excessive alcohol intake also leads to an increased incidence of unintentional injuries such as falls, burns, drownings and car crashes and other behavioral problems like suicides, sexual and other assaults and poor academic performance.[19] It is also related to the development of many mental diseases including depression and psychosocial disorders.[20] Overall mortality is increased in these people.[21,22]

Alcohol abuse is also associated with cardiovascular diseases.[23,24] It increases the propensity to develop atrial fibrillation[25] and alcohol related cardiomyopathy.[26-28] Binge drinking (heavy episodic drinking) has been associated with an increased risk of myocardial infarction[29] and cardiac death.[30]

Alcoholism also increases the risk of stroke[31-33] and stroke related mortality.[34]

Yoga and alcoholism

Yoga practice is a feasible adjunct in the treatment of alcohol dependence.[35] In a study involving 126 individuals who practiced transcendental meditation and 90 individuals in a matched control group, the continued use of alcohol was examined. There was no discontinuation reported in the control group, for beer or wine consumption, while the meditation group reported a 40% discontinuation within the first 6 months. After 25-39 months of meditation, 54% of the meditators reported discontinuation of hard liquor consumption, compared to only 1% in the control group.[36] In women, age 18 to 65 years, suffering from PTSD, yoga intervention consisting of 12 Kripalu-based Hatha yoga sessions of 75 minutes each, resulted in a trend toward decreased alcohol use, when compared to the control group.[37]

3. Antioxidants

Reactive oxygen species play critical roles in the regulation of various cell functions and biological processes[1] – however, uncontrolled production of reactive oxygen species and the inability of the endogenous anti-oxidants to counter them results in oxidative stress[2] and vascular injury - a major hallmark of cardiovascular diseases.[3]

Oxidative stress has been implicated as one of the underlying cause[4-6] and consequence.[7] of hypertension. Oxidative stress contributes to decreased nitric oxide, endothelial dysfunction, inflammation, hypertrophy, apoptosis, cell migration, fibrosis, and angiogenesis in the vasculature.[8-10] Increased oxidative stress on the vasculature is also seen in diabetes,[11] obesity,[12,13] smoking,[14] excessive air pollution,[15] dyslipedemia[16] and with aging.[17]

Oxidative vascular damage results in the development and progression of atherosclerosis.[18] Oxidation of low density lipoprotein (LDL)-cholesterol[19] leads to recruitment of monocytes and the formation of oxidized-LDL laden foam cells which go on to form the lipid core of the atherosclerotic plaque.[20] Oxidation of LDL also promotes the growth and migration of smooth muscle cells and fibroblasts, which contribute to the atherosclerotic process.[21] These atherosclerotic processes induced by oxidative stress play important pathologic role in coronary artery disease.[22]

Oxidative stress is also seen in the myocardium in heart failure,[23-25] resulting in left ventricular (LV) dysfunction.[26] It also plays a role in ischemic stroke,[27] peripheral artery disease,[28] and erectile dysfunction.[29]

Yoga and Oxidative Stress/Anti-oxidants

In a review of 97 studies, Pal and Gupta concluded that regular yogic practices enhance antioxidant status and reduce oxidative stress in healthy, (decreased malondialdehyde and increased superoxide dismutase, catalase, glutathione and ascorbic acid levels) diabetic, (increased glutathione, vitamin C content, superoxide dismutase activity and decreased malondialdehyde content) prediabetic, (reduced malondialdehyde content) hypertensive (reduced malondialdehyde content) and renal disease (decreased protein oxidation, and increased superoxide dismutase activity) patients.[30]

4. Atherosclerosis

Arterial atherosclerosis, along with superimposed thrombosis, is the main underlying pathology behind heart attacks and strokes – the most common of all cardiovascular diseases.[1] More than 95 percent of all coronary artery disease is due to atherosclerosis.[2] Extracranial and intracranial large vessel atherosclerosis account for about 20% of ischemic stroke cases.[3] Atherosclerosis also plays a major causal role in peripheral arterial disease[4] and erectile dysfunction.[5,6]

Chronic low grade vascular inflammation[7,8] of medium-sized and large arteries[9] fueled by abnormal lipid metabolism[10] results in the development of atherosclerosis.[11] Inflammation causes endothelial (the inner lining of blood vessels) dysfunction, allowing excess circulating small low-density lipoprotein cholesterol particles in the blood to enter and get trapped inside of the arterial wall[12] where they get oxidized, under conditions of chronic oxidative stress – such as seen in smokers.[13,14] This attracts macrophages,[15,16] which then swallow these oxidized low-density cholesterol particles.[17] The macrophages get loaded with fat – and become 'foam cells'.[18] These fat laden cells continue to accumulate inside the arterial wall – the macrophage foam cells undergo apoptosis and this contributes to the formation of a lipid core.[19] As the foam cells grow in volume, the lipid core collection ultimately encroaches the inner lumen of the artery, and forms a plaque.[20] LDL oxidation also stimulates smooth-muscle cells to migrate[21] both into the necrotic lipid core and also to form a fibrous cap on the plaque.[22] However, due to smooth muscle apotosis,[23,24] or intense inflammation,[25] or a combination of other factors,[26] the covering wall of the plaque may rupture and open a wound inside the artery.[27,28] This erosion sets into motion a cascade of events – platelets and clotting proteins rush to this area to heal the wound by forming a blood clot.[29] This unfortunately cuts off the blood supply further down – resulting in a heart attack (damaged or dead heart muscle) or stroke (damaged or dead brain tissue).[30] These events may occur suddenly and are often fatal. It is estimated that approximately 76% of all fatal coronary thrombi are precipitated by plaque rupture. Atherosclerotic lesions can also become problematic through stenosis or embolic occlusion[31] throughout the human vasculature.[11]

Yoga and atherosclerosis

In a prospective, randomized, controlled trial, 42 men with angiographically proven coronary artery disease were randomized to control (n = 21) and yoga intervention group (n = 21). At the end of one year, data revealed that the yoga group (along with lifestyle interventions) required less revascularisation procedures (coronary angioplasty or bypass surgery- one versus eight patients in the control group). There was also more regression of coronary atherosclerotic lesions (20% versus 2%) and less progression of lesions progressed (5% versus 37%) in the yoga group on repeat angiography.[32]

In another prospective, controlled, open trial of angiographically proven coronary artery disease patients (71 patients in study group and 42 patients in control group), yoga (with lifestyle interventions) for one year resulted in regression of disease (70.4% in study group v/s 28% in control group on angiography) arrest of progression on myocardial perfusion imaging (MPI) (46.5% in study group v/s 33.3% in control group) and progression (9.9% in study group vs 35.7% in control group) on MPI and 29.6% in study group v/s 60.0% in controls on angiography).[33]

In a study of carotid intima media thickness (cIMT - a measure of atherosclerosis), researchers randomized 100 adult patients with metabolic syndrome to yoga and control groups. At the end of 1 year, the yoga group showed a significant regression of cIMT (0.842 to 0.808) whereas there was no significant change in cIMT in the control group (0.831 to 0.834).[34]

5. Autonomic Nervous System

The autonomic nervous system (ANS) is a part of the peripheral nervous system and regulates physiological processes without conscious control.

The ANS connects the central nervous system (brain and spinal cord) with most organs and controls important physiological and behavioral processes.[1] The organs/organ systems innervated and regulated by ANS include: circulatory - heart, blood vessels, digestive -gastrointestinal tract glands and sphincters, kidney, liver, salivary glands, endocrine - adrenal glands, integumentary - sweat glands, reproductive - uterus, genitals, respiratory - bronchiole smooth muscles, urinary - sphincters, and visual - pupil dilators and ciliary muscles.

The two major divisions of ANS are the sympathetic nervous system (SNS) and the parasympathetic nervous system (PNS). The sympathetic nervous system (SNS) originates from the thoracolumbar region of the spinal cord while the parasympathetic nervous system originates from cranial nerves III, VII, IX, and X and the sacral nerves S2-S4.[2] The two most common neurotransmitters released by neurons of the ANS are norepinephrine. (postganglionic neurons of the sympathetic nervous system) and acetylcholine (postganglionic neurons of the parasympathetic nervous system). The autonomic nervous system is also involved in the functioning of several hormonal systems including: the hypothalamic-pituitary-adrenal (HPA) axis, the reninangiotensin-aldosterone system (RAAS), and the endocannabinoid system. The SNS system is responsible for the 'fight and flight' response (the "emergency system"), while the PNS is responsible for the 'rest and digest' functions ("resting or recovery system").

The ANS plays an important role in disease.[3] ANS dysfunction is associated with a host of disorders, such as diabetic autonomic neuropathy,[4] hyperhidrosis,[5] orthostatic intolerance/postural tachycardia syndrome,[6] and vasovagal syncope.[7] It has also been noted in conjunction with neurodegenerative diseases such as Alzheimer's disease,[8] and Parkinson's disease;[9] neurodevelopmental disorders such as autism spectrum disorders;[10] autoimmune diseases such as rheutmatoid arthritis,[11] systemic lupus erythematosus,[12] multiple sclerosis,[13] inflammatory bowel diseases;[14] metabolic disturbances such as metabolic syndrome,[15] diabetes,[16] dyslipidemia,[17] and obesity;[18] and mental disorders such as generalized anxiety,[19] major depression,[20] and schizophrenia.[21] Abnormal ANS function has also been noted in cancer patients.[22] Abnormal ANS function, is also predictive of increased mortality in healthy populations.[23,24]

The ANS system also plays an important role in modulating heart function, both in health and disease.[25] The heart is innervated by both parasympathetic and sympathetic fibers.[26] The sympathetic system acts on β1 adrenergic receptors in the heart to increase chronotropy (changes in heart rate), dromotropy (conduction in the tissues of the heart) and inotropy (contractility of heart muscle) of the heart. The parasympathetic system acts via cholinergic action on cardiac M2 receptors to decrease chronotropy, dromotropy, and inotropy.[27] As far as the vascular system is concerned, increased sympathetic activity causes vasoconstriction while increased parasympathetic activity causes vasodilation of blood vessels.[28]

Besides its direct neural effects on the heart and the vasculature,[29] autonomic dysfunction via its hormonal effects, can promote oxidative stress, reduce vasodilation, increase inflammation, and accelerate atherosclerosis progression leading to vascular disease.[30]

Scientific studies documenting the significant impact of ANS dysfunction (particularly increased sympathetic activity) on the heart and the vascular system are numerous.[31-44] The deleterious impact of a low parasympathetic tone and high sympathetic tone is on several risk factors for atherosclerosis, including hypertension,[31,32] diabetes,[33-35] dyslipidemia,[36,37] arterial siffness,[38,39] stress,[40] anxiety,[41] inflammation[42,43] and thrombogenesis.[44]

The negative contribution of autonomic dysfunction to the development of cardiovascular diseases has been well documented in published research.[45-47] It not only stimulates vascular atherosclerosis[48-50] but also promotes its progression, including in the coronary arteries.[51,52] Impairment of the vagal cardiac tone is associated with coronary artery diseases[53] and its severity.[54] It also prognosticates adverse future events – angioplasty and coronary artery bypass grafting,[55] and mortality.[56] ANS hyperactivity also plays a crucial detrimental role in heart failure[57] and is also associated with increased mortality in these patients.[58] Treatement with beta blockers, which inhibit the cardiac sympathetic drive, helps these patients.[59] Its role in cardiac arrhythmias is also recognized – a relative increased SNS and decreased PNS status, contributes to the development, progression, and maintenance of atrial fibrillation.[60] Ventricular arrhythmias are also strongly associated with abnormal ANS activity.[61]

Ischemic stroke is also related to ANS dysfunction.[62] Patients with high sympathetic activity in acute ischemic stroke exhibit more instances of sudden death.[63] High sympathetic activity also prognosticates post-stroke health – including a higher incidence of future cardio- and cerebrovascular events.[64]

As mentioned before, autonomic dysfunction is associated with an increased risk of cardiovascular mortality.[65-68]

ANS and Erectile dysfunction

Autonomic dysfunction is also related to erectile dysfunction,[69] especially in diabetics, where it works in concert with vascular atherosclerosis.[70,71]

Yoga and the ANS

Almost every scientific study on the physiological effects of yoga modalities on the human body suggest that part or most of the beneficial effect is mediated via a reduction in the sympathetic and an increase in the parasysmpathetic activity (of the autonomic nervous system) Some relevant studies:

Multi-modal yoga helps improve the autonomic system imbalance[72] by tilting toward a healthy parasympathetic predominance.[73]

Several yogic breathing exercises (*pranayama*) help improve parasympathetic activity in the practitioners.[74,75] These include slow breathing,[76] bhramari breathing,[77] and alternate nostril breathing.[78] Parasympathetic activity increases and sympathetic activity decreases has also been noted following Sudarshan Kriya Yoga breathing exercises.[79]

Meditation also favorably modulates the autonomic nervous system with a gradual decrease in sympathetic dominance, resulting in a better balance between the sympathetic and the parasympathetic activity.[80,81]

Yoga *nidra* independently increases heart rate variability indicating a favorable shift in autonomic balance to the parasympathetic side.[82]

A study of 65 males (24–60 years in age) who underwent yoga practice for 12 weeks reported (Male Sexual Quotient questionnaire) improvement in erectile function, in addition to other domains of sexual function.[83]

6. Biochemicals

Several endogenous biological chemicals (such as hormones and neurotransmitters) directly or indirectly influence the heart and the vascular system in the human body.

BDNF (depression hormone)

Brain derived neurotrophic factor (BDNF) is a major growth factor in the central nervous system[1]. It is essential for the development of the CNS and for neuronal plasticity.[2] Low circulating BDNF levels are associated with neurological disorders such as dementia[3] and Parkinson's disease.[4] Low BDNF levels are also associated with many psyhiatric disorders, such as schizophrenia[5] and depression.[6,7] Depression plays a major role in the development and progression of heart and vascular disease.[8-11]

High serum BDNF is associated with a decreased risk of CVD.[12] In a study by Kaess and group, individuals in the highest quartile of BDNF had a 25% to 30% lower adjusted risk for future CVD events compared with those in the lowest quartile.[13] High levels also provide plaque stability in established coronary artery disease.[14] They are also associated with decreased cardiovascular mortality.[15]

Yoga and BDNF

In one study, 20 healthy physically active male volunteers in 3 age groups (20-39;30-39;40-50 years) were randomly selected from a pool of 124 volunteers. They practiced yogasana, *pranayama*, and meditation daily for 1 h, 6 days a week, for a period of 3 months in the morning. BNDF levels (pg/ml) increased significantly in these volunteers following yogic practice (in all age groups).[16]

Fifty-four drug-naïve consenting adult outpatients with Major Depression (32 males, 22 females) received antidepressants only (n = 16), yoga therapy only (n = 19), or yoga with antidepressants (n = 19). Serum BDNF were obtained before and after 3 months using a sandwich ELISA method. An increase in BDNF levels with yoga was associated with an improvement in depression scores in these pateints.[17] Other studies have revealed similar results – yoga practice increases BDNF levels.[18-20]

Exercise improves BNDF levels.[21,22] and yoga is a low intensity exercise.[23-25]

Cortisol (stress hormone)

Cortisol is a glucocorticoid hormone that gets synthesized from cholesterol in the adrenal cortex.[1] Cortisol levels exhibit a circadian rhythm – very low or undetectable cortisol levels are present at midnight and gradually build up overnight, being high on waking, surging 50%-60% in the first 30-40 minutes and then dropping during the day to the nadir at night.[2,3] Cortisol helps regulate metabolic,[4,5] cardiovascular[6] and immunological[7] physiological equilibrium. It also helps regulate the stress response.[8]

Cortisol levels (especially a flattened diurnal variation) have been implicated in the pathogenesis of several mental and physical health outcomes.[9-12] Abnormal cortisol levels affect the development of insulin resistance[13,14] and high cortisol levels are linked with diabetes mellitus,[15] central adiposity,[16] high blood pressure[17,18] and inflammatory processes.[19] Elevated levels are also related to increased anxiety,[20] depression[21] and fatigue.[22] Cortisol behaves as a stress hormone.[23,24] Chronic stress by activating the hypothalamic–pituitary–adrenal axis in the brain, leads to secretion of corticotrophic releasing hormone (CRH) from the hypothalamus. CRH stimulates the pituitary gland in the brain to produce adrenocorticotropic hormone, which in turn stimulates the release of cortisol from the adrenal glands.[25] Increased stress is associated with coronary heart disease.[26]

Several studies have documented a link between cortisol and endothelial dysfunction,[27-31] subclinical atherosclerosis,[32-34] overt atherosclerosis,[35-39] in the vascular bed as well as in the coronary circulation.[40-46] High levels of hair or fingernail cortisol are associated with two- to three-fold increased risk of acute coronary syndrome in patients, compared to those with low levels.[47] Flattened diurnal serum cortisol profile is seen in patients with post-myocardial infarction related depression.[48] Depression during myocardial infarction has been associated with an increased mortality.[49]

In general, high cortisol levels are associated with increased cardiovascular events,[50] and negative cardiovascular outcomes.[51,52] Data from the Whitehall II study found that flatter cortisol slopes across the day were associated with higher cardiovascular disease related mortality.[53] Another prospective study reported an association between higher levels of urinary cortisol and CVD mortality.[54] Researchers have also found that high levels of serum cortisol were independent predictors of cardiac events and mortality among patients with chronic heart failure.[55,56]

Elevated cortisol after stroke is associated with increased dependency, morbidity, and mortality.[57]

Yoga and cortisol

Multiple studies show that yoga helps to decrease cortisol levels.[58-60] In a meta-analysis of forty-two studies, Pascoe and associates reported that yoga *asanas* were associated with reduced evening cortisol and waking cortisol levels.[61] In a recent study of fifteen patients with chronic fatigue syndrome, sitting isometric yoga (biweekly 20 min practice with a yoga instructor and daily home practice) for eight weeks resulted in reduction of cortisol levels.[62]

Reduction of cortisol levels have also been noted with laughter yoga,[63] SKY breathing exercises,[64] and meditation.[65,66]

DHEA (longevity hormone)

The human body naturally produces the hormone dehydroepiandrosterone (DHEA) in the deep layer of adrenal cortex called zona reticularis.[1] Dehydroepiandrosterone sulfate, acts as a neurosteroid, cardioprotective, antidiabetic, antiobesity, and immuno-enhancing agent.[2]

The blood levels of DHEA peak at approximately 20–25 years of age and decline rapidly and markedly after the age of 30 years,[3] reaching a low of 10%–20% (of those encountered in young adults), at 70-80 years of age.[4] DHEA is therefore often considered a youth hormone.[5-7] 'Youth' effects include providing promnestic benefits (improves memory by increasing acetylcholine release from the hippocampus),[8] helping buffer the negative effects of stress[9] and reducing fatigue.[10] DHEA also helps decrease depression.[11]

Many studies have demonstrated an inverse association between levels of DHEA and atherosclerosis.[12,13]

Low DHEA levels are associated with an increase in cardiovascular risk, morbidity, and mortality.[14-17] They not only predict ischemic heart disease in men[18] and but also more severe coronary atherosclerosis on coronary angiography.[19] Low levels are also linked with higher mortality in men - those with lower DHEA sulphate levels (< 3.8 μmol/L) exhibit a 3.3-fold higher risk to die of cardiovascular disease, particularly ischemic heart disease.[20] Mortality is also increased in post-menopausal women (greater than two-fold increased risk of CVD mortality).[21] Low DHEA levels are also detrimental in patients with heart failure[22,23] and those with heart transplants.[24] In general, published data clearly indicates that DHEA is cardioprotective[25] but the prognostic value of levels in patients with cardiovascular disease is still unclear.[26]

Low DHEA levels have also been implicated in an increased risk of stroke in women.[27] DHEA levels may also help predict functional outcome 1 year after stroke.[28]

Low DHEA levels have been related to a higher risk for erectile dysfunction,[29-32] even in people younger than 60.[33] DHEA supplementation has been related to an improvement of erectile function, but also of desire, sexual interest, sexual activity, arousal, and fantasy.[34,35]

Yoga and DHEA

Long-term combined practice of yoga (*asana*, *pranayama*, and *dhyana*) produces an increase of dehydroepiandrosterone sulfate (DHEAS) level compared to control group – in one study, DHEAS level in the yoga group was 137.15 ± 53.08 ug/dL while in the control group it was 118.18 ± 58.86 ug/dL.[36]

In another study, 12 weeks of yogic training produced a significant increase in DHEAS for both male and female groups as compared to their baseline data, whereas no as such changes were observed in the control group.[37]

Meditation also raises DHEA levels. Dehydroepiandrosterone sulfate was measured in 270 male and 153 women who were experienced practitioners of the transcendental meditation (TM) and TM Sidhi Programme. The mean DHEAS levels were found to be higher in all the age groups, when compared with age-sex matched non-meditators – in the males, there was a 6% elevation in the 42–44 year group; 13% in the 45–49 year group and 54% in the 50–55 year group, whereas in the female group elevation was reported as 28% in the 35–39 year group; 28% in the 40–44 year group; 34% in the 45–49 year group, 54% in the 50–54 year group and 29% in the 55–59 year group.[38]

Dopamine (reward hormone)

Dopamine is an endogenous catecholamine and has widespread effects both in neuronal (as a neurotransmitter) and non-neuronal tissues (as an autocrine or paracrine agent).[1]

In the brain, dopamine plays a critical role in anhedonia (diminished interest or pleasure in response to stimuli that were previously perceived as rewarding) – often noted in major depressive disorders.[2-4] These patients have significantly lower dopamine transporter binding compared with healthy subjects,[5,6] sugesting lower dopamine concentrations.[7-9] The connection between depression and increased cardiovascular and cerebrovascular disease is well established.[10,11] Depression is also related to peripheral artery disease[12] and erectile dysfunction.[13] The brain dopamine system is also involved in various neurological and psychiatric disturbances such as Parkinson's Disease,[14] schizophrenia,[15] and cocaine addiction.[16]

Peripheral dopamine receptors are present in the kidneys, pancreas, lungs, and in numerous blood vessels.[17] Dopamine may therefore influence the vascular system indirectly through its actions in the brain and the peripheral arterial system.

Yoga and dopamine

In one study, 20 healthy physically active male volunteers in 3 age groups (20-39;30-39;40-50 years) were randomly selected from a pool of 124 volunteers. They practiced yogasana, *pranayama*, and meditation daily for 1 h, 6 days a week, for a period of 3 months, in the morning. Dopamine levels (nanogram per milliliter) increased in all age groups: 20-29 years: before 910.4 ± 79.07 to after 1,321.9 ± 64.64 : 30-39 years: before 863.5 ± 108.30 to after 1,218.8 ± 54.11 and 40-50 years: before 760.7 ± 116.35 to after 922.1 ± 65.92.[18]

Kjaer and colleagues demonstrated an increase in endogenous dopamine release in the ventral striatum during Yoga *Nidra* meditation.[19]

GABA (anti-anxiety hormone)

Gamma-aminobutyric acid (GABA) is the major inhibitory neurotransmitter[1] with high concentrations in the hypothalamus.[2] Reduced activity in GABA systems has been found in many mood disorders,[3] anxiety disorders,[4] and epilepsy.[5] An increase in GABA levels is associated with improved mood and decreased anxiety.[6]

Decreased GABA related inhibition in the hypothalamic paraventricular nucleus is associated with sympatho-excitation – contributing to the pathogenesis of cardiovascular-related disorders such as hypertension,[7-9] diabetes,[10] and heart failure.[11-12]

Yoga and GABA

GABA levels in the brain determined using magnetic resonance spectrocopy demonstrated that experienced yoga practitioners had a significant (27%) increase in whole-slab GABA levels after a 60-minute session of yoga postures compared to no change in GABA levels in controls after a 60-minute reading session.[13]

In another study of healthy subjects, yoga subjects showed an increase in GABA levels which was associated with an improvement in mood and a decrease in anxiety (when compared to a walking group).[14]

Growth Hormone (anti-aging hormone)

Human growth hormone (GH) is secreted from anterior pituitary and plays an important role in growth in children and adolescents.[1-3] Its levels are relatively low before puberty but with sexual maturations and adolescence there is a period of high GH output - stimulating somatic growth.[4] It also plays an important role in tissue metabolism in adults.[5] This includes helping maintain the structure and function of the normal adult heart.[6]

Growth hormone deficiency has significant association with several vascular disease risk factors – including higher insulin resistance,[7,8] increased serum low density lipoprotein (LDL)-cholesterol concentration,[9] decreased fibrinolysis,[10] increased sympathetic nervous activity,[11] and raised C-reactive protein.[12] Low growth hormone levels may accelerate the development of atherosclerosis.[13]

Growth hormone deficiency is associated with an increased prevalence of coronary artery disease and stroke.[14-16] Low growth hormone levels may also play a role in the pathogenesis/treatment of heart failure.[17] A retrospective study by Rosén and Bengtsson showed that hypopituitary status (low GH) in adults doubled overall mortality due to increased cardiovascular mortality, as compared with the normal population.[18]

Low levels of GH are also linked with peripheral arterial disease.[19]

Yoga and growth hormone

In one study, 12 weeks of yoga training produced a significant increase in GH in both male and female groups as compared to their baseline levels, whereas no as such changes were observed in the control group.[20]

Yoga training significantly increased circulating GH (control: -3%; yoga: +22%) in 79 centrally obese metabolic syndrome subjects aged 58 ± 8 years after a year of training. The study compared GH levels in 39 subjects who received yoga training with 40 subjects who received no training.[21]

Regular moderate exercise helps improve/increase basal levels of GH in the human subjects.[22,23] Yoga is considered a low intensity exercise[24-27] and this may positively influence the basal level of GH in the plasma blood.

Melatonin (rest/sleep/heal hormone)

Melatonin is a neurohormone produced by the pineal gland[1] and enters the cerebrospinal fluid through the pineal recess.[2] It protects against oxidative stress,[3,4] regulates energy metabolism,[5] modulates the immune system,[6,7] reduces inflammation[8] and postpones the aging process.[9] It also plays a significant role in regulating the sleep-wake cycle.[10] It has low daytime circulating levels and elevated nocturnal levels that coincide with the sleep phase – or in other words, it influences and helps maintain the circadian sleep-wake cycle, also known as the 'circadian rhythm'.[11,12]

Melatonin has been found useful in treating jet lag[13] and insomnia.[14] It has beneficial effects in diabetes,[15] obesity,[16] cancer[17] and mood disorders.[18] It also reduces peri-operative anxiety.[19,20]

Melatonin reduces inflammation,[21] has cardiac and vascular antioxidant actions,[22-24] and helps reduce the atherosclerotic process.[25,26] It may have beneficial anti-hypertensive effects.[27]

Melatonin also protects the heart.[28-30] Decreased melatonin levels are seen in coronary heart disease[31] and melatonin helps limit the loss of tissue following ischemia and reperfusion injury.[32,33] It may also play a postive role in heart failure[34,35] and in abrogating drug mediated cardio-toxicity.[30]

Melatonin is also beneficial in ischemic stroke.[36]

Yoga and melatonin

Yoga practice has been noted to increase nighttime melatonin secretion.[37] Meditation is also associated with a rise in melatonin levels.[38]

Norepinephrine/Epinephrine (catecholamines)

There are two main peripheral catecholamines - norepinephrine (noradrenaline) and epinephrine (adrenaline).[1] Elevated levels of peripheral catecholamines are associated with hypertension[2-4] and sustained elevation can result in cardiac hypertrophy and heart failure.[5] A massive surge of plasma catecholamines is responsible for the takotsubo syndrome – a stress induced cardiomyopathy.[6,7]

Yoga and catecholamines

Yoga practice reduces catecholamine levels. In one study, 20 healthy physically active male volunteers in 3 age groups (20-39;30-39;40-50 years) were randomly selected from a pool of 124 volunteers. They practiced yogasana, *pranayama*, and meditation daily for 1 h, 6 days a week, for a period of 3 months in the morning. There was insignificant reduction in norepinephrine levels of 22.42 and 22.16 % in group A (age 20-29 years) and B (age 30-39 years), respectively, following yoga practice. However, significant reduction of 28% in the levels of norepinephrine was observed in group C (age 40-50 years) following yogic practice. Levels of epinephrine decreased significantly following yogic practice in all age groups.[8]

In another study, 25 university students, divided into two groups: a control (no yoga intervention, n=13) group and a yoga (n=12) group, underwent yoga practice was with an instructor for 90 minutes once a week spread over 12 weeks, with recommendations to practice daily at home for 40 minutes with the help of a DVD. Yoga practice significantly reduced the plasma levels of epinephrine, compared to the controls.[9]

In a study which compared norepinephrine levels between two groups of heart failure patients—one which practiced meditation and another which attended weekly meetings, it was found that the group practicing meditation displayed lower levels of norepinephrine in their blood samples compared to the non-meditation group.[10]

Researchers also found that regular meditators utilizing either transcendental meditation (TM) or Sidhi-TM techniques expressed lower norepinephrine levels than a control group of healthy subjects, when their plasma catecholamine levels were measured in mornings and evenings.[11]

Oxytocin (cuddling/love hormone)

Oxytocin is a hypothalamic hormone that enters the peripheral circulation through the posterior pituitary gland.[1,2] It stimulates uterine contractions during parturition and promotes milk ejection during lactation.[3] It plays an important role sexual activity, maternal behaviour and bonding between mothers and infants.[4] It helps social functioning[5,6] by decreasing cortisol release in response to social stress[7] and reduces amygdala activity to fearful or threatening visual images.[8] It also regulates eating behaviour and metabolism[9] – reducing caloric intake.[10,11]

Oxytocin is also cardioprotective[12-15] with several beneficial cardiovascular effects (oxytocin receptors are present in the heart and vascular beds) – these include lowering blood pressure, reducing heart rate, inflammation and oxidation, and favorably modulating several other cardiovascular metabolic processes.[16] The reduction in fear-related activation in the amygdala and the reduction in cortisol levels in response to social distress – are all vascular beneficial effects.[17-19]

Higher levels of oxytocin are associated with higher heart rate variability and reduced risk of cardiovascular diseases.[20]

Yoga and oxytocin

In a study in schizophrenic patients, subjects were randomized to either a yoga group (N=15) or to a waitlist group (N=28). Yoga consisted of loosening exercises, breathing practices, *suryanamaskar*, sitting, supine and prone *asanas* along with *pranayama* and relaxation techniques. After one month (15 in the yoga group and 12 in the waitlist group finished the study) a significant improvement in plasma oxytocin levels in the yoga group, but not in the waitlisted group, was noted.[21]

Prolactin

Prolactin is an anterior pituitary hormone - it helps support lactation and several metabolic, osmoregulatory, and immunoregulatory functions.[1] Prolactin levels also play a role in vascular health, and high prolactin levels are associated with incident hypertension, diabetes, and low levels of high density lipoprotein cholesterol.[2]

High prolactin levels also affect mortality – in one study with 3929 individuals (1946 men and 1983 women), aged 20-81 (mean 50.3 years), revealed that individuals with prolactin concentrations in the highest tertile (when compared with lowest prolactin tertile) experienced the highest all-cause mortality risk (men: HR, 1.75; women: HR, 1.66), with cardiovascular death in both sexes following a similar pattern.[3]

Yoga and prolactin

Sitting isometric yoga in fifteen patients with chronic fatigue syndrome (biweekly 20 min practice with a yoga instructor and daily home practice) for eight weeks resulted in a decrease in serum prolactin levels.[4]

In another study, 126 patients with menstrual problems were subjected to yoga *nidra* for 35-40 minutes/day, five times/week, for 6 months. Prolactin levels decreased significantly at the end of the study.[5]

Serotonin (happiness neuro-transmitter)

Serotonin (5-hydroxytryptamine, 5-HT) is a neurotransmitter that is produced in the raphe nuclei of the brainstem and hypothalamus,[1] and helps regulate mood (enhnaces feelings of happiness),[2,3] sleep-wake behavior,[4] and food intake.[5] Serotonin is also available in the peripheral tissues, being mainly produced in the gut.[6-12]

Low concentrations of serotonin are associated with many negative emotions, including aggressiveness,[13] melancholic depression,[14] panic disorder[15] and suicidal thoughts and attempts.[16] Negative emotions have deleterious cardio-vascular and cerebro-vascular effects.[17-23]

Yoga and serotonin

In one study, 20 healthy physically active male volunteers in 3 age groups (20-39;30-39;40-50 years) were randomly selected from a pool of 124 volunteers. They practiced yogasana, *pranayama*, and meditation daily for 1 h, 6 days a week, for a period of 3 months. Yoga practice resulted in an increase in serotonin levels (nanogram per milliliter) in all age groups: age 20-29 years, before 209.6 ± 26.88 and after 315.8 ± 27.84; age 30-39 years, before 163.7 ± 25.04 and after 261.4 ± 20.23; ages 40-50 years, before 105.32 ± 11.17 and after 203.4 ± 16.9.[24]

In another study, healthy volunteers were recruited from among university students, and divided into two groups: a control no yoga intervention (n=13) group and a yoga (n=12) group. Yoga practice was given with an instructor for 90 minutes once a week spread over 12 weeks, with recommendations to practice daily at home for 40 minutes with the help of a DVD. At the end of the study, the yoga group demonstrated an increase in the plasma serotonin levels compared to the control group.[25]

In one study of Transcendental Meditation practitioners, the urine samples were analyzed for serotonin, and the meditators exhibited a higher level before meditation when compared to the controls, and a much higher level after meditation.[26]

7. Blood Pressure/Hypertension

Blood pressure is the pressure of the blood in the circulatory system and is related to the force and rate of the heart beat and the diameter and elasticity of the arterial walls. Blood pressure is recorded as two numbers: the systolic and the diastolic. The systolic blood pressure (SBP) – the first number, reflects the pressure exerted against the artery walls by the blood when the heart beats (pumps the blood out). The diastolic blood pressure (DBP) is the second number and indicates how much pressure the blood is exerting against the artery walls when the heart is resting between beats. Blood pressure can be measured by a sphygmomanometer, either manually or electronically. Home monitors are available for self-use – automatic finger-tip and wrist monitors are somewhat less reliable than upper arm cuff monitors.[1]

The American College of Cardiology and the American Heart Association defined new numbers concerning normal, elevated and hypertensive levels of blood pressure in 2017:[2]

Normal blood pressure (normotensive) in humans is defined less than 120/80 - (systolic blood pressure <120 mm Hg and diastolic blood pressure <80 mm Hg). It is considered elevated if the systolic is between 120–129 mm Hg and the diastolic is less than 80 mm Hg. It is considered hypertensive if the systolic blood pressure is between 130–139 mm Hg or the diastolic blood pressure is between 80–89 mm Hg. This is categorized as Stage 1 hypertension. If the systolic blood pressure is more than 140 mm Hg or the diastolic blood pressure is more than 90 mm Hg, the hypertension is categorized as Stage 2. In about 90% of all high blood pressure cases, no specific cause can be isolated, and this is usually referred to as essential hypertension.

Hypertension is common - data from 135 population-based studies (N=968,419 adults from 90 countries), indicated that 31.1% of the world's adult population had hypertension in 2010.[3] Hypertension causes ongoing damage to the heart and the vascular system, and is also often accompanied by several other risk factors, which are common in these patients:

- Current cigarette smoking, secondhand smoking
- Diabetes mellitus
- Dyslipidemia/hypercholesterolemia
- Overweight/obesity
- Physical inactivity/low fitness
- Unhealthy diet
- Psychosocial stress

High blood pressure (hypertension) greatly increases the risk of several cardiovascular diseases.[4]

In an observational study including >1 million adult patients ≥30 years of age, higher SBP and DBP were associated with increased risk of cardiovascular disease incidence, including angina, myocardial infarction, heart failure, stroke, peripheral artery disease, and abdominal aortic aneurysm, with each being evaluated separately.[5] Hypertension is also a major cause of cardiac arrhythmias. Besides troublesome symptoms, irregular heart rhythm is dangerous and may result in strokes or sudden death.[6] It raises the risk of vascular dementia - high blood pressure is associated with a 62 per cent higher risk of vascular dementia between the ages of 30-50.[7] It is also associated with several types of visual disturbances,[8] and erectile dysfunction.[9]

Hypertension increases cardiovascular related mortality. This has been increasing - from 2005 to 2015, the actual number of hypertension related deaths rose by 37.5%.[10] The higher the blood pressure, the greater the risk of cardiovascular mortality. Researchers have indicated that each difference of 20 mm Hg usual SBP or, 10 mm Hg usual DBP at ages 40 – 60 years, is associated with more than a twofold difference in the death rate from stroke, ischemic heart disease and other vascular causes.[11] Even people with elevated high blood pressure have a greater risk of having a heart attack, a stroke, or heart failure than those with normal blood pressure levels.[12,13]

Several large clinical studies have shown that reducing blood pressure in hypertensive patients reduces the risk of cardiovascular events.[13,14,15] Benefit results even with small reductions. This was seen in the Framingham Heart Study/National Health and Nutrition Examination Survey II. In white men and women aged 35 to 64 years, a 2 mmHg decrease in diastolic blood pressure reduced the risk of coronary heart disease by 6%, and stroke by 15%.[16]

Reductions in blood pressure also influence mortality, favorably. In a meta-analysis of 61 observational studies of blood pressure and mortality (1 million adults) a small 2-mmHg fall in mean SBP was associated with a 7% lower risk of ischemic heart disease related death and a 10% lower risk of stroke related death.[17]

Hypertension is primarily treated with pharmaceuticals.[18] Lifestyle changes (salt and alcohol reduction, calorie restriction and physical exercise) are also included in most guidelines,[19] and widely accepted as being beneficial.[20] Despite these measures, a significant number of patients do not reach goal, and are labelled resistant.[21]

Resistant hypertension, is present in about 10-15% of all hypertensive patients.[22-25] It is defined as blood pressure that is uncontrolled despite the use of 3 or more antihypertensive agents from different classes or blood pressure controlled with the use 4 or more agents.[26] Patients with resistant hypertension are at a higher risk to develop complications such as stroke, heart disease or congestive heart failure.[27,28]

The SPRINT trial suggested a lower treatment goal in hypertensives - reducing systolic blood pressure to 120 mm Hg decreased heart attacks, heart failure and stroke by one third and mortality by a quarter when compared to a goal of 140 mm Hg.[29]

Hypertension and peripheral arterial disease

High blood pressure is associated with an increased risk of peripheral arterial disease.[30,31] In one study, a 20 mm Hg higher than usual systolic blood pressure resulted in a 63% higher risk of peripheral arterial disease.[32]

Hypertension and erectile dysfunction

In a meta-analysis of 40 studies including 121,641 subjects, researchers found that hypertension was closely related to ED.[33] Systolic blood pressure elevation also increases the risk of erectile dysfunction in diabetic patients.[34] Further, several anti-hypertensive drugs, such as central-acting, β blockers and diuretics[35] may also contribute to erectile dysfunction.

Yoga and blood pressure

Complementary and alternative medicine interventions, including yoga, are commonly used by patients for blood pressure control.[36,37] Yoga positively modulates hypertension and appears to have a feasible role as an adjunct intervention in hypertensive patients.[38,39]

In 64 healthy participants (25 males and 39 females), regular practice of yoga for 1 month decreased the SBP by approximately 4 mmHg (136.9 mmHg to 133 mmHg) and the DBP by approximately 2 mm Hg (84.7 mmHg to 82.34 mmHg).[40] A meta-analytic review of 17 studies (22 trials), yoga practice was associated with a decline in both systolic (−4.17) and diastolic blood pressure (-3.26 mmHg) in patients with hypertension.[41]

In a study to review the benefits of meditation, researchers selected 19 eligible studies. In the meta-analysis of these 19 studies, Yang and group reported that yogic meditation was noted to reduce systolic and diastolic blood pressure by a mean of 4.02 mmHg.[42] Breathing exercises taught by yoga also play a role in decreasing blood pressure. Fifteen minutes of alternate-nostril yoga breathing in fifteen healthy male volunteers significantly decreased systolic blood pressure (average SBP: -4 mm Hg; average DBP: -2 mm Hg).[43]

A systematic review of all published studies on yoga and high blood pressure (cohort studies, 30 nonrandomized, controlled trials, 48 randomized, controlled trials (RCTs), and 3 case reports), involving 6,693 subjects and with durations ranging from 1 week to 4 years, revealed that in most studies yoga effectively reduced blood pressure in both normotensive and hypertensive populations.[44]

Continuing yoga practice is associated with a continuing decline in blood pressure. In a study of 50 healthy volunteers (30 males and 20 females), yoga practice was continued for six months. Devasena and Narhare noted that the mean systolic blood pressure before yoga practice was 131.4 ± 10.2 mmHg. After 2 months, systolic blood pressure was reduced to 130.3 ± 9.9, after 4 months, it was

126.4 ± 9.8, and after 6 months, it was further reduced to 123.5 ± 9.9. A similar trend was noted with diastolic blood pressure. The mean diastolic blood pressure before yoga practice was 85.6 ± 6.8 mmHg. After 2 months, it was reduced to 85.2 ± 6.7, after 4 months, it was 81.8 ± 6.8, and after 6 months, it had further reduced to 79.6 ± 7.3.[45]

Yoga also improves the quality of life in hypertensive patients.[46,47]

8. Blood Sugar/Diabetes

Diabetes mellitus-type II or 2 (DM) is unfortunately, a common disease – there were 30.3 million (9.4% of the population) Americans affected in 2015. Of this number, 23.1 million were diagnosed while 7.2 million remained undiagnosed.[1] Worldwide, it is also a major health issue, with its prevalence expected to continue rising[2,3] - to an estimated 552 million diabetic adults by 2030.[4] It is estimated that 21% of the US population will be diabetic by the year 2050.[5] It is a leading cause of death and disability both in the USA and the rest of the world.[6]

Type I diabetes accounts for 5%-10% of subjects diagnosed with diabetes[7] and is mainly the result of destruction of β cells of the pancreas via autoimmune mechanisms.[8] Type 1 diabetes accounts for 80%-90% of diabetes in children and adolescents.[9]

Type II diabetes mellitus, commonly seen in adults, indicates impaired insulin action as well as its secretory failure.[10] This form of diabetes, accounts for 90–95% of those with diabetes in adults.[11]

Diabetes is diagnosed when:[12]

- the fasting (no caloric intake for at least 8 hours.) blood sugar level is 126 mg/dL or higher on two separate tests.
- a random blood sugar level of 200 mg/dL or higher also suggests diabetes, especially in a patient with symptoms of hyperglycemia or hyperglycemic crisis.
- a glycated hemoglobin (A1C) measurement with a level of 6.5 percent or higher on two separate occasions.
- an abnormal glucose tolerance test. After an overnight fast, the fasting blood sugar level is measured. After drinking a sugary liquid (containing 75 g of anhydrous glucose dissolved in water), blood sugar levels are tested periodically for the next several hours. A reading of more than 200 mg/dL after two hours indicates diabetes.

Another 'type' of diabetes now gaining increasing attention is 'pre-diabetes' – because it burdens the sufferer with high cardiovascular complication burden and because it usually progresses to overt diabetes mellitus type 2.[13] Prediabetes affects about 84.1 million Americans,[14] who are 18 or above in age. Pre-diabetes is diagnosed if the tests fall in the following range:

Fasting plasma glucose: 100 mg/dl (5.6 mmol/l) to 125 mg/dl (6.9 mmol/l)
2-h plasma glucose in the 75-g oral glucose tolerance test: 140 mg/dl (7.8 mmol/l) to 199 mg/dl (11.0 mmol/l)
A1C: 5.7–6.4%

Individuals with prediabetes exhibit an elevated risk of damage to the micro-vasculature and macro-vasculature, resembling the long-term complications of diabetes.[14]

Diabetes causes several complications in the body - it is associated with:

Cancer: According to the American Cancer Society, people with type 2 diabetes are at an increased risk for many types of cancer.[15]

Pregnancy related problems: Gestational diabetes mellitus can lead to fetal macrosomia, hypoglycemia, hypocalcemia, and hyperbilirubinemia.[16]

However, the major complications of diabetes mellitus are vascular.[17] These are both microvascular and macrovascular. Microvascular damage includes:

Diabetic retinopathy: a major cause of blindness in adults aged 20-74 years in the United States. Diabetic retinopathy accounts for 12,000-24,000 newly blind persons every year.[18]

End-stage renal disease (ESRD): It is estimated that diabetes accounts for 44% of new cases of ESRD.[19]

Neuropathy: Diabetes mellitus is the leading cause of nontraumatic lower limb amputations in the United States, with a several fold increase in risk when compared to the nondiabetic population.[20]

Macrovascular complications of diabetes relate to the cardiovascular, cerebrovascular and peripheral vascular systems.

Type II diabetes patients exhibit a higher cardiovascular morbidity.[21] This is partly because a large percentage of these patients share a cluster of risk factors for cardiovascular disease. These include hypertension (prevalence of 75% to 85% of hypertension), elevated LDL cholesterol (prevalence of 70% to 80%) and obesity (prevalence of 60% to 70%).[22]

The incidence of cardiovascular disease is two- to eightfold higher in patients with type 2 diabetes than in those without diabetes.[23] The lifetime risk for developing cardiovascular disease is about 67% in men and 57% in women at age 50 years.[24] Diabetics account for approximately one third of all percutaneous coronary intervention procedures, and more than 25% of patients undergoing coronary artery bypass graft surgery.[25] Diabetic patients also do not thrive well compared to patients without diabetes following an acute myocardial infarction or major cardiovascular procedures.[26,27]

Coronary heart disease is the main cause of death in diabetics (both type 1 and type 2).[28,29] It is estimated that 68 percent of people age 65 or older with diabetes die from some form of heart disease; and 16% die of stroke.[30] DM is associated with a 2 to 4-fold increased mortality risk from heart disease and stroke.[31] In a meta-analysis of 37 prospective cohort studies of fatal coronary heart disease among a total of 447,064 people, the rate of fatal coronary heart disease was about 3.5-fold higher in patients with diabetes than in those without.[32] The relative risk for diabetes related fatal coronary heart disease is 50% higher in women than it is in men.[33]

In 1998, Haffner and group noted that adults with diabetes had the same risk for future myocardial infarction as adults with previous myocardial infarction and without diabetes.[34] Subsequent data has confirmed that diabetes patients requiring glucose-lowering therapy and nondiabetics with a prior myocardial infarction carry the same cardiovascular risk[35] - diabetes is now considered a 'coronary heart disease equivalent'.[36] Diabetes mellitus type 2 and heart failure also frequently co-exist (30–40% of patients) and this is also associated with a higher risk of heart failure hospitalization, all-cause and cardiovascular mortality.[37]

Prediabetic patients also share several cardiovascular risk factors, specifically abdominal obesity, hypertension and low high-density lipoprotein cholesterol levels – and suffer from a higher risk of cardiovascular disease when compared to normal people.[38] It has been estimated that in individuals with no history of diabetes, every 18 mg/dl higher fasting glucose above 100 mg/dl increases the risk of coronary heart disease by about 12%. In established prediabetics, (fasting glucose 100-125 mg/dl) the risk of coronary heart disease is increased by 15% in women and 7% in men.[39] Similar findings were reported earlier in a review of 18 studies by Yamini and group.[40] This increased risk also applies to increased all-cause and cardiovascular mortality.[41] Strokes are also more common in prediabetes patients. In a study by Fonville and group, almost 50% of the 'nondiabetic' patients with a recent transient ischemic attack or stroke had prediabetes.[42]

Diabetes is also major risk factor for peripheral artery disease(PAD).[43] PAD is a severe disease of the legs (untreated can lead to gangrene and amputation), and its presence is often associated with significant disease in other arterial vasculature as well,[44] especially the coronary arteries and cerebral arteries.[45] Observational studies has revealed that PAD is a strong independent predictor of coronary and cerebrovascular events.[46] People with peripheral arterial disease have significant more risk of heart attack or stroke.[47] These patients also increase their risk of cardiovascular and all-cause mortality by about 3 times when compared to those without PAD.[48-50]

Men with DM have a higher prevalence of erectile dysfunction (ED) compared with the general population – in one study, of 7,689 patients (6,719 (87%) in a stable sexual relationship), Giuliano and group reported that erectile dysfunction was present in 71% of the patients with diabetes alone (n = 2,377).[51] The duration and severity of diabetes correlates with the severity of ED.[52] ED also confers an elevated risk of cardiovascular events in diabetic men.[53]

Data is persuasive that lowering of blood sugar in diabetics reduces the incidence and progression of microvascular disease, such as retinopathy, neuropathy, and nephropathy.[54] It is estimated that every 1% reduction in Hemoglobin A1c (HbA1c) decreases the risk of developing eye, renal and nerve disease by 40%.[55]

Several large-scale clinical trials show that the improvement of glycemic control is associated with a reduction in the incidence of major macrovascular events. The reduction in cardiovascular events has varied from 41% in type I diabetes[56] to 42% for nonfatal myocardial infarction and stroke.[57] In another study, there was a 16% reduction in myocardial infarction in type II diabetes patients.[58]

However, intensive lowering of blood sugar does not appear to alter the incidence of macrovascular disease and the recommended goal is to get HbA1c to only below 7%.[59] Intense control of diabetes has shown mixed results in preventing cardiovascular complications. Although initial studies suggested reduction in cardiovascular events with intensive control,[60] subsequent studies[61] and meta-analysis[62] have indicated higher episodes of hypoglycemia and congestive heart failure in these patients. Adverse cardiovascular effects of some anti-hyperglycemic medications[63] may further counter-balance or even reverse any cardiovascular risk benefit derived from a good glycemic control.[64]

The data therefore suggests that intensive glycemic control of type 2 DM by lowering HbA1c levels to <6.5% may not be beneficial in preventing diabetes-related CVD. However, several newer medication classes (SGLT2 inhibitors and GLP-1 receptor agonists) are associated with low risk for hypoglycemia and have favorable effects on weight and are associated with improved cardiovascular disease outcomes – data on these are accumulating and may change the therapeutic paradigm. The American Diabetic Association at this time recommends that a reasonable A1C goal for many non-pregnant adults with type 2 diabetes be less than 7 percent.[59]

Insulin resistance (resistance to insulin-stimulated glucose uptake) is the major underlying defect in the development of cardiovascular disease in patients with diabetes mellitus.[65] However, many diabetics also share many other risk factors that increase the incidence and severity cardiovascular disease,[66] including dyslipidemia, hypertension, obesity, abdominal obesity, lack of adequate physical exercise, stress, cigarette smoking, autonomic dysfunction, low anti-oxidant status and several inflammatory, hematological and thrombogenic abnormalities.

Certain interventions can help prevent the onset of diabetes in patients with impaired glucose intolerance. Proper lifestyles play an important role in warding off diabetes mellitus.[67] The major beneficial non-drug interventions are proper nutrition/weight loss[68] and exercise.[69] Physical activity should be at a goal of at least 150 min/week (moderate activity including aerobic, resistance, and flexibility training) Losing 5 to 7 percent of the starting weight helps reduce the chance of developing the disease. Bariatric surgery also improves cardiovascular risk factors and long-term cardiovascular events in type 2 diabetes.[70] Metformin, a medicine used to treat diabetes, could delay the onset of diabetes.[71] Metformin worked best for women with a history of gestational diabetes, younger adults, and people with obesity.[72]

Yoga and diabetes:

Multi-modal yoga practice has been associated with improvements in fasting blood sugar,[73] post prandial sugar,[74] HbAic,[75] fasting insulin levels[76] and anti-diabetic medication usage.[77]

Several systemic reviews and meta-analysis have determined that:

- yoga was associated with a 5.4 to 33.4% reduction in fasting glucose, 24.5 to 27.0% reductions in postprandial glucose, and 13.3 to 27.3% reduction in glycohemoglobin.[78]

- yoga modalities improved glycemic control and decreased insulin resistance in 2,170 participants (several trials).[79]

- yoga practice significantly decreased fasting blood sugar (−23.72 mg/dL), post-prandial blood sugar (−17.38 mg/dL) and HbA1c (−0.47%) in 12 randomized controlled trials with a total of 864 patients.[80]

Yoga also improves other comorbid/causative factors associated with diabetes, including atherogenesis,[81] dyslipidemia,[82] high blood pressure,[83] body weight,[84] visceral adiposity,[85] impaired fibrinolysis,[86] hypo-coagulability,[87] inflammation,[88] endothelial dysfunction,[89] oxidative stress,[90] stress,[91] and autonomic system imbalance.[92]

Besides improving diabetes and reducing the risk factors for cardiovascular disease, yoga also has a beneficial effect on the quality of life of these patients.[93]

9. Cardiac arrhythmias

Cardiac arrhythmia occurs when there is any change from the normal sequence of heart beats - too fast, too slow, or erratic.[1] This usually results from abnormal initiation or conduction of the cardiac electrical impulses.[2] Besides uncomfortable feelings experienced by the patient,[3,4] irregular heart rhythm can result in low cardiac output,[5] blood clots in the heart (and embolized - like to the brain)[6] and even death.[7]

Atrial fibrillation (AF) is a common cardiac arrhythmia[8,9] and is associated with significant morbidity and mortality, especially from embolic stroke.[10-13] Patients with AF patients also experience an impaired quality of life, mainly due to depression and anxiety.[14] Treatment includes antiarrhythmic drugs[15] and catheter ablation,[16] but results are often variable and suboptimal.[17]

Ventricular arrhythmias originate in the ventricles.[2] Malignant ventricular arrhythmias like ventricular tachycardia and ventricular fibrillation often lead to death.[18,19] Coronary heart disease remains the main cause of fatal ventricular arrhythmias.[20] Negative emotions often precipitate dangerous ventricular arrhythmias.[21-23] Treatment of dangerous ventricular arrhythmias is not perfect and is usually limited to drugs[24,25] or an implantable cardioverter-defibrillator.[26]

Yoga and cardiac arrhythmias

Yoga has shown several benefits in patients with atrial fibrillation.[27-29] Yoga reduces both symptomatic and asymptomatic episodes of atrial fibrillation.[30] The autonomic nervous system appears to play a role in the onset of paroxysmal atrial fibrillation[31] and yoga helps down-regulate the hypothalamic-pituitary-adrenal axis, reducing sympathetic nervous system activity and increasing parasympathetic activity in the heart.[32]

Several other lifestyle modalities[33] have been linked with atrial fibrillation and modifying these to a healthier level helps reduce atrial fibrillation.[34-36] Yoga practice can also help ameliorate most of these.[37] These include alcohol intake,[38] diabetes mellitus,[39] diet,[40,41] exercise,[42] hypertension,[43] negative emotions,[44] obesity,[45] sleep deprivation,[46] smoking[47] and stimulant intake.[48] Yoga also helps calm the emotions (depression, anxiety and fear) related to symptoms experienced by these patients.[49,50] Quality of life is also improved in these patients (with yoga practice).[51]

Yoga practice may also be beneficial for ventricular ectopics.[52-55] Yoga is known to down-regulate the hypothalamic-pituitary-adrenal axis, reducing sympathetic nervous system activity and increasing parasympathetic activity.[52] This beneficially modulates the cardiac autonomic function.[53] This may help ameliorate ventricular ectopy – and this has been noted with yogic breathing[54,55] The appreciable benefit of yoga practice on coronary heart disease[56,57] – a common cause of complex arrhythmias may further help reduce malignant ventricular arrhythmias in this population, and help decrease mortality. Yoga also helps reduce negative emotions which often are triggers for ventricular arrhythmias.[58-61]

10. Cardiac output

Cardiac output is the amount of blood the heart pumps in 1 minute, and it is dependent on the heart rate, contractility, blood pressure and several peripheral regulatory mechanisms. An adequate cardiac output provides adequate tissue perfusion and adequate oxygenation – or proper nourishment of the tissues of the body. The normal range for cardiac output ranges from 4 to 8 L/min and varies depending on the body's metabolic needs. For example, during exercise, cardiac output goes up linearly as the oxygen consumption goes up.[1]

A low cardiac output at rest or during stress indicates heart failure.[2] and is associated with increased cardiovascular morbidity and mortality.[3]

Yoga and cardiac output

Yoga practice increases cardiac output, both acutely and over a period. In a study of thirty-six apparently healthy, nonobese, sedentary, or recreationally active individuals from the community, yoga was performed for one session with a series of 23 hatha-based yoga postures. Both novice and advanced yoga practitioners demonstrated an increase in cardiac output.[4] Yoga practitioners for over 2 years not only have a higher resting cardiac output when compared to those without yoga practice, but also exhibit a greater increase in cardiac output with exercise.[5]

Yoga also increases the cardiac output in patients with heart failure,[6] while also improving subjective (including quality of life) parameters in these patients.[7-10] It may therefore have value in cardiac rehabilitation in these patients.[6]

11. Cardiac Rehabilitation

Cardiac rehabilitation programs are complex interventions prescribed in cardiac patients and include health education, advice on cardiovascular risk reduction, increased physical activity and stress management.[1-3]

Most patients enter cardiac rehabilitation after a myocardial infarction, acute coronary syndrome[4], coronary artery bypass grafting, percutaneous coronary intervention,[5] heart failure[6] or heart or heart/lung transplant.[7] Cardiac rehabilitation is designed to stabilize, slow down or even regress cardiovascular disease.[8] It is effective in reducing major events (revascularization, unstable angina, and heart failure), even up to ten years following an attack,[9] Meta-analytic studies indicate that with rehabilitation, cardiovascular deaths are reduced by about 20% and sudden death by about 37% during the first year after an acute myocardial infraction.[10] There is also a reduction in anxiety and depression which are common among these patients.[11] Patients also experience an improved exercise capacity and functionality, and a better quality of life and well-being.[12-14]

Yoga and cardiac rehabilitation

Complementary and alternative medicine modalities have been used for cardiac rehabilitation.[15-17] Yoga has also been suggested for cardiac rehabilitation[18] and has shown clinical effectiveness in this group.[19]

In a study of 45 patients referred for cardiac rehabilitation (18 female and 27 male), researchers assigned them into 3 groups (relaxation, meditation and control). At the end of the study, there was a significant reduction in depression, systolic and diastolic blood pressure and heart rate in the meditation group when compared with the control group.[20]

In another study, 250 male participants (35–65 years), who had undergone coronary bypass grafting, were recruited. The yoga group were exposed to three modules (30 min each): the first module (up to 6th week) included MSRT (Mind Sound Resonance Technique), breath awareness and DRT (deep relaxation technique), all done in supine posture. Physical postures and *pranayama* practices were added in the second (6th week to 6th month) and third (6th month to 12th month) yoga module. Non-yogic intervention for the control group was designed to match the duration (30 min), and the level of physical activity as tolerated. At the end of the study, researchers found that the yoga group had significantly better left ventricular ejection fraction, body mass index and blood glucose. They also exhibited a better positive affect. There was a decrease in perceived stress, depression, and negative affect.[21]

In a meta-analysis,[22] the authors reviewed two studies investigating the benefits of yoga in patients with chronic heart failure. There were a total of 30 yoga and 29 control patients. They found that yoga compared with control had a positive impact on peak oxygen consumption and health related quality of life.

12. Congestive Heart Failure

Congestive heart failure (CHF) is a common cardiac disease.[1] It is estimated that it effects over 5.8 million people in the USA and over 23 million worldwide.[2,3] An American has a one in five risk of developing heart failure during his/her lifetime.[4,5] Heart failure is a deadly disease, with substantial morbidity and mortality. It is estimated that following a diagnosis, 30-day mortality is around 10%, 1-year mortality is 20–30%, and 5-year mortality is 45–60%.[5] As the heart failure gets severe, life expectancy of CHF patients becomes comparable to those with aggressive cancers.[6] Patients with heart failure have multiple symptoms, including fatigue, dyspnea, fluid retention, and cachexia. Despite symptomatic treatment to relieve symptoms and the use of several classes of drugs to improve the prognosis, including implantable devices,[7,8] heart failure continues to be responsible for almost 1 million hospitalizations annually, accounting for over 6.5 million hospital days.[9] Worldwide, the prevalence of heart failure has continued to increase, and it has become a major global health problem.[10] Complementary and alternative medicine has been used by patients with heart failure.[11,12]

Yoga and congestive heart failure

The role of yoga in the management of heart failure has also been investigated in several trials.[13]

When yoga was combined with standard care, an 8-week regimen of yoga in patients with CHF resulted in significant improvements. The study involved 19 patients with Grade I-III heart failure (with a mean ejection fraction of 25%). Nine patients were randomized to yoga and ten to standard medical care. At the end of the study, patients in the yoga group showed significantly improved graded exercise time and peak vo2 (maximal oxygen consumption which reflects exercise capacity). The yoga group patients also had significant reductions in serum levels of IL-6 and hsCRP (markers of inflammation) and an increase in extracellular superoxide dismutase (antioxidant). Minnesota Living with Heart Failure Questionnaire scores improved by 25.7% in the yoga group and by only 2.9% in the medical treatment group.[14]

In a study of 15 stable heart failure patients, given 8 weeks of yoga classes, the researchers reported a significant improvement in endurance and strength. Balance and overall mood/wellbeing also improved. Symptom stability, a subscale of quality of life, improved significantly. No adverse effects were noted.[15]

Pullen and group recruited 38 African Americans (plus one Asian and one Caucasian) with heart failure and randomly assigned them to a yoga group (21 patients) and a control group (19 patients). Both groups also followed a home walk program. At the end of the study, the yoga group showed improvements in flexibility, treadmill time, peak vo2, and IL-6, CRP biomarkers. Quality of life was also improved in the yoga group.[16]

A meta-analysis of two major studies revealed a 22% improvement in peak vo2 during cardiopulmonary exercise testing in the yoga group, indicating an increased exercise capacity. There was also a major improvement noted in the quality of life by 24% using the Minnesota Living with Heart Failure Questionnaire.[17]

In a recent study of 130 (NYHA I-II) heart failure patients, randomization was done either to the 12-week yoga plus standard therapy (65 patients) or standard therapy (65 patients). In the yoga group, 44 patients and in the control group, 48 patients completed the study. The yoga group were noted to have a significant decrease in heart rate, blood pressure and rate pressure product compared to control group. Also, LFnu and LF-HF ratio decreased significantly and HFnu increased significantly in yoga group compared to control group. (spectral heart rate variability measures low-frequency (LF)nu and high-frequency (HF)nu) These changes are consistent with an improvement in the parasympathetic activity and a decrease in the sympathetic activity in the yoga group patients.[18]

13. Coronary Artery Disease

Cardiovascular disease is the leading cause of death in the world. It is responsible for 31% of all global deaths.[1] It is estimated that in the year 2030, cardiovascular diseases will be responsible for 23.6 million deaths worldwide.[2,3] Cardiovascular disease is also the leading cause of death in the USA.[4]

In the USA, coronary artery disease (CAD) is the most common form of cardiovascular disease.[5] It caused approximately 1 of every 6 deaths in the United States in 2010.[6] It is estimated that one American has a coronary event approximately every 34 seconds and one American will die from it approximately every 1 minute 23 seconds.[6] Coronary artery disease is responsible for about 370,000 deaths annually in the United States.[7] More than 95 percent of all coronary artery disease is due to atherosclerosis.[8] Atherosclerosis is a chronic inflammatory disease,[9] and causes plaque formation inside the coronary arteries. Cardiovascular risk factors may aggravate vascular inflammation, and thus contribute to the pathogenesis of coronary artery disease.[10]

The major risk factors include hypertension, cigarette smoking, diabetes mellitus or elevated glucose levels, abnormal cholesterol levels, inactivity and obesity/overweight.[11,12] Genetics and some other still unidentified risk factors also play a role.[13]

Patients with CAD can present with stable angina pectoris, unstable angina pectoris, or a myocardial infarction.[14] Sudden death may also be the first manifestation of coronary artery disease.[15] Novel biomarkers[16] and advanced invasive[17] and non-invasive[18] techniques have been instrumental in reaching an accurate diagnosis of CAD. Treatment is aimed at improving lifestyle,[19] and may include medications, stenting and bypass surgery.[20,21]

Cardiac rehabilitation also has been beneficial in its management.[22-24] Complementary and alternative therapies are popular,[25-27] and yoga appears appealing.[28]

Yoga and coronary artery disease

Yoga and yogic lifestyle have been shown to reduce most risk factors for coronary artery disease. These include reductions in high blood pressure, obesity, hypercholesterolemia, diabetes mellitus, smoking and inactivity.[29]

Yoga practice has been consistently associated with a decrease in blood pressure. In a meta-analytic review of 17 studies (22 trials), yoga was associated with a small but significant decline in both systolic and diastolic blood pressure (−4.17 and −3.26 mmHg respectively).[30] Several other analyses have reached similar conclusions.[31-33]

Yogic lifestyle also results in weight loss. In a coronary artery disease study involving 42 men with angiographically proven CAD, a yoga intervention (along with diet control, control of other risk factors and moderate aerobic exercise) group was compared with a control group. Interventions for one year in 21 men in the yoga group resulted in a decrease in body weight, when compared to the 21 men in the control group.[34] Several other studies have confirmed weight loss associated with yoga practice.[35-38]

Many studies have reported that yoga improves lipid profiles in not only healthy individuals,[39,40] but also in hypertensive patients.[41] It also improves the lipid profiles in people at risk for coronary artery disease[42] and in those with diabetes mellitus.[43] In a meta-analysis, Innes and group reported that in 8 non-randomized control trials (N = 737 participants) yoga participants registered significant improvements in lipid profiles. These included reductions in levels of total cholesterol, low-density lipoprotein cholesterol, very low-density lipoprotein cholesterol, and triglycerides, and increases in high-density lipoprotein cholesterol, relative to standard care.[44]

Yoga may play a complementary role in reducing the risks associated with prediabetes,[45] and established diabetes.[46] Yoga is beneficial even if the diabetes is poorly controlled.[47]

Yoga practice in several studies has helped patients stop smoking.[48] In a review of four studies, Todd and associates found that the practice of yoga helped smokers quit.[49] The yoga practitioners had increased desire and motivation to quit smoking. They had fewer urges to smoke and had reduced temptations to smoke.[50] Yogic breathing has also shown to reduce the craving for cigarettes.[50] In a review of 19 randomized controlled trials, Klinsophon and group concluded that yoga, when combined with cognitive-behavioral therapy, demonstrated a positive effect on smoking cessation.[51]

Physical inactivity has deleterious health effects, comparable to smoking and obesity,[52] with a major percentage of individuals developing cardiovascular diseases.[53] Yoga is a low intensity and low impact exercise.[54] Yoga, using the body's own weight and the natural gravity, puts the body through a wide range of motion.[55,56] Yoga routines, despite their low energy expenditure[56], improve many cardiorespiratory fitness parameters, and could be used in place of other aerobic activities recommended by current guidelines for cardiovascular disease prevention.[57]

Several studies have also reported an improved heart rate variability due to increased parasympathetic and reduced sympathetic activity in the yoga patients. There are also reductions in inflammatory biomarkers such as C-reactive protein (CRP), interleukin IL-6 and tumor necrosis factor TNF-a.[58,59] Biomarkers of stress, namely, cortisol and beta-endorphin are also reduced.[60,61] These positive modulations suggest a potential role in primary prevention of coronary artery disease. Its role is secondary prevention has also been suggested.[62]

Studies have also shown an improvement in several pulmonary parameters in patients with coronary artery disease with *pranayama* practice.[63] In a study of 80 patients with coronary artery disease, yoga practice (40 patients) resulted in statistically significant improvements in slow vital capacity, forced vital capacity, peak expiratory flow rate, maximum voluntary ventilation, and diffusion factor/transfer factor of lung for carbon monoxide after 3 months of yoga regimen, when compared to patients in the usual care group (also 40 patients).[64]

Studies have also reported a regression in coronary atherosclerosis with yoga and yogic lifestyle intervention.[34] In one study of coronary artery disease patients (71 patients in study group and 42 patients in control group), the study group was given a family based yoga program which included, control of risk factors, dietary modifications and stress management for a period of one year. At the end of the study, the yoga group showed statistically significant reductions in serum total cholesterol and serum low density lipoprotein cholesterol. These patients also demonstrated regression of disease, arrest of progression and limited progression in many patients in the yoga group, when compared to the controls.[65]

Depression is pathological in patients with coronary artery disease,[66] and yogic techniques have demonstrated effectiveness in improving mood in these patients.[67] Yoga practice also improves functionality as well as mentation in patients following a heart attack.[68,69]

14. Diet

Diet plays a crucial role in the prevention, development and progression of heart and vascular disease.[1] Several dietary ingredients and habits are either beneficial or detrimental to the human vascular system.

Red/Processed meat

Ninety-three percent of Americans are omnivores. Omnivores eat food of both plant and animal origin. In other words, they also eat meat. Meat is usually categorized as red, white or processed. Red meat is usually referred to muscle meat such as that from beef, veal, pork, lamb, horse, deer and some types of game. Certain parts of chicken and the muscle tissue of ducks and geese are also considered red meat. Red meat is usually made of slow twitch fibers. It has a myoglobin count higher than 65%. White meat usually refers to poultry, fish, amphibians, and reptiles, is lighter in color and is mainly made of fast twitch fibers. "Processed meat" refers to meat, with added water, salts and other compounds, mainly to extend their shelf life. These include bacon, hot dogs, sausages, cold cuts and other predominantly red meats.

Red processed meat is linked with an increased risk of obesity,[2] colorectal cancer[3-6] and type II diabetes mellitus.[7-9] Red meat, especially processed red meat, consumption increases all-cause mortality.[10-12]

There is also an increased risk of cardio-neuro-vascular disease,[13-18] and cardiovascular mortality.[19,20]

The association of red meat intake and high blood pressure has been reported in several publications. Lajous and associates reported in 2014 that in women who consumed ≥5 servings. (50 g = 1 serving) of processed red meat/week, there was a 17% higher rate of hypertension when compared to women who consumed <1 serving/week.[13]

Micha and group[14] found no significant association between unprocessed red meat consumption and coronary heart disease risk - however, each 50 g serving/day of processed meats was associated with 42 % higher risk of coronary heart disease. Deleterious effects on the heart with processed meat intake was also seen in a prospective follow-up trial on 37,035 Swedish men – the study revealed that there was a 28% increase in heart failure in men consuming 1.2 servings/day of processed red meat and a 43% more increase in heart failure related deaths in those consuming 0.2 servings/day.[15] In another study, 2,806 women with heart failure, followed for a mean of 13.2 years, showed that in women who consumed ≥ 50 g/day processed red meat compared to those who consumed < 25 g/day, there was a statistically significant 23% higher risk of heart failure.[16]

Increased consumption of red meat is associated with an increase in ischemic strokes. In a meta-analysis of five prospective cohort studies, involving a total of 239, 251 subjects and 9,593 stroke events, Chen and associates found that the relative risk for ischemic stroke were 15% higher for total meat consumption (red and processed meat combined), 9% higher for red meat consumption and 14% higher for processed meat consumption, in the high meat consumption group when compared to the low meat consumption group.[17] A meta-analysis of prospective cohort studies suggests that higher consumption of total, red, and processed meats is associated with an 18%, 11%, and 17% increase in the risk of stroke, while higher intake of white meat is related to a 13% reduction in stroke incidence.[18]

In a meta-analysis of two cohort studies, Pan and his group followed 37,698 men from the Health Professionals Follow-up Study (1986-2008) and 83,644 women from the Nurses' Health Study (1980-2008). In this analysis, the cardiovascular mortality was increased by 13% for a 1-serving per day increase in consumption of unprocessed red meat, and by 12% for a similar increase in the consumption of processed red meat.[19] In a meta-analysis of several cohort studies (1,674,272 individuals), Abete and group noted a 16% higher risk of cardiovascular mortality with red meat consumption, and a 18% higher risk of cardiovascular mortality in those with the highest category of processed meat consumption.[12]

There are many pathways by which red meat consumption (especially processed red meat) can increase the risk of developing cardiovascular diseases. These include higher levels of total serum cholesterol,[21] low-density-lipoprotein cholesterol,[22] and triglycerides.[23] in meat eaters when compared with individuals who consumed no meat. Red meat is also high in heme iron, which may potentiate oxidation.[24] Processed meats are higher in dietary sodium[25] and nitrates.[26] On an average, processed meats contain about 400 % more sodium and 50 % more nitrates per gram and these are vascular unfriendly.[27-29] Several studies point that elevated plasma trimethylamine N-oxide (TMAO), a gut bacteria metabolite, which is high in red meat eaters, may be involved in the etiology of hypertension, atherosclerosis and coronary artery disease.[30]

Fast food/Junk food

The United States Department of Agriculture describes fast food as "food purchased in self-service or carry-out eating places without wait service". It is usually caloric dense and is rich in refined sugars, sodium and saturated fats, including trans-fats – all dietary components that are detrimental for the cardiovascular health. Fast foods unfortunately, continue to grow in popularity. Fast food is high in sodium,[31] in saturated fat and trans-fatty acids[32] and consumption results in weight gain[33] and insulin resistance.[34] Fast foods are also rich in processed meats (like hot dogs) and low in fiber, fruits and vegetables. Processed meat consumption increases cardiovascular disease.[35] There is a higher risk of dying from coronary heart disease by 20 percent in people who eat fast food once a week, when compared to people who avoid fast food. The risk increases by 50%, for people eating fast food two-three times each week and climbs to nearly 80 percent, for people who consume fast food items four or more times each week.[36]

Carbonated drinks/Sugar sweetened beverages

Carbonated beverages and sugar sweetened beverages are available everywhere in the world and are routinely consumed. Unfortunately, these beverages increase the risk of diabetes mellitus,[37,38] coronary artery disease[39] and strokes.[40] In an analysis of 40,389 healthy men from the Health Professionals Follow-Up Study, during a 20-year monitoring period, a causal link was noted between soda intake and diabetes mellitus. Sugar sweetened beverage drinkers had a 24% higher risk of developing diabetes mellitus.[41] In this study, the risk of developing diabetes mellitus fell by 17% if one serving of sugar-sweetened beverage was replaced with 1 cup of coffee. In the Nurses' Health Study, a positive association between sugar sweetened beverage intake and risk of coronary heart disease (nonfatal myocardial infarction or fatal coronary heart disease) was observed in over 88,000 women followed for 24 years. Nurses who consumed ≥ 2 sugar sweetened beverages per day had a 35% greater risk of developing coronary heart disease compared to those who consumed <1 sugar sweetened beverage per month.[42] Soda intake is also associated with a higher risk of stroke. This was evident from the Nurses' Health Study (a prospective cohort study of 84,085 women followed for 28 years), and the Health Professionals Follow-Up Study (a prospective cohort study of 43,371 men followed for 22 years). There were 1,416 strokes in men during the 841,770 person-years of follow-up and 2,938 strokes in women during 2,188,230 person-years of follow-up. Greater drinkers of sugar-sweetened and low-calorie sodas experienced a 16% higher risk of stroke.[42] Mechanisms for this cardiovascular damage include hyperglycemia, dyslipidemia, inflammation, or endothelial dysfunction.[43]

A recent study has further highlighted the increased cardiovascular mortality in women with increased sugary drink intake.[44]

Energy drinks

Energy drinks usually contain caffeine, sugars, herbal extracts, taurine, and amino acids. Caffeine, a natural stimulant, is the main active ingredient and most energy drinks contain 80–150 mg of caffeine per 8 ounces.[45] Their intake can have deleterious effects on the heart and the vascular system. Energy drinks can increase the heart rate and raise the arterial blood pressure.[46] Habitual use may increase caloric intake and result in obesity.[47] Irregular heart rhythms have also been reported.[48] Abnormal vascular endothelial function has been seen[49] and other arterial vascular damages has been reported.[50]

Plant based diets

Plant based foods provide macronutrients (carbohydrates, protein, and fats), micronutrients (vitamins and minerals), and bioactive compounds (such as flavonoids, plant sterols, polyphenols). They are also low in fat, cholesterol, salt, animal products, and sugar. It is therefore no surprise that a high daily intake of plant-based foods promotes good health.[51]

Scientific evidence has demonstrated that eating more fruits and vegetables protects against many chronic diseases,[52] including type 2 diabetes,[53,54] dementia,[55] and some cancers.[56] There is also a reduction in all-cause mortality.[57]

Plant based diets are also cardioprotective.[58,59] A Cochrane review of 10 trials with a total of 1,730 participants, concluded that increased intake of fruits (and vegetables) has favorable effects on cardiovascular risk factors.[60] People eating more plant based foods when compared with people who frequently consume red meat, have less obesity,[61] lower blood pressure,[62] less diabetes,[63] lower serum levels of LDL,[64] and more elastic arteries.[65] They also have less oxidative stress and less micro-inflammation compared with a meat-centric diet.[66] Several other cardioprotective effects have been noted,[67] including anti-oxidant,[68] and anti-platelet actions.[69] Plant based diets can help prevent and reverse atherosclerotic CAD.[70,71] The beneficial results of these actions are reflected in many cardiovascular end points.

In a prospective population-based cohort study, 20,069 men and women aged 20 to 65 years, free of cardiovascular disease, were monitored via a 178-item habitual food consumption questionnaire. The data showed that those with a higher vegetable intake had reduced coronary heart disease.[72] A reduction was also noted with higher fresh fruit consumption.[73]

He and his colleagues observed that participants consuming more than 391 g/day of fruit and vegetables had a 17% lower risk of non-fatal and fatal coronary heart disease incidence than those who consumed less than 235 g/day.[74,75]

He and another group of associates studied data from eight studies. These included 257,551 individuals (sustaining 4,917 stroke events) for an average follow-up of 13 years. Compared with individuals who had less than three servings of fruit and vegetables per day to those with consumption of more than five servings per day, the latter group had a reduced risk of stroke.[76]

Plant-based nutrition includes several substances which provide additional cardio-protection due to their high concentration of phytochemicals. These include berries,[77,78] legumes,[79] whole grains,[80-82] and nuts.[83,84] Plant based diets are also rich in cardioprotective fiber.[85] Plant based foods are also provide adequate amounts of potassium,[86,87] and magnesium.[88]

Diet and Peripheral vascular disease

High intake of fruit and vegetables is associated with decreased peripheral atherosclerosis[89] and less peripheral arterial disease.[90]

Yoga and diet

Yoga practitioners are more likely to follow a vegetarian diet as noted in the Australian Longitudinal Study on Women's Health (ALSWH). In one part of this study, 11,344, 8,200, and 9,151 women aged 19-25 years, 31-36 years, and 62-67 years, respectively, were included. In these three groups, 29.0%, 21.7%, and 20.7%, of women, respectively, practiced yoga/meditation. Women practicing yoga/meditation were significantly more likely to follow a vegetarian (OR=1.67-3.22) or vegan (OR=2.26-3.68) diet.[91]

A survey of 4,307 randomly selected individuals from 15 US Iyengar yoga studios, 1,087 individuals responded, with 1,045 (24.3%) surveys completed. Data revealed that 9.6% of yoga practitioners were vegetarian compared to 2.7% in the general population.[92]

Data on yoga practitioners and fast food/soda/sugary drinks and energy drinks is not available, although yogic teachings may result in a lower consumption in yoga practitioners when compared to the non-yogic community.

15. Drug Abuse/Addiction

Addiction to recreational drugs has become a major health problem.[1] Heroin, cocaine and amphetamines are the most common illegal drugs used in the United States.[2] There is a high rate of drug related deaths in young people.[3] Cardiovascular system involvement often plays a critical role in these deaths.[4]

Heroin (a semisynthetic analogue of morphine) is a narcotic analgesic that is commonly abused by oral ingestion, smoking or by an intravenous injection. Heroin abuse may be responsible for almost half of the drug related deaths in some countries.[5] Heroin increases the parasympathetic activity and reduces the sympathetic activity – this results in slow heart rate, low blood pressure and often irregular heart rhythm, while withdrawal symptoms are associated with increased sympathetic nervous system activation, decreased parasympathetic nervous system activation, and/or decreased cardiac vagal activity.[6] Life threatening bacterial infection of the valves of the heart can also occur due to intravenous narcotic abuse. Heroin overdose may also cause the lungs to fill up with fluid (non-cardiogenic pulmonary edema) – another potentially fatal condition.[7] Cocaine ingestion may raise the levels of circulating catecholamines by as much as 5 times.[8] It does this by both a peripheral action (inhibiting norepinephrine reuptake in peripheral sympathetic nerve terminals) as well as a central action (stimulating central sympathetic outflow).[9] The resultant high sympathetic activity may lead to coronary artery spasms, myocardial infarction and even death. A dilated cardiomyopathy may also occur.[10] Sudden cardiac death has also been seen.[11] Amphetamines abuse can cause similar cardiovascular complications as cocaine.[12]

Yoga and drug abuse

Yoga practitioners are less likely to be involved in drug abuse. Yoga teaches avoidance of recreational drugs. Yogi Bhajan[13] states:

"If you have to be addicted to something, be addicted to doing sadhana daily. Otherwise, addiction is not a source of freedom. And you are not free by taking drugs. The neurons of the brain will become feeble. You will lose your nostril pituitary sensitivity. You can never smell the subtlety of life. You'll always be dragging your life."

Yoga helps reduce stress,[14,15] depression,[16,17] achieve a higher state of consciousness,[18,19] improve self-awareness, self-compassion and self regulation[20,21] and increase self-esteem.[22-24] These benefits help patients with drug addiction.[25-27]

Yoga therapy may be viable complementary therapeutic modality for drug abuse.[28-30]

16. Erectile Dysfunction

Erectile dysfunction (ED) is a common problem in men.[1] It is more common with increasing age – erectile dysfunction increases from 5% to 15% between ages 40 to 70 years.[2] It affects about 30 million men in the US.[3] It also has a high prevalence worldwide.[4]

Erectile dysfunction in caused by an organic etiology in more than 80% of cases.[5] Non-endocrine causes include vasculogenic – the most common cause, (affecting both inflow and outflow of blood),[6-8] neurogenic (affecting innervation and nervous function)[9] and iatrogenic (relating to a medical or surgical treatment)[10,11] Endocrine causes include reduced serum testosterone levels.[12] However, in many cases, there is also a frequent coexistence of psychological components - interpersonal relationships, mood and quality of life.[13-15]

Erectile dysfunction often represents widespread vascular dysfunction[16] and most cases are related to atherosclerotic disease.[17-19] It is therefore strongly associated with and often a marker of cardiovascular disease.[20-25] Its severity also correlates with the severity of heart disease - compared to men without erectile dysfunction, men with severe erectile dysfunction had almost one and a half to twice the relative risk for ischemic heart disease, peripheral vascular disease, combined CVD events, and all-cause mortality.[26-30]

Although numerous investigative methods are available, penile duplex ultrasonography to evaluate blood flow direction and velocity, is commonly used for assessing both arterial insufficiency and veno-occlusive dysfunction in these patients.[31] Weight loss and physical activity improves erectile function in obese men.[32] Besides lifestyle changes, appropriate medical therapies (depending on the etiology) include testosterone supplementation, (in hypogonadal men) phosphodiesterase type 5 inhibitors, and transurethral or intra-cavernosal therapies. Surgical intervention via revascularization or penile prosthesis placement may be required in men demonstrating a lack of response to medical therapy.[33]

Yoga and erectile dysfunction

There are limited number of studies on the role of yoga in the treatment of sexual dysfunction, especially erectile dysfunction in men.[34] Yogic philosophy and yogic practice may be conducive to better sexual functioning and satisfaction.[35,36]

Yoga however, helps improve many other domains of sexual functions (desire, intercourse satisfaction, performance, confidence, partner synchronization, erection, ejaculatory control, orgasm) – as studied by the Male Sexual Quotient after 12 weeks session of yoga.[37] In a comparative trial with fluoxetine in 68 patients (38 yoga group; 30 fluoxetine group), yoga practice was significantly more effective in delivering an improvement in premature ejaculation.[38]

Reduction of stress improves sexual function.[39] Yoga is helpful in reducing stress and anxiety.[40,41]

17. Exercise

Exercise is good for the human health. The famed Indian physician Susruta, in 600 BC, prescribed exercise to his patients. Hippocrates (460–377 BC) praised the health benefits of physical exercise. Both Plato (427–347 BC) and Galen (129–217 AD) referred to exercise as an important complement to medicine and important for maintaining good health.[1]

Leisure time exercise is prophylactically beneficial against many health maladies,[2-7] including metabolic syndrome,[8] obesity,[9] insulin resistance,[10] prediabetes,[11] type 2 diabetes,[12] non-alcoholic fatty liver disease,[13] cognitive dysfunction,[14] depression,[15] anxiety,[16] osteoporosis,[17] osteoarthritis,[18] balance,[19] bone fractures/falls,[20,21] rheumatoid arthritis,[22] colon cancer,[23] breast cancer,[24] endometrial cancer,[25] gestational diabetes,[26] preeclampsia,[27] polycystic ovary syndrome,[28] pain,[29] diverticulitis,[30] constipation,[31] gout[32] and gallbladder disease.[33] It also diminishes sarcopenia,[34] improves cardiorespiratory fitness,[35] enhances the quality of life,[36] decreases aging, prevents premature death and improves longevity.[37]

Exercise has many physiologic benefits affecting the heart and the vascular system.[38-47] There is a reduction in blood pressure.[48-50] The lipid profile is improved with a reduction in triglyceride levels, increase in high-density lipoprotein cholesterol levels and a decrease in the low-density lipoprotein to high-density lipoprotein ratio.[51-53] Obesity is reduced.[54,55] Exercise improves sugar metabolism and insulin sensitivity,[56,57] improves metabolic profile,[58] and reduces systemic inflammation.[59,60] There is an improvement in autonomic tone,[61,62] and a decrease in blood coagulation.[63] The endothelial function[64] and vascular elasticity[65-67] is better. Exercise helps improve coronary blood flow[68] and augments cardiac function.[69] Many psychological risk factors (stress, anxiety and depression) for vascular diseases are also improved by routine physical activity.[70-72]

Exercise reduces coronary artery disease and myocardial infarction.[73,74] It also helps reduce mortality in patients with established coronary artery disease[75] – in one study improvement in the cardio-respiratory fitness reduced cardiovascular mortality risk by 52%.[76]

Exercise has been shown to be beneficial for coronary heart disease in several studies.[88,89] The advantages of mild, moderate and severe exercise include risk reduction of about 30-50% in coronary heart disease, in both men and women.[90-93] A meta-analysis by Sofi et al[94] revealed that moderate and high levels of physical activity were associated with 12% and 27% reductions in coronary heart disease incidence, respectively. A subsequent meta-analysis by Li and Siegrist[95] demonstrated that in men, moderate and high levels of leisure-time physical activity had 20% and 24% reductions in coronary heart disease risk, respectively, while in women, they were associated with 18% and 27% reductions in coronary heart disease risk, respectively. Even low levels of exercise are beneficial when it comes to cardiovascular diseases.[96,97] The Honolulu Heart Study, documented that elderly men walking more than 1.5 miles per day (a low intensity exercise) reduced their risk of coronary disease.[98]

Exercise is beneficial in heart failure, both for primary prevention (exercise provides protective benefit in preventing heart failure)[77-80] as well as secondary prevention (exercise training provides benefits in established heart failure).[81-82]

The benefits of regular exercise have also been noted on cardiac arrhythmias.[83] Increased walking greatly reduces the risk of atrial fibrillation.[83]

Exercise also reduces the incidence of stroke.[84] In one study, compared with no exercise category, the middle categories of exercise frequency (3-4 or 5-6 times/week) showed the lowest risk of stroke - a decrease of about 20%.[85] Exercise also helps in improving functionality, cardiorespiratory fitness and other health outcomes following a stroke.[86,87]

Exercise, strenuous or light, helps reduce mortality.[76] Low exercise status is associated with a higher lifetime risk of cardio-neuro vascular mortality.[99] Katzmarzyk and colleagues observed that in men with metabolic syndrome (n=3,757), a low level of cardiorespiratory fitness was associated with a 2.6-fold higher cardiovascular mortality risk compared to men with a higher level of cardiorespiratory fitness.[100] In the MRFIT Study, leisure time exercise reduced cardiovascular mortality (during a 16 year follow up) in men with a high risk of coronary heart disease.[101] A meta-analysis by Kodama et al[102] revealed that a 1 MET increase in CRF was associated with a 15% reduction CVD/CHD mortality. In a recent study, Lee and group[103] found that minimal running of 5 to 10 min/day (15-year follow-up of 55,137 adults) was associated with a 45% reduced mortality from cardiovascular disease. Low levels of exercise in the elderly and frail people, also helps reduce mortality.[104]

The American Heart Association also recommends physical activity incorporating 150 minutes per week of moderate exercise (thirty minutes a day five times a week) or 75 minutes per week of vigorous exercise (or a combination of moderate and vigorous activity) for cardiovascular health benefits.[105]

The ACSM recommends that most adults engage in 'moderate-intensity cardiorespiratory exercise training for ≥30 min/d on ≥5 d/wk for a total of ≥150 min/wk, vigorous-intensity cardiorespiratory exercise training for ≥20 min/d on ≥3 d/wk (≥75 min/wk), or a combination of moderate-intensity and vigorous-intensity exercise to achieve a total energy expenditure of ≥500-1000 MET/wk'. They also recommend resistance exercises for each of the major muscle groups, flexibility exercises for each major muscle-tendon group, and neuromotor exercise involving balance, agility, and coordination.[106]

Exercise and PAD

In patients with peripheral vascular disease, treadmill exercise increases maximal treadmill walking distance by 50% to 200%.[107] Home based walking programs also help these patients in improving their endurance.[108]

Exercise and Erectile Dysfunction

Erectile dysfunction is inversely associated with physical activity.[109,110] Exercise has shown to benefit erectile function not only in healthy people,[111,112] but also in obese individuals[113] and in those with hypertension.[114]

Yoga and exercise

Yoga practice is an exercise and improves fitness.[115] Most yoga *asanas/pranayamas* are considered low impact in nature and fall into the category of mild intensity exercise,[116,117] Yoga uses the body's own weight and the natural gravity, putting the body through a wide range of motion.[118] Yoga routines, improve cardiorespiratory fitness parameters,[119] and can therefore be used in place of other aerobic activities recommended by current guidelines for cardiovascular disease prevention.[120] According to Larson-Meyer,[116] METs in *surya-namaskar* (sun salutation) routines are usually higher, ranging from 3-6 (METS), and therefore meet the criteria for moderate-intensity physical activity. Many other researchers have reached similar conclusions.[121-123]

18. Heart Rate

The first organ to form and begin working in an embryo during pregnancy is the heart. The human heart starts beating as early as 16-21 days after conception.[1] At around 9 to 10 weeks, this heart beat is audible. The normal heart beat, as mentioned earlier, varies according to age: 0-3 months of age - 99-149 per minute; 3-6 months of age – 89-119 per minute; 6-12 months of age – 79-119; 1-10 years of age - 69-129; 10-adulthood – 60-100. Most endurance athletes gradually develop an efficient heart which generates a greater stroke volume. This allows the heart to circulate the same amount of blood with fewer contractions. Their resting heart rate may vary between 40-60 BPM.[2]

The heart rate is easy to measure at the wrist or the neck. It can also be reliably measured by common commercial electronic devices such as a fingertip monitor, a watch, wrist band etc. Health care providers can measure the heart rate at many different sites such as the groin, back of the knees or the dorsal aspect (top) of the feet – besides using electronic instruments. The electrocardiographic recording is one common instrument used for getting an accurate heart rate.

High resting heart rate is not healthy for the heart and circulation. In one study, it was estimated that the risk of a heart attack increased by 10% with an increase of 10 beats per minute (bpm).[3] It is also associated with an increased risk of stroke in patients with stable cardiovascular disease.[4] In patients with heart failure, one study calculated that cardiovascular death or hospital admission for worsening heart failure increased by 3% with every beat increase from baseline heart rate and 16% for every 5 bpm increase.[5]

Several major studies have demonstrated increased mortality with increased resting heart rate.[6] A large study involving 5,070 subjects free of cardiovascular disease (with a 30 year follow up and biennial heart rate measurements) revealed that, all-cause, cardiovascular, and coronary mortality rates increased progressively in relation to antecedent heart rates – in both sexes and at all ages.[7] A second study demonstrated that middle aged men with no ischemic heart disease and a resting heart rate of more than 90 bpm exhibited a threefold increased mortality risk when compared to those with a rate lower than 60 bpm.[8] In another study, researchers looked at the heart rate reserve (HRR) and mortality. HRR is calculated by deducting the resting heart rate from the maximum heart rate. The maximum heart rate is the number arrived at by deducting the age from 220. The higher the heart rate reserve, the lower the cardiovascular and all-cause mortality.[9]
In general, an increase of 15 bpm was associated with a 24% increased risk in men and 32% increased risk in women of death.[10] High resting heart rate raises vascular morbidity and mortality by several complicated mechanisms, including causing increased arterial stiffness, raising blood pressure,[11] and increasing myocardial oxygen demand while impairing delivery.[12]

Endurance athletes enjoy lower resting heart rates (40-60 beats per minute) because the heart becomes more efficient. This translates into improved longevity. In a study of 15,174 Olympic athletes, tracked between 1896 and 2010, a low heart rate in this group was associated with 2.8 years of longer life than the general population of the same age, gender and nationality.[2]

Lowering the heart rate in patients with certain cardiovascular diseases (coronary heart disease and heart failure) with drugs, such as beta-blockers and ivabradine, reduces overall and cardiovascular-related mortality.[13]

Yoga and heart rate:

Yoga decreases the resting heart rate, and this has been seen in several published studies.

A decrease of 9 bpm was reported following 6 weeks of multimodal yoga in 33 patients.[14] In another study, 50 healthy male subjects (18–25 years age), subjected to Mukh Bhastrika (a breathing technique) for 12 weeks experienced a reduction in heart rate – in the bhastrika practitioners, the resting pulse rate reduced from 73.3 bpm to 59.9 bmp after 12 weeks.[15]

In one study involving *pranayama* and meditation practice for 15 days – there was a reduction of about 4 bpm in resting pulse rate in 50 normal healthy individuals.[16]

The heart rate reduction with yoga practice continues to progress with continuing yoga practice. In a study by Devasena and Narhare, 50 healthy volunteers (30 men/20 women) had a mean resting heart rate before yoga practice of 77.8 bpm. Following 2 months of practice, it reduced to 77.1 bpm; after 4 months it reduced to 73.5 bpm and after 6 months to 71.3 bpm.[17]

Yoga practice modulates the resting heart rate in many ways. For example, yoga is a low intensity exercise[18] and exercise is known to decrease the resting heart rate.[19] *Pranayama* stimulates the pulmonary stretch receptors which reduce sympathetic tone, lowering the heart rate.[20] Meditation also improves the autonomic system balance – it reduces the sympathetic tone and increases parasympathetic activity.[21]

19. Heart Rate Variability

Heart rate variability (HRV) is the physiological phenomenon of variation in the time interval between heartbeats. HRV reflects autonomic nervous system functioning, particularly the parasympathetic branch. The major control is via the baroreceptors – mechano-receptors located inside the large arteries (carotid sinus and the aortic arch) that sense changes in blood pressure. An increase in pressure results in slowing of the heart rate while a decrease results in an increase. There is also input from the pulmonary stretch receptors and arterial chemoreceptors. These changes occur from beat to beat. Normally, a greater heart rate variability is associated with a better overall health.[1-4]

Reduced heart rate variability (decreased cardiac vagal or parasympathetic control) is not healthy and is associated with several medical disorders. These include diabetes mellitus,[5] end stage renal disease[6] and anxiety/stress.[7,8] It is also related to increased mortality – one study reported a 70% increase in the risk of death in the elderly from any cause.[9]

Heart rate variability reduction is also an important finding in many serious disorders of the heart and circulation.[10-14]

In a study of 2,061 examinees from the biracial Atherosclerosis Risk in Communities (a study cohort), researchers found that reduced vagal activity (decreased HRV) and an imbalance of sympatho-vagal function was associated with the risk of developing hypertension.[15] Newly diagnosed patients with early hypertension demonstrate reduced HRV.[16,17] In a meta-analysis of eight studies with a total number of 21,988 participants, low HRV was associated with a 32–45% increased risk of a first cardiovascular event in populations without known cardiovascular disease.[18]

People with reduced HRV (one standard deviation decrement in the standard deviation of total normal RR intervals) are at a 47% increased risk for new cardiac events (such as heart attacks and heart failure).[19] In a study of 2,252 people free of coronary heart disease at baseline, when followed for three years, scientists found that when comparing heart rate variability between those with high numbers to those of lower numbers, the increased risk of developing coronary heart disease in people with low HRV, can be as high as 39%.[20] Patients with heart failure also have a reduced HRV, with the sickest patients having more reduced heart rate variability.[21]

Lower HRV is also associated with increased cardiovascular deaths. When 808 patients with a heart attack were followed for an average of 31 months, Kleiger and group found that the relative risk of mortality was 5.3 times higher in the group with HR variability of less than 50 ms than the group with HR variability of more than 100 ms.[22] Sudden death is also increased. Sudden death is usually due to cardiovascular causes – in unknown coronary artery disease patients, it is the first presentation in about 20% to 30% of the deaths.[23] In a study of 325 elderly followed for 10 years – 29 of the 164 deaths noted were sudden. Persons with low

HRV were more likely to have experienced sudden death in this study.[24]

Yoga and heart rate variability

Yoga practitioners exhibit higher HRV at rest in general.[25] Several studies have shown that yoga practice improves parasympathetic activity[26] and increases HRV in healthy individuals. In sedentary office workers subjected to a 10-week, worksite-based yoga program during lunch hour, increased heart rate variability was noted.[27] In another study of 32 healthy male volunteers in the age group of 30–60 years, multi-modal yoga for one month resulted in an increase in HRV.[28]

Several individual yoga modalities also help improve HRV. These include alternate nostril breathing, [29] slow breathing at 6 times per minute,[30] yoga *nidra*,[31] Burmese Buddhist Vipassana meditation,[32] and laughter yoga.[33]

A major meta-analysis of 42 randomized control trails concluded that yoga practice improves heart rate variability (besides improving many other cardiovascular risk factors).[34]

20. Lipids

An abnormal lipid profile is associated with the development of vascular atherosclerosis.[1] It is estimated that more than 95 percent of all coronary artery disease is due to atherosclerosis.[2]

The relationship between high cholesterol and coronary artery disease has been well recognized in both middle aged people[3] and older people.[4] In the latter study by Houterman and group , when the highest to the lowest serum total cholesterol quartile was compared in subjects aged 55 years and older, the relative risk of myocardial infarction in the group with high serum total cholesterol was 1.9 times more in men and 3.2 times more in women. In men and women aged 70 years and older, the increased risk was 3.2 in men and 2.9 in women. The association of increased serum cholesterol with premature cardiovascular disease has also been noted in young subjects in 1993 – in a study of 1,071 young male medical students with a mean age of 22 years.[5] In a more recent study, Su-Min Jeong and group examined 2,682,045 young adults (aged 20–39 years) - increased cholesterol levels were significantly associated with elevated ischemic heart disease risk of twenty one percent.[6] In the Prospective Studies Collaboration (a meta-analysis of individual participant data on 892 337 persons without cardiovascular disease at baseline, enrolled in 61 prospective cohort studies, with 33 744 ischemic heart disease deaths, over nearly 12 million person-years of follow-up) a linear association between total plasma cholesterol and the risk of ischemic heart disease mortality was noted.[7] In a large recent study, data from 97 cohorts, 1,022,276 individuals, and 20,176 coronary heart disease and 13,067 stroke cases were included. Results showed that coronary heart disease was increased as the total cholesterol levels increase - a 1-mmol/L increase in total cholesterol was associated with a coronary heart disease risk increase of 1.20 (20% more) in women and 1.24 (24% more) in men. No effect of increased total cholesterol was noted on the risk of total stroke in both sexes.[8]

High total cholesterol also raises the risk premature mortality. In one study, cholesterol levels were measured (from 1951 to 1955) in 1,959 men and 2,415 women (aged between 31 and 65 years) who were free of cardiovascular disease and cancer. In subjects under the age of 50 years, cholesterol levels were directly related with subsequent 30-year overall mortality. Death from any cause increased by 5% for each 10 mg/dL increase in total cholesterol levels. The cardiovascular mortality increased by 9% for each 10 mg/dL increase in total cholesterol levels.[9] Higher cardiovascular related mortality was also confirmed in a large subsequent study involving 23,000 men and 26,000 women (aged 30-54 years) who were monitored between 1974 and 1980. This study showed that the relative risk for mortality from any cause as well as from cardiovascular disease was markedly elevated when the highest fifth of the cholesterol distribution was compared with the lowest fifth. Overall, all-cause mortality was three times higher in men and 3.8 times higher in women. Mortality from any cardiovascular disease was 2.8 times higher in men and 2.9 times higher in women.[10]

Lowering cholesterol levels are beneficial - for every 1% reduction in cholesterol, an estimated 2.5% reduction in coronary heart disease incidence is noted.[11]

Cholesterol lowering with statins has shown to reduce cardiovascular events in meta-analysis studies. [12,13]

LDL

The LDL cholesterol levels in newborns is only 20–40 mg/dL.[14] As the LDL levels increase above these levels, the initiation of atherosclerosis occurs and progressive development of the atherosclerotic plaque increases in a dose-dependent manner.[15,16]

The association of elevated LDL cholesterol levels and coronary heart disease has been well documented by genetic, epidemiological and clinical studies.[17,18] In a meta-analysis of 68 studies with 302,430 participants without known vascular disease at the time of enrolment, 8,857 non-fatal MI and 928 coronary heart disease deaths occurred over 2.79 million person-years of follow-up. Researchers reported that the plasma LDL-C concentration was log-linearly associated with increased risk of non-fatal myocardial infarction or coronary heart disease death.[19]

Lowering LDL cholesterol levels, either by diet/exercise, genetic intervention or drugs, helps decrease vascular events.[20] The drug related improvement was demonstrated in several clinical trials, namely the Scandinavian Simvastatin Survival Study,[21] Heart Protection Study,[22] Prospective Study of Pravastatin in the Elderly at Risk,[23] Antihypertensive and Lipid-Lowering Treatment to Prevent Heart Attack Trial - Lipid-Lowering Trial,[24] and the Anglo-Scandinavian Cardiac Outcomes Trial - Lipid-Lowering Arm.[25] Reductions were seen in all vascular events such as angina, non-fatal heart attacks and stroke and also in cardiovascular mortality.

Even small reductions result in significant clinical benefits. In primary prevention (patients without evidence of cardiovascular disease), there was a 1.5% lower event rate per each 1-mmol/L lower LDL-C level reduction; and in secondary prevention (patients with established cardiovascular disease) there was a 4.6% lower event rate per each 1-mmol/L lower LDL-C level reduction.[26] Additional reductions in LDL cholesterol with more intensive therapy appear to further reduce the incidence of major vascular events.[27]

HDL

In 1977, the Framingham study (The Framingham Heart Study was started in 1948 with 5,209 adult subjects in the town of Framingham. It is still ongoing and is now on its third generation of participants) reported that low levels of HDL were a major risk factor for coronary artery disease.[28]

Numerous studies since then have confirmed the harmful effects of low HDL levels. Low HDL-C is now considered an independent risk factor for cardiovascular disease.[29,30]

Low HDL is also associated with increased mortality – in a 12 year follow up study of 2,748 Framingham Heart Study participants ages 50 to 79, low levels of high-density lipoprotein cholesterol (HDL-C) and its relationship to mortality was studied. Mortality was increased for both men and women with low HDL-C levels. When the first HDL-C quintile (less than 35 mg/dl) was compared to the top quintile (greater than 54 mg/dl), death was increased (in the low HDL-C group) in men to 1.9 for all causes, and 3.6 and 4.1 for death due to cardiovascular and coronary heart disease, respectively, after adjustment for standard cardiovascular risk factors. In women, comparing the bottom HDL-C quintile (less than 45 mg/dl) to the top quintile (greater than 69 mg/dl), death rate (in the lower HDL-C group) was 1.5 for all causes and 1.6, and 3.1 for death due to cardiovascular and coronary heart disease, respectively.[31]

High levels of HDL cholesterol are associated with a lower risk of coronary heart disease.[32] Gordon and colleagues noted a 2–3% decrease in coronary artery disease risk with each increase by 10 mg/dL in HDL-C.[33] In the Coronary Primary Prevention Trial and Multiple Risk Factor Intervention Trial (both randomized trials in middle-age high-risk men) a 1-mg/dl increment in HDL-C was associated with a significant coronary heart disease risk decrement of 2% in men. In the Framingham Heart Study, there was a reduction in heart disease risk of 3% in women with a 1 mg/dL increment in HDL-C.[34] In Lipid Research Clinics Prevalence Mortality Follow-up Study, a 1 mg/dl increment in HDL-C was associated with significant 3.7% (men) and 4.7% (women) decrements in cardiovascular disease mortality rates.[34]

However, medications such as niacin and CEPT inhibitors (known to raise HDL levels) have been unable to improve cardiovascular morbidity and mortality in patients with low HDL.[35] Genetic studies manipulated to increase HDL-C have also failed so far. Some suggestions have been made that phytochemical intake (high in plant-based diets) may help alter the biochemical HDL composition – reducing cardiovascular disease.[36]

Triglycerides

Several epidemiological studies have revealed strong associations of triglyceride concentration with risk of cardiovascular and neurovascular disease.[37,38] In a meta-analysis of 17 population-based prospective studies of triglyceride and cardiovascular disease, the authors indicated that hypertriglyceridemia increases the incidence of CVD by 32% in men and 76% in women.[39] Elevated triglyceride levels are now considered an independent risk factor for cardiovascular disease.[40-42] High triglyceride levels also raise cardiovascular disease related mortality.[43]

Reducing triglyceride levels is beneficial. In a review of 18 trials involving 45,058 participants, fibrate therapy (to reduce triglyceride levels) produced a 10% risk reduction for major cardiovascular events and a 13% risk reduction for coronary events but had no benefit on stroke.[44] In a controlled trial with 555 consecutive post-myocardial infarction patients, reduction of triglycerides with the use of two drugs – fibrates and niacin, reduced the all-cause mortality by 26%, and ischemic heart disease mortality by 36%.[45]

Lipids and peripheral arterial disease

Decreasing low density lipoprotein-cholesterol levels to target (<2.6 mmol/l; 100 mg/dl), or lower, is associated with improvement of symptoms and a reduction in vascular events in patients with PAD.[46]

Lipids and venous disease

Lipid lowering with the use of lipid-lowering drugs results in a decreased risk of venous thrombosis.[47-49] However, controversial results have emanated from several epidemiological studies.[50-53] and the lipid-venous disease connection remains unclear.

Yoga and blood lipids

Yoga is beneficial for improving lipid profiles in healthy and unhealthy subjects. In one study of twenty healthy football players, yoga resulted in a reduction in total cholesterol, LDL cholesterol and triglycerides.[54] In a Chinese study of 30 healthy female students, twice weekly (8 weeks) yoga reduced total cholesterol from 4.13 to 3.75 and LDL cholesterol from 2.14 to 1.81.[55] A meta-analysis of forty four randomized control trials with a total of 3,168 participants showed positive effects of yoga practice on blood lipids (mean difference compared to usual care or no intervention): total cholesterol decreased by 13.09 mg/dl, HDL increased by 2.94 mg/dl, and triglycerides decreased by 20.97 mg/dl.[56] Another meta-analysis of 32 trials published in 2016, reported that yoga practice was associated with a reduction in total cholesterol by 18.48 mg/dl, low-density lipoprotein cholesterol by 12.14 mg/dl and, triglycerides by 25.89 mg/dl. The high-density lipoprotein cholesterol increased by 3.20 mg/dl.[57]

Cardiovascular disease is the major cause of death in patients with diabetes mellitus.[58] One of the major risk factors for cardiovascular disease in these patients is dyslipedimia.[59] In a meta-analysis, Innes and group reported that in 8 trials (N = 737 participants) yoga participants registered, significant improvements in lipid profiles in diabetics. These included reductions in levels of total cholesterol, low-density lipoprotein cholesterol, very low-density lipoprotein cholesterol, and triglycerides, and increases in high-density lipoprotein cholesterol relative to standard care.[60] In another meta-analysis of patients with type 2 diabetes, twenty-three studies with 2,473 participants (mean age = 53 years; 43% women) were analyzed and yoga practice (12 weeks average – 50 sessions average) was associated with significant improvements in the lipid profile. Compared to controls, participants in the yoga intervention reduced their total cholesterol, low-density lipoprotein, and triglyceride levels and increased high-density lipoprotein levels.[61] In another meta-analytic review involving 864 diabetics (total of 12 randomized controlled trials), Cui and group reported that there was marked benefit of yoga practice on lipid levels in these patients: reductions were −18.50 mg/dL for total cholesterol, +4.30 mg/dL for high-density lipoprotein cholesterol, −12.95 mg/dL for low-density lipoprotein cholesterol and −12.57 mg/dL for triglycerides.[62]

Yoga has modulating effects on several lipid influencing factors – including loss of weight, improved insulin resistance and decreased stress, and these may be responsible for a positive lipid profile attributed to a regular yoga practice.[63]

21. Lymphedema

Lymphedema is a chronic, incurable condition resulting from impaired drainage of the lymphatic system.[1] It can be caused by the anomalous development of the lymphatic system (primary lymphedema) or injury to the lymphatic vasculature (secondary lymphedema) – such as trauma, malignancy, infection or surgery.[2] Primary lymphedema is seen in children but is rare, affecting about 1/100,000 children.[3] Secondary lymphedema is mostly seen in adults,[4] especially in patients infected with lymphatic filariasis (a parasitic disease not uncommon in the developing world)[5] or with breast cancer (usually following surgery) in the developed world.[6,7] Globally, filariasis-related lymphedema is estimated to affect 16.7 million people,[8] while cancer-related lymphedema is estimated to affect between 15% and 80% of all breast cancer survivors.[9]

It is estimated that nearly 5 million Americans suffer from lymphedema of the extremities or genitalia.[10] It is clinically characterized with swelling, localized pain, atrophic skin changes and secondary infections.[11] It usually does not improve and continues to gradually worsen – the accumulating interstitial lymphatic fluid causes continuous subcutaneous fibro-adipose production[12-14] - eventually, the affected limb becomes disfigured.[15] This causes significant physical[16] and psychological morbidity[17] and greatly diminishes the quality of life in these patients.[18]

Treatment is based on the etiology. In filariasis related lymphedema, improvement in hygiene with meticulous skin care, prevention of secondary infections, passive elevation and range of motion exercises, and the use of oral antibiotic or anti-inflammatory medications during acute events is recommended by the World Health Organization.[19] Self-massage and compression bandaging is also useful.[20] For cancer related lymphedema, specialized lymphatic massage by a therapist and multilayer compression bandaging to reduce limb size is recommended along with meticulous skin care and specific physical exercises.[21]

Yoga and lymphedema

Yoga has been used to relieve lymphedema.[22,23] In one study, yoga was used as a major component of modified integrative treatment protocol in 425 lymphatic filariasis patients. The patients noted an improvement in their gait. Their disability was reduced, and their quality of life also improved.[24]

Another study was done in patients with breast cancer related lymphedema (BCRL). The yoga practice included breathing exercises for 10 minutes and 17 yoga postures for 25 minutes, followed by 10 minutes of meditation and 10 minutes of deep relaxation. After 8-weeks, researchers noted reduced tissue induration of the affected upper arm and improved the quality of life in these patients.[25]

In a study of six women with BCRL, modified Hatha yoga for 8 weeks (3 times a week), with compression sleeves, resulted in major improvements in the arm swelling – with a significant decrease in arm volume from baseline.[26]

22. Metabolic Syndrome

Metabolic syndrome is a cluster of metabolic abnormalities which include impaired glucose metabolism, dyslipidemia, abdominal obesity, and elevated blood pressure.[1,2] Diagnosis is made if the patient has 3 of the following 5 abnormalities: Waist circumference for males >40 in, females>35 in, fasting TG≥150mg/dL or treatment of this lipid abnormality, HDL<40mg/dL in males and <50mg/dL in females or treatment for this lipid abnormality, hypertension with BP>130/85mm Hg or taking medication for hypertension and fasting glucose >100mg/dL or taking medicine for high glucose.[3,4] It is estimated that based on these criteria, almost 35% of US adults, and 50% of those older than 60 years, have metabolic syndrome.[5]

Metabolic syndrome results in a 5-fold increase in the risk of type 2 diabetes mellitus.[6] It also increases the risk of non-alcoholic fatty liver disease.[7] Its presence increases all-cause mortality,[8] both in those over the age of 21[9] and in the elderly.[10]

Metabolic syndrome increases cardiovascular disease[11-14] and each of its component is also an independent risk factor for cardiovascular disease.[15,16] However, the clustering of these in the metabolic syndrome results in an overall cardiovascular risk that is higher than the individual components – resulting in a 2.59-fold greater likelihood of experiencing a cardiovascular event in the next 10 years.[17] Metabolic syndrome doubles the risk of mortality from vascular diseases such as, coronary heart disease, stroke, and vascular dysfunction,[18,19] particularly in women.[20] There is also an increase in sudden cardiac death in these patients.[21]

Treatment (with pharmacotherapy) is aimed at the major risk factors - elevated LDL cholesterol levels, hypertension, and diabetes[22] but benefits also accrue by targeting each of the five components.[23,24] Lifestyle changes, weight loss, prudent diet, adequate exercise and CAM modalities also help, both in its prevention and in its treatment.[25,26]

The Cardiovascular Health Study recognized that metabolic syndrome increases the risk of peripheral vascular disease (PAD).[27] Metabolic syndrome is common in patients with peripheral arterial disease.[28] In one study, metabolic syndrome was present in >50% of PAD patients.[29]

Metabolic syndrome (in men older than 50 years) results in an increase in moderate to severe erectile dysfunction.[30] Patients with erectile dysfunction also have a higher prevalence of metabolic syndrome than control subjects.[31]

Yoga and metabolic syndrome

Several trials have looked at the benefits of yoga practice in patients with metabolic syndrome.[32-35]

A randomized case control study has demonstrated that 3-month of yoga intervention in 101 middle aged adult patents induced significant improvements of metabolic syndrome parameters including waist circumference, systolic/diastolic

blood pressure, fasting blood sugar level, HbA1c, serum triglyceride and high-density lipoprotein-cholesterol from baseline to the end of the study period.[36] Tyagi and associates noticed reduced oxygen requirements during resting conditions and greater metabolic flexibility in yoga practitioners, compared to non-yoga practitioners and metabolic syndrome patients.[37] In a study of 283 adults, participants were randomized and assigned to a control group of 137 and a yoga group of 146. The study was completed by 182 participants. After a year of yoga intervention, there was improvement of waist size and systolic blood pressure in the yoga group.[38] Another study also noted improvement in several metabolic parameters after a 12-week Hatha yoga intervention. 173 Chinese men and women aged 18 or above were assigned to two groups: yoga intervention group (n = 87) or the control group (n = 86). At the end of the study, yoga group participants achieved greater decline in waist circumference, fasting glucose and triglycerides, when compared to the control group.[39] Yoga training also improved
quality of life in these patients. Improvement in the quality of life in patients with metabolic syndrome was also reported by another study.[40]

Paul-Labrador and colleagues reported beneficial effects of transcendental meditation - at the end of the study, the participants in the transcendental meditation group, when compared to a health education group, revealed improvements in blood pressure, plasma glucose and insulin levels.[41] Stress is also reduced in these patients, with the practice of yoga.[42]

23. Negative Emotions

Negative emotions and positive emotions co-exist in our lives. The ability of humans to handle them well is associated with an improved physical health.[1] Inability to accept them or an attempt to suppress them is associated with poor health,[2] and increased mortality.[3,4]

Negative emotions are also detrimental for the heart and circulatory health.[5] Longitudinal studies of more than 3000 European adults found that chronic stress for a period of several years predicted high blood pressure during 3 to 7 years of follow-up.[6] Similar findings were noted in the fifteen year Coronary Artery Risk Development in Young Adults study.[7] Exaggerated cardiovascular responses to mental stress tasks also increase the risk for developing hypertension in subsequent years.[8]

Negative emotions are also potentially important risk factors for coronary heart disease (CHD).[9] In the Normative Aging Study, negative emotions were not only associated with an incidence of coronary heart disease, but participants who had the highest level of negative emotions also experienced the greatest incidence of CHD.[10] The INTERHEART study of 24,767 adults in 52 countries showed that chronic psychosocial stress was associated with increased incidence of myocardial infarction, irrespective of the country of residence.[11]

General psychological distress increases the risk of ischemic stroke.[12] In marriage, relationships with high levels of hostility and low levels of warmth induce an approximately 8.5% increased risk for myocardial infarction and stroke – when compared to those in a positive marital relationship.[13] Negative emotions also raise cardiovascular mortality.[14]

The harmful cardiovascular response is primarily mediated via the autonomic nervous system (stimulation of the sympathetic nervous system),[15] but also results from an increase in systemic inflammation.[16] Increased inflammation leads to enhanced atherosclerosis and cardiovascular disease.[17] Negative emotions are associated with an increase in carotid intima media thickening.[18] Carotid intima media thickness is a surrogate marker for cardiovascular disease and a recent meta-analysis reported a 17% increase in the risk of myocardial infarction and stroke with only a 0.1 mm difference (increase) in common carotid intima media thickness during a 4 years of follow-up.[19]

Severe life stress is often associated with the development of depression.[20,21] Depression, has been shown to be independently associated with a higher risk of cardiovascular disease and cardiovascular mortality - in a meta-analysis of sixteen studies, depressed patients had a 39% increased risk of cardiovascular mortality.[22]

Major negative emotions include anger/hostility, anxiety/stress, and depression.

Anger/Hostility

Anger, an intense emotional reaction, can be both constructive (problem solving) and destructive (self-justification and assigning blame elsewhere; holding grudges and intensifying long term animosity). Anger, especially the destructive kind, stimulates the hypothalamic–pituitary–adrenal axis and results in increased levels of adrenaline and noradrenaline – causing harmful physical responses such as an increased heart rate and elevated blood pressure, narrowing of the coronary arteries in diseased areas and a reduction in the amount of blood pumped by the heart.[23] Anger also induces increased platelet aggregability.[24] Several research publications have firmly established the negative association between anger and coronary heart disease.[25]

The Framingham Heart Study in 1980 reported that suppressed anger independently predicted the 8-year incidence of coronary heart disease among both men and women.[26] In a 3-year follow-up study of 3,750 Finnish men aged 40 to 59, high ratings of hostility in men with preexisting heart disease were associated with an increased coronary heart disease mortality.[27] Men with a high potential for hostility, studied in the Multiple Risk Factor Intervention Trial, had a 50% higher risk of coronary heart disease.[28] Episodes of anger were 2.3 times more likely to trigger a heart attack in the Determinants of Myocardial Infarction Onset Study.[29] The Normative Aging Study examined whether problems controlling one's anger would predict coronary heart disease events among men. These prospective data, based on a study of a total of 1,305 men, indicate that anger is associated with a twofold to threefold increase in the risk of total coronary heart disease and angina pectoris.[30]

Hostility is characterized by frequent, intense bouts of anger and aggression towards other people.[31,32] This emotion is particularly harmful for the heart and circulation.[33-37] A meta-analysis of research on hostility and physical health that included 45 studies indicated that hostility was an independent risk factor for coronary heart disease.[38] In the Kuopio Ischemic Heart Disease Risk Factor Study of 2,125 men, aged 42-60 years, men with hostility scores in the top quartile were at more than twice the risk of all-cause mortality (relative hazard - RH 2.30), and cardiovascular mortality (RH 2.70), when compared to men with scores in the lowest quartile.[39]

Anger proneness is also associated with the occurrence of peripheral arterial disease.[40]

Yoga and anger/hostility

Yoga interventions have shown to diminish aggression in normal healthy individuals. In one study involving 38 healthy females with more than 2 years of experience with yoga (long-term yoga group) and 37 age-matched healthy females who had not participated in yoga (control group), using the Profile of Mood States (POMS) questionnaire, researchers found that the average self-rated mental disturbance, tension-anxiety, anger-hostility, and fatigue scores were lower in the yoga group.[41] In another study, involving 160 participants (eighty each in the yoga group the control group), *asanas*, *pranayama*, meditation, and yogic theories were taught to the yoga group for ten weeks. Mild to moderate physical exercises and management theories were taught to the control group. At the end of the study, yoga group scores were significantly lower for aggression.[42] Yoga has been shown to decrease anger/aggressive behavior in students[43] and at work place.[44] Yoga intervention also improves the behavior of prisoners.[45,46]

Anxiety/Stress:

Anxiety, is a common emotion, usually in response to (and/or associated with) stress.[47,48] If protracted or severe, both stress and anxiety can cause considerable physical harm.[49] Examples include reactivation of latent viruses (e.g., Epstein Barr virus and herpes simplex)[50] and increased vulnerability to infections,[51] such as HIV,[52] sleep disorders[53] digestive problems,[54] progression of cancer,[55,56] and higher all-cause mortality.[57,58] There is often considerable associated mental co-morbidies,[59] especially depression.[60] It is a known risk factor for suicide.[61] Persistent anxiety is a pathological psychiatric diagnosis – generalized anxiety disorder.[62] Anxiety is also an important component of panic attacks and obsessive-compulsive disorder.[63] Fear of social situations is often due to social anxiety disorder.[64] Anxiety also plays a major role in post-traumatic stress disorder.[65]

Several scientific studies have reviewed the negative association between anxiety and cardiovascular disease.[66] The strongest association is with ischemic heart disease.[67] Researchers doing a meta-analysis of several studies involving almost 250,000 persons followed for an average of 11 years, estimated that anxiety was associated with a 26% increased risk of coronary heart disease.[68] The risk is as high as 79% in patients with high levels of health related anxiety.[69] In a survey of 49,321 young Swedish men, 18 to 20 years of age, who were medically examined for military service in 1969 and 1970, the diagnosis of anxiety independently predicted subsequent coronary heart disease events.[70] Anxious patients with established cardiovascular disease also have higher number of hospitalizations.[71] In a meta-analysis, researchers found that post-traumatic stress disorder appears to impart a twofold risk of recurrent acute coronary syndrome.[72] In a second meta-analysis, generalized anxiety disorder was associated with a 21 % increase in the risk of sustaining a major adverse cardiac event.[73] Another meta-analysis of twenty studies involving 249,846 persons with a mean follow-up period of 11.2 years for incident coronary heart disease showed that anxiety was an independent risk factor for cardiac mortality.[74,75]

Stress adversely influences the health status and quality of life of patients with PAD above and beyond the influence of clinical indicators.[76]

Yoga and anxiety/stress

A multitude of studies have demonstrated the effectiveness of yoga in reducing anxiety and stress in humans[77-79] including a systemic review.[80] Recent studies in 63 female community residents in New Taipei City aged 40-60 years revealed that an eight-week hatha yoga intervention decreased perceived stress.[81]

Major reduction in work-related stress with mindfulness meditation, yoga, and physical exercise was demonstrated by de Bruin and associates.[82]

Benefits with yoga practice have also been seen in PTSD patients[83,84] and in prisoners.[85]

Depression

Major depression is a common mental disorder.[86,87] Worldwide, it is a major cause of disease burden[88] and the second-leading cause of years lived with disability.[89] The lifetime prevalence in the United States is 19.2%.[90] and is a common reason for primary care visits.[91]

Depression is associated with increased absenteeism from work and reduced productivity.[92] Other negative consequences include disruption of family life, alcohol, drug and smoking addictions, and sexual dysfunction.[93-96] Crime and suicidal behaviors are common in depressed patients.[97,98] Patients with major depression also experience accelerated aging, premature mortality, and overall reduced life expectancy.[99,100]

Major depression also has a high rate of co-morbidity and increases the risk of developing or worsening cardiovascular diseases.[101] Many studies have reported a higher incidence of hypertension in patients with depression.[102] Depression is also associated with a higher risk of incident coronary heart disease.[103] A meta-analysis in 2004 of 11 studies showed that major depression conferred an overall relative risk of 1.64 for developing coronary heart disease, with the risk increasing with increasing levels of depression.[104] It is estimated that approximately 20 to 50% of patients who die from myocardial infarction may have experienced an episode of depression prior to the infarction.[105]

One in five patients with coronary artery disease or heart failure is depressed.[106,107] Patients with established cardiovascular disease fare poorly if there is comorbid depression with an increased risk for recurrent cardiovascular events and an increased cardio-neuro vascular mortality.[108-110] The presence of depression doubles the risk that patients with newly diagnosed cardiovascular disease will experience an adverse cardiovascular event within one year.[111] A study in 2006 estimated the increase in relative risk for mortality in patients with coronary heart disease with comorbid depression as being 1.8.[112] Following a heart attack, major depression increases the risk of cardiac mortality within 6 months by almost five times.[113] This risk continues up to 10 years following the diagnosis of established cardiovascular disease, relative to non-depressed control subjects.[114]

Depressed patients also exhibit a higher risk of stroke.[115] It is estimated that one in three patients with stroke, is depressed,[116] and experience a higher mortality.[117]

Yoga and depression:

There are innumerable scientific studies validating the beneficial effects of yoga in ameliorating depression.[118-123] A recent 12 week study confirmed the depression ameliorating effects of yoga.[124] Several mechanisms play a role in this beneficial effect.[125,126] These include down-regulation of the hypothalamic-pituitary-adrenal axis and reduced sympathetic nervous system activity,[127] increase in vagal tone,[128] increase in serotonin, gamma-aminobutyric acid and brain-derived neurotropic factor,[125] and enhancement of cerebral alpha wave activity.[129] Mindfulness aspects of yoga may reduce negative ruminations in depression[130] and initiate reduced stress/distress.[131]

Negative emotions and PAD

Depression has been related to an increased risk of diabetic vascular complications,[132] including foot ulcers.[133] Depression is also associated with obesity[134] and metabolic syndrome,[135] both with increased risk of peripheral artery disease.[136-138]

Negative emotions and ED

Depression is commonly associated with erectile dysfunction.[139,140] Anxiety can also play an important role in sexual functioning, especially in men.[141,142]

24.   Obesity

Obesity is a global problem.[1] It is estimated that over 2.1 billion people – nearly 30% of the world's population – are either obese or overweight and unfortunately, these numbers are on the increase.[2] In the US, the prevalence of obesity was 39.8% in 2015-2016 - with about 93.3 million of US adults affected.[3]

According to the Centers for Disease Control and Prevention, obesity can be diagnosed from the Body Mass Index (BMI), which is a person's weight in kilograms divided by the square of the body height in meters.[4] A normal BMI is between 18.5 to <25, overweight between 25.0 to <30, and obese between 30.0 or higher. Underweight refers to a BMI of less than 18.5. Obesity is further categorized as Class 1: if the BMI is 30 to < 35; Class 2: if the BMI is 35 to < 40 and Class 3 ("extreme" or "severe" obesity) if the BMI is 40 or higher.

Body mass index, however, does not consider the distribution of fat around the body – especially visceral fat or abdominal fat around the organs.[5] Visceral fat greatly increases the risk and incidence of cardiovascular diseases and cardiovascular death.[6]

Three measurements are commonly used to diagnose excessive visceral fat:

Waist size: Typically, the smallest waist size is measured, usually just above the belly button for women and just below the belly button for men. According to the National Heart, Lung, and Blood Institute, men who have a waist circumference greater than 40 inches (102 cm) and women who have a waist circumference greater than 35 inches (88 cm) are at higher risk of cardiovascular diseases.[7]

Waist–hip ratio is the ratio of the circumference of the waist to that of the hips. A waist–hip ratio above 0.85 in females and above 0.9 is males is indicative of obesity – especially visceral obesity.[8] These people are often described as "apple-shaped" and have high amounts of visceral abdominal fat and suffer from greater health risks[9] than those with a "pear-shaped" body, which carries more weight around the hips.

Waist-to-height ratio, is defined as waist circumference divided by height. Higher values are recorded in people with increased visceral abdominal fat stores and this prognosticates a higher risk of obesity-related cardiovascular diseases.[10]

Obesity is associated with a plethora of health problems.[11] These include: diabetes mellitus,[12] hypoventilation syndrome,[13,14] kidney diseases,[15] liver diseases such as non-alcoholic fatty liver,[16] subfertility/infertility,[17] gastrointestinal reflux,[18] gall bladder disease,[19] arthritis,[20] and several cancers.[21] There are also several emotional issues that occur in obese people,[22] and include poor self-esteem,[23] and depression.[24] Obese patients also experience a diminished functional status.[25] Obesity also results in an increased medication burden for associated pain, psychiatric disorders, and co-morbid disorders.[26,27]

Obesity also increases overall mortality rate.[28-30] and this is mainly due to comorbidities such as type 2 diabetes mellitus, dyslipidemia, hypertension, obstructive sleep apnea, certain types of cancer, steatohepatitis, gastroesophageal reflux, arthritis, polycystic ovary syndrome, and infertility.[31] In a meta-analysis study of 2.88 million individuals, obesity was associated with an increase in mortality rate of 18% compared to non-obese individuals.[32]

Obesity is also associated with an increase in risk factors for heart and circulatory disease.[33] Obese patients are 3.5 times more likely to have hypertension, while 60–70% of hypertension in adults may be attributable to adiposity.[34] Obese individuals also have abnormal lipid profiles.[35,36] and more type 2 diabetes mellitus. The risk of developing diabetes increases by 20% for each 1 kg/m2 increase in the BMI.[37] Obesity increases the risk of depression.[38] Obesity is also associated with an increase in several other cardiovascular risk factors.

The higher the BMI, the higher the systolic and diastolic blood pressure. It is estimated that almost 78 percent of primary hypertension in men and 65 percent in women can be ascribed to excess weight.[39] Obesity is also an independent risk factor for coronary artery disease.[40,41] Data from 97 prospective cohort studies that collectively enrolled 1·8 million participants between 1948 and 2005 revealed that in obese patients CHD increased by 50% and stroke increased by 69%.[42] Obese children and obese adolescents also face a twofold or higher risk of suffering from hypertension, coronary heart disease, and stroke, when they reach adulthood.[43] Obesity is also detrimentally associated with cardiomyopathy,[44] worsening of cardiac function. [45,46] and atrial fibrillation.[47]

Cardiovascular mortality is also increased. This has been recognized as far back as 1959.[48] Several subsequent studies have confirmed this.[49,50] In a pooled analysis of 11 cohort studies with over 650,000 adults, Cerhan and associates found that men experienced a reduction of 3 years and women a reduction of 5 years in life expectancy, due to earlier mortality, when those with the highest versus lowest waist circumference were compared.[50]

Being overweight or obese in middle age also shortens life expectancy by an estimated 4–7 years.[51]

Obesity also increases the risk for peripheral artery disease – in a recent study - the Atherosclerosis Risk in Communities Study, which began in 1987, researchers found that people who were obese were 1.5 times more likely to develop peripheral artery disease than those who were normal weight.[52]

Erectile dysfunction is also common in obese people.[53] Skrypnik reported that 79% of men presenting with erectile disorders are either overweight or obese (BMI of 25 kg/m2 or greater). Being overweight (BMI 25-30 kg/m2) is associated with 1.5 times and being obese (BMI over 30 kg/m2) with 3 times greater risk of sexual dysfunction.[54]

Patients who are obese increase their risk for all types of lower limb venous disease.[55] Venous disease is also clinically worse in these patients.[56]

Intentional weight loss helps improve several vascular risk factors such as hypertension,[57] diabetes,[58] metabolic syndrome,[59] and abnormal blood lipid levels,[60] – leading to improved long-term outcomes,[61,62] especially in patients with coronary artery disease.[63] The America Heart Association and American College of Cardiology practice guidelines recommend an initial 10% body weight loss for patients with CAD who are overweight or obese, with the goal of achieving a body mass index (BMI) <25 kg/m2.[64] Bariatric surgery offers an alternative treatment for those with BMI ≥ 40 or 35–40 kg/m2 with other significant co-morbidity[65] and this procedure has been associated with an improvement in several obesity related medical disorders.

Yoga and weight

Several studies have demonstrated weight loss with the practice of multi-modal yoga.[66-70] In a study involving sixteen healthy postmenopausal obese women (8 yoga group and 8 control group), yoga exercise for 16 weeks was associated with a significant decrease in body weight, percentage of body fat, lean body mass, body mass index, waist circumference, and visceral fat area.[66] In another study, a total of 80 male subjects with BMI between 25 to 35 kg/cm2 were enrolled (72 completed the study). After training for 14 weeks, the yoga group continued the practice for the next 3 months. The control group was not given any specific physical activity. The researchers noted a statistically significant weight loss in the yoga group.[67] A 12-week yoga program in 40 obese women also demonstrated a reduction in central obesity, when compared to 20 obese controls. The yoga group achieved a reduction in the waist-hip ratio, body weight, BMI, and percentage of body fat and also increased the percentage of body muscle.[68] In a study by Siu and group, yoga practitioners lost an average of 3 inches of waist circumference at completion of the 1-year experimental period when compared to the control group which did not show any decrease in waist size.[69] Mindfulness meditation is also effective as a compliment to traditional weight loss programs, as was seen in 13 of the 19 studies reviewed.[70]

Yoga is also associated with a lesser weight gain, particularly for overweight young adults. Among overweight young adults in the EAT-III trial, subjects who regularly practiced yoga showed a non-significant increase in their BMI (-0.60 kg/m2), while those who did not regularly practice yoga showed significant increases in BMI (+1.37 kg/m2).[71] In a study of 15,550 adults (Vitamin and Lifestyle cohort study), aged 53 to 57 years, four or more years of yoga practice was associated with a 3.1-lb lower weight gain among normal weight participants and an 18.5-lb lower weight gain among overweight participants.[72]

Weight loss with yoga practice is safe. In a meta-analysis of thirty trials with a total of 2,173 participants, Lauche and others confirmed the safety of yoga as an effective intervention to reduce the BMI in overweight and obese individuals.[73]

Several factors associated with yoga help the positive weight change in its practitioners. Yoga is an exercise. It helps burn calories.[74] METs for individual *asanas* averaged 2.2 ± 0.7, whereas that for *pranayamas* averaged 1.3 ± 0.3. *Surya namaskars* were consistent with moderate intensity exercise. On the basis of ACSM/AHA classification, the majority of yoga modalities were classified as light intensity exercise (less than 3 METs).[75] Yoga also helps increase other moderate to vigorous physical activity in its practitioners.[76] Yoga practitioners also lead healthier lifestyles, including practicing better nutrition,[77] They eat more fruits and vegetables, eat less fast food and processed snacks and drink less sugary drinks.[78] They are also more relaxed and exhibit increased positivity[79] leading to a reduction in overeating.[80]

25. Peripheral artery disease

Peripheral artery disease (PAD) is an atherosclerotic occlusive disease that affects the arteries of the lower extremities.[1] It is a common malady, with about 202 million people having PAD in the world in 2010 (up from 164 million in 2000).[2] Its prevalence rises with increasing age – 1% at ages 40-49 years to 22.4% at age 80 or older.[3] The atherosclerotic narrowing usually involves the iliac bifurcation, and the iliofemoral and popliteal arteries.[4] Intermittent claudication, or pain in the leg muscles during walking, is one of the its most common clinical presentation.[5] Diabetes is a major risk factor[6] – patients with type 2 diabetes mellitus have a 3–4 times higher relative risk of developing PAD than normal subjects.[7] Hypertension is another risk factor, with a 20 mm Hg higher than usual systolic blood pressure being associated with a 63% higher risk of PAD and a 10 mm Hg higher diastolic blood pressure associated with a 35% increase.[8] Smoking is the third important risk factor for this disease.[9] Obesity is also causally linked with PAD.[10] Other risk factors include dyslipidemia, inflammation, hypothyroidism, elevated fibrinogen levels and hyperhomocysteinemia.[11] Genetic factors also play a role.[12]

PAD is a powerful predictor of atherosclerotic disease in other arterial beds[13] and a strong independent predictor of coronary and cerebrovascular events.[14] PAD patients have four to five times more risk of suffering a heart attack or stroke,[15] and experince increased mortality.[16] It is estimated that the risk of cardiovascular and all-cause mortality remains about 3 times higher in PAD patients compared to those without PAD, despite therapy.[17] The disease can also lead to non-healing wounds, gangrene and amputation, especially if left untreated.[18] PAD patients have a poor quality of life.[5,19]

Measurement of the ratio of the systolic blood pressures in the ankle and the arm (the ankle brachial index or ABI), is used both for screening and confirmation of PAD. An ABI < 0.9 in one lower limb extremity (measurement taken at rest under standard conditions) is considered diagnostic of PAD, with an ABI between 0.9 and 1.0 considered borderline.[20]

Treatment is usually aimed at reducing cardiovascular risk factors, smoking cessation, loss of body weight, pharmaceuticals, increased physical activity, and surgical intervention.[21,22]

Yoga and PAD

Yoga helps decrease most of the risk factors for peripheral arterial disease,[23-31] including hypertension,[23] dyslipidemia,[24] diabetes mellitus,[25] obesity,[26,27] atherosclerosis,[28,29] and smoking.[30,31] It seems logical to presume that yoga practice will be prophylactically and therapeutically beneficial in these patients. However, no specific published literature on the direct beneficial effect of yoga in preventing or treating PAD was found.

26. Positivity/Happiness/Laughter

Positivity, or positive orientation, refers to "a general tendency to view life and experiences with a positive outlook."[1,2] It is a common component of self-esteem, life satisfaction, and optimism.[3] Positivity is associated with happiness[4] and being happy is an important objective of life.[5] Happiness appears to depend both on inherited factors as well as on external or environmental factors.[6-10] Genes, especially *5-HTTLPR* and *MAOA*. have an influence of about 33%, on our happiness.[6] Exogenous factors include a multitude of behavioral, socio-cultural, economical, and geographical life events.[7-10] Happiness has beneficial health effects.[11-13] Positive/happy people have higher quality relationships, improved physical health, better work performance and higher income.[14] They are more resilient to illness and disease,[15-17] and live longer.[18] In a meta-analysis of twenty-six studies of initially healthy populations and 28 studies targeting people with an established illnesses such as HIV/Aids, positive affect and positive traits such as optimism and hopefulness were associated with reduced mortality.[18]

They also have lower heart and vascular disease risk factors.[19-34] Greater life satisfaction is also associated with decreased hypertension.[19] People living in happier nations have lower hypertension.[20] Happy people are less likely to eat unhealthy food,[21] and more likely (especially in men) to have a smaller waist circumference.[22] In general, happy people are less likely to be obese.[23,24] Positivity in women is associated with lower concentrations of inflammatory markers (C-reactive protein and fibrinogen).[22] Happy people maintain healthy lifestyles – non-smokers and ex-smokers are happier than smokers.[25,26] They have lower triglyceride levels[22] – triglycerides have been linked to poorer physical health– notably a higher risk of metabolic syndrome, cardiovascular diseases, and type 2 diabetes mellitus.[27] Happiness is a positive emotion and happy people are therefore less likely to have negative emotions such as depression, anxiety, stress, anger and hostility – emotions that are detrimental to the cardiac health.[28-32] They have what is commonly considered 'cardioprotective' personality traits - optimism, conscientiousness, openness to experience, and curiosity.[33,34]

Positive people have less heart and vascular disease.[35-38] They have less coronary disease – in one study of 6,025 men and women aged 25–75 years (free of coronary heart disease at baseline) when followed for an average 15 years, revealed a 26% reduction in relative risk of coronary heart disease between the highest and lowest tertile of emotional vitality.[36] In another study of 1739 adults (862 men and 877 women) researchers found that a positive affect reduced the hazard rate of incident coronary heart disease by 27% over a 10 year period.[37] Having a strong sense of purpose in life, is also a part of happiness, and this was associated with reduced cardiovascular events in a Japanese study involving a prospective cohort of 2,959 Japanese subjects.[38]

Positivity, especially happiness, is associated with many neuro-hormonal changes that are cardioprotective. These include lower blood pressure, better sleep, lesser inflammation, lower norepinephrine levels and better heart rate variability in people. The protective para-sympathetic tone is also increased.

Laughter

Laughter is also a positive emotion and signals happiness.[39] Besides uplifting the mood in otherwise healthy situations,[40] it can provide a positive respite from the adverse emotional effects associated with illness.[41,42] It helps reduce depression,[43-44] and improves life satisfaction[45] and the quality of life.[42] These effects have been demonstrated whether laughter has been spontaneous or simulated[45,46] Simulated laughter (Laughter Yoga) is usually conducted in a group setting and incorporates clapping, arm and leg movement, deep breathing exercises, gentle neck and shoulder stretches as well as simulated laughter and smile exercises.[47,48] Although unnatural, forced laughter reduces anxiety and stress and improves life satisfaction, subjective wellbeing, and mood, even in healthy participants.[49]

Emerging data also substantiates the role of humor and mirthful laughter (natural or simulated) in beneficially modulating general health, including cardiovascular health.[50] It has been associated with improvement in several risk factors for cardiac and vascular diseases.[51-58] Although blood pressure may initially increase following a bout of laughter, it is followed by a decrease. In a study involving 200 individuals involved in a regular practice of mirthful laughter, there was a 6.18 mm/Hg reduction in systolic blood pressure and a 3.82 mm/Hg reduction in diastolic blood pressure.[51] Mirthful laughter is associated with short term 'aerobic exercise' like effects, as evidenced by muscle contractions, fast and sporadic deep breathing, increased heart-rate and improved oxygen consumption.[52] Controlled studies in healthy students have demonstrated that laughter is associated with improved heart function, as evidenced by increases in stroke volume and cardiac output.[53] Positive emotions like laughter improve the endothelial (inner lining of the blood vessels) function.[54] Laughter also helps motivate the elderly to participate in physical activity and to adhere to exercise programs.[55] Laughter reduces stress and anxiety in sick patients.[56] Stress related cardiovascular damaging hormones such as cortisol, growth hormone and plasma dopamine, show a decrease after watching humorous movies.[57] It is beneficial in patients with depression.[45] There is also an improvement in social life.[58]

Yoga and positivity/happiness/laughter

Yoga improves subjective well-being.[59,60] In a study of 200 young participants (ages 17 to 27 years), 100 yoga practitioners when compared to 100 non practitioners, the former demonstrated higher levels of happiness.[61] In a survey of 4307 randomly selected individuals from 15 US Iyengar yoga studios (n = 18,160), representing 41 states (with 1045 surveys completed) revealed that 86.5% of the yoga practitioners agreed or strongly agreed that 'I am happier because of yoga'.[62] Many yoga practitioners join laughter clubs and participate in group laughter yoga for its benefits.[49,63,64]

27. Sedentary behavior/Excessive sitting

Sedentary behaviors (from the Latin *sedere*, "to sit") such as sitting, lying down, watching television, writing and reading, do not increase energy expenditure above the resting level of 1.0–1.5 METs (metabolic equivalents).[1] An average American spends about 7.7 h per day in sedentary behavior, primarily sitting.[2] Sedentary behavior is also common in the young - they spend 2-4 hours per day in screen-based behaviors and 5-10 hours per day sedentary.[3]

Excessive leisure time sitting is unhealthy,[4] and increases the risk of several major diseases, such as obesity,[5] diabetes,[6] low back pain[7] and cancer.[8] It also increases mortality.[9] Physical inactivity or sedentary behavior is estimated to result in a 9% premature mortality, from all causes, worldwide.[10]

Sedentary behavior is also detrimental to the cardiovascular system.[11] Excessive sitting increases the risk of several cardiovascular risk factors.[12] Sitting increases obesity, especially juvenile obesity.[13] Uninterrupted long periods of sitting may increase hyperglycemia - a recent randomized clinical trial (Diabetes Prevention Program) showed that an intensive lifestyle modification (healthy diet and moderate physical activity of 30 minutes a day for 5 days a week) reduced the incidence of type 2 diabetes by 50% as compared with placebo.[14] Inactivity also decreases high-density lipoprotein cholesterol levels[15] and is associated with high blood pressure.[16] Prolong sitting also worsens endothelial function.[17]

Sedentary behavior also increases the risk of cardiovascular diseases.[18,19] In a retrospective study of 5,159 men aged 40 to 59 years and with no history of coronary heart disease and followed for 16.8 years, physical activity was inversely related to coronary heart disease.[20] It also increases cardiovascular mortality.[21-23] A study based on 21 yr of follow-up of 7744 men found that those who reported spending more than 10 h a week sitting in automobiles (compared to less than four hours a week), and more than 23 h of combined television time and automobile time (compared to less than 11 hours a week) had an 82% and 64% greater risk of dying from cardiovascular disease, respectively.[22] In the NIH-AARP study, when 240,819 US participants, aged 50–71 years, were monitored for 8.5 years, sedentary time was found to be directly related to cardiovascular mortality.[23]

On the other hand, decreased sitting time/increased physical activity has been associated with a reduction of cardiovascular risk factors.[24,25] There is a reduction in coronary heart disease - women in the Nurse's Health Study (n=88,393) who were moderately active (1–3.49h/week) and extremely active (≥3.5h/week), had 43% and 58% lower risk of CHD, respectively, compared to sedentary women (<1h/week).[26] The mortality rates also go down.[27]

Sitting and peripheral arterial disease (PAD) of the legs

Accumulating evidence demonstrates that prolonged exposure to the sitting position (e.g., from 1 to 6 h) impairs endothelial function in the leg vasculature, including the popliteal and femoral arteries[28,29] and this has been implicated as a principal feature of the initiation and progression of obstructive atherosclerotic lesions in the legs – the main cause of PAD.[30,31] Excessive sitting is also associated with faster functional decline, in patients with PAD.[32]

Fidgeting[33] and other physical activity, such as standing,[34] help prevent this physical stress on the leg vasculature – and help PAD. Exercise also helps walking performance and quality of life in these patients.[35] Greater quantities of accelerometer-measured physical activity are also associated with lower all-cause and CVD mortality among people with PAD.[36]

Sedentary behavior and erectile dysfunction

Erectile dysfunction is influenced by physical activity,[37] and higher physical activity levels are associated with a lower risk for erectile dysfunction.[38] The reverse is also too - Japanese men with type 2 diabetes have more erectile dysfunction if they had higher sitting times.[39]

Sitting and venous disease

In normal healthy individuals, blood is pumped out the legs by calf muscle action.[40] Prolonged sitting or standing and inactivity contribute to venous blood pooling due to inadequate calf muscle pumping.[41] This raises the venous pressure and leads to chronic venous insufficiency.[42] The resultant venous hypertension disturbs the venous integrity and function, resulting in varicose veins, chronic inflammation, leg swelling, or even skin alterations and ulceration.[43]

Prolonged cramped sitting during long-lasting air travel also increases the risk of deep vein thrombosis of the legs and pulmonary embolism.[44] Increased risk of venous thromboembolism also occurs in individuals in jobs unrelated to air travel, but, involving prolonged and cramped sitting.[45]

Sitting and lymphatic flow

Normal lymphatic flow is probably the result of the intrinsic contractions of the lymphatics,[46] but is also dependent on calf muscle contractility.[47]

Yoga and sedentary behavior

The CDC defines physical activity as "Any bodily movement produced by the contraction of skeletal muscle that increases energy expenditure above a basal level".[48] Yoga is a low intensity exercise,[49] and many postures engage the calf muscles (and thereby activate the calf muscle pump).[50]

Young adult yoga practitioners are non-sedentary – they report higher levels of physical activity than non-practitioners.[51] Yoga also encourages older adult practitioners to exercise more, despite many of them suffering from chronic health conditions.[52,53]

28. Sleep

Adequate sleep is necessary for good health[1] and survival.[2] The amount of sleep each person needs each day depends on many factors, including age.[3-5] Adults average about 7- 8 hours of sleep per day,[3] while the average level of sleep is about 9 hours per night for adolescents.[4] Women in the first 3 months of pregnancy and infants generally require more sleep than adults.[5]

Sleep is composed of rapid eye movement (REM) and non-rapid eye movement (NREM) sleep. REM sleep is defined by a rapid and low-voltage EEG, with rapid, random movement of the eyes and a low muscle tone.[6] NREM sleep is further subdivided into stages 1, 2, and slow-wave sleep (SWS). Stage 1 is the period of transition between wakefulness and sleep, whereas stage 2 coincides with sleep onset with spindles and K-complexes appearing on the electroencephalogram (EEG). SWS sleep phase of NREM is characterized by a preponderance of high-amplitude, low-frequency components on the EEG. Healthy nighttime sleep consists of four to five 90-min cycles of NREM and REM per night. The NREM is more prevalent in the beginning and REM more prevalent towards the end of the night.[7]

Disturbed sleep quantity and quality is associated with a plethora of health problems.[8,9] It affects hunger and appetite[10-14] and increases obesity in these individuals.[15,16] Inadequate sleep increases insulin resistance[17,18] inadequate beta-cell compensation[19] and an increased the risk of developing diabetes[20] and prediabetes.[21] The immune system is compromised[22,23] and there is an increases susceptibility to infection.[24,25] Sleep deprivation increases the risk of developing certain cancers.[26,27] It affects the pituitary hormone levels.[28] It affects the emotional status, and is associated with anxiety and depression.[29,30] There is cognitive decline with chronic insomnia.[31] It reduces the quality of life.[32] Sleepiness is also responsible for many car accidents and fatalities.[33] Chronic inadequate sleep is also related to a higher all-cause mortality.[34,35] Higher mortality is also seen with higher sleep duration (>9h/night).[36]

Inadequate sleep also affects the heart and the vascular system.[37-39] Sleep deprivation is closely connected with an increased incidence of hypertension.[40] Individuals sleeping less than 6 hours/night are 20–32% more likely to develop hypertension compared to those sleeping 7–8 hours.[41,42] It is also associated with an attenuated nocturnal dipping in blood pressure, which prognosticates cardiovascular disease.[43] Sleep deprivation is associated with increased inflammation,[44,45] increased sympathetic activity[46,47] and higher cortisol levels[48] – all factors associated with increased cardiac and vascular diseases.[49,50]

Short and fragmented sleep is independently associated with an increased risk of subclinical atherosclerosis in the entire arterial bed.[51] There is also an increased rate of coronary artery calcification.[52] Coronary artery calcification prognosticates future cardiovascular events.[53,54] Compared to 7–8 hours/night, sleep of less than 5 hours was associated with a 25% raised risk for coronary heart disease in a large study of postmenopausal women.[53] People with short sleep times have higher rates of myocardial infarction.[54] Overall, they have more cardiac events[55] and suffer from an increase in cardiovascular mortality.[56] In the National Institutes of Health-AARP Diet and Health Study, (239,896 US men and women aged 51–72 years and free of cancer, CVD, and respiratory disease) there were 44,100 deaths over a 14 year follow up period. Compared with 7–8 hours of sleep per day, both shorter and longer sleep durations were associated with higher total and CVD mortality in this population.[57]

Short sleep duration is also associated with an increased risk of stroke.[58] A study of 93,175 postmenopausal women found that both self-reported short (≤6 hours/night) sleep duration was significantly associated with ischemic stroke, (including fatal and non-fatal events) during a 7.5-year follow-up.[59]

Poor sleep duration and quality in night shift workers is also harmful to the health.[60] It is associated with higher levels of obesity,[61] type 2 diabetes[62] and cardiovascular diseases.[63]

Sleep and Peripheral vascular disease

PAD is more common in patients with obstructive sleep apnea – a pulmonary disease resulting from repetitive upper airway occlusion and causing episodes of hypoxia, disturbed sleep, and daytime somnolence.[64] PAD patients with abnormal sleeping or lying down habits (more or less than 8–9 hours per day) demonstrate higher all-cause and cardiovascular disease mortality compared to people who reported sleeping or lying down 8–9 hours per day.[65]

Sleep and Erectile dysfunction

ED is common in patients with obstructive sleep apnea.[66,67]

Sleep and Venous Disease

Obstructive sleep apnea may also be an independent risk factor for venous thrombo-embolism.[68]

Yoga and sleep

Yoga practice helps sleep quantity and quality in several human groups - both healthy and unhealthy, and under different conditions.

Yoga practice improves sleep in healthy individuals – in a study of 12 healthy newly recruited students were trained to do yogic relaxation for 1 month, 20 min per day – they reported a reduction in sleep disturbances and improved quality of sleep.[69] In a national survey of yoga practitioners, Ross and group reported that 68.5% of the respondents reported better sleep with yoga.[70]

In 20 participants with chronic insomnia, after an 8-week yoga intervention, significant improvements were noted in several sleep measures as compared with pretreatment values.[71] Nurses, with considerable work stress, when performing yoga more than two times every week for 50-60 minutes each time after work hours, reported sleeping better.[72] Obese urban men showed improvement in parameters of sleep quality after 14 weeks yoga.[73] Elderly men and women (over 60 years of age) with insomnia, given 12 weeks of yoga showed significant improvements in a range of subjective factors of sleep quality.[74] A study involving yoga interventions for 8 to 16 weeks in women during and after menopause showed significant improvements in self-reported sleep outcomes.[75,76] Sicker patients, like those with rheumatoid arthritis,[77] diabetes mellitus,[78] and breast cancer, also report better sleep with yoga.[79]

29. Smoking/Tobacco Use

It is estimated that in 2015, 20.1% U.S. adults (an estimated 48.7 million) used tobacco products. Of these, 15.1% (36.5 million) used cigarettes, 3.5% (7.9 million) used e-cigarettes, 3.4% (7.8 million) used cigars, cigarillos or filtered little cigars, 2.3% (5.1 million) used smokeless tobacco, and 1.2% (2.7 million) used pipes, water pipes, or hookahs.[1] E-cigarettes were the most commonly used tobacco products among middle school and high school students.

Tobacco smoke is a complex mixture of over 7,000 identified chemicals, many of them toxic and carcinogenic – the main active compound is a para-sympathomimetic stimulant alkaloid, called nicotine. Nicotine is highly addictive.[2] Second hand smoke (mixture of side-stream smoke) also contains thousands of chemicals, many of which are known or suspected contributors to adverse health effects.[3] Third hand smoke refers to residual tobacco pollutants that remain on surfaces and in dust after tobacco has been smoked, and are re-emitted into the environment as pollutants[4] leaving a foul odor and also bringing ill health to nonsmokers.[5]

Smoking is associated with a plethora of deleterious health conditions,[6] including chronic obstructive pulmonary disease,[7] lung and other cancers,[8,9] diabetes mellitus,[10] dental ailments,[11] rheumatoid arthritis[12] and cataracts.[13] It also affects men's fertility[14] and assisted reproduction[15] and can cause significant problems during pregnancy.[16-18] It is responsible for increased mortality all over the world.[19-22]

Smoking is also a major and independent risk factor for cardiovascular disease.[23-25] Smoking is associated with atherosclerotic vascular disease (smoking causes endothelial dysfunction, increased arterial stiffness, increased oxidative stress, and decreased nitric oxide bioavailability),[26,27] hypertension,[28-31] increased resting heart rate,[32] coronary artery disease,[33,34] unstable angina,[35] myocardial infarction,[36,37] sudden cardiac death,[38] and overall increased cardiovascular mortality.[39]

Women may be more susceptible to the harmful effects of smoking. A meta-analysis of 75 cohort studies (almost 2.4 million individuals) demonstrated a 25% greater risk for coronary heart disease in female smokers when compared with male smokers.[40]

A recent study (290,215 US adults) showed that consistent light smoking (even smoking less than one cigarette per day) throughout a lifetime also results in an excess risk for cardiovascular disease mortality.[41] On an average, smoking reduces the human life span by about 10 years.[42]

Cigarette smoking is also an independent risk factor for both ischemic stroke (both in men and women).[43-45] Smoking increases the risk of stroke by 2 to 4 times.[46-48]

Second hand smoke:

Second hand is also known as environmental tobacco smoke. It is a combination of mainstream smoke which is exhaled by a smoker and side stream smoke that is emitted from the end of a lighted cigarette/cigar etc. Second hand smoke is toxic[49] and exposure results in premature death and disease, especially from respiratory disease and lung cancer.[50] Harmful effects also occur in children and these include increased lower respiratory infection, asthma, acute otitis media, sudden infant death syndrome, and higher school absenteeism.[51] Adolescents exposed to second-hand smoke are more likely to use tobacco.[52] Mortality is also higher in people exposed to second hand smoke.[53]

Second hand smoke is also harmful to the cardiovascular system.[54,55] A meta-analysis of 19 studies revealed that exposure to second hand smoke increased the risk of ischemic heart disease by 30%.[54] An epidemiological review found that nonsmokers exposed to environmental smoke had a 25% increased risk of coronary heart disease as compared with nonsmokers not exposed to smoke.[55]

In an analysis of 21,743 participants, aged 45 or older, in the Reasons for Geographic and Racial Differences in Stroke study, second hand smoke raised the risk of a stroke by 30%.[56]

Second hand smoke also raises cardio-vascular mortality rates.[57] Data from a recent meta-analysis of 23 prospective and 17 case-control studies of cardiovascular risks associated with second-hand smoke exposure demonstrated an increased risk of 18%, 23%, 23%, and 29% for total mortality, total cardiovascular disease, coronary heart disease and stroke, respectively, in those exposed to secondhand smoke.[58]

Third hand smoke

Residual tobacco smoke (third-hand smoke), refers to tobacco smoke pollutants that are absorbed, attached, or stacked on the surface of substances and dust.[59] Third hand smoke is an environmental and public health hazard, as it becomes a continuous and unseen pollutant reservoir.[60] Exposure to third hand smoke is associated with pathological changes in the liver, lungs, and skin[61,62] and several ailments, including insulin resistance and diabetes, lipid abnormalities and metabolic syndrome – all with an injurious cardiovascular effect.[63]

Cigar smoking carries similar risks as cigarette smoking.[64]

Quitting smoking at any age significantly lowers morbidity and mortality from smoking-related diseases.[65] The risk of smoking related cardiovascular disease appears to approach that of nonsmokers after about 10 years of cessation. In a meta-analysis of 17 studies (10 from North America, 6 from Europe and 1 from Australasia) researchers concluded that there was a 10% reduction in the incidence of acute coronary events following the introduction of smoke-free legislation.[66] Quitting smoking also results in a rapid decrease in the risk for ischemic stroke.[67]

Cessation of smoking reverses the trend of increased heart attack/stroke and premature mortality.[68] Smokers who quit smoking at 25 to 34 years of age gained 10 years of life compared with those who continued to smoke. Those aged 35 to 44 years gained 9 years and those aged 45 to 54 years gained 6 years of life, on average, compared with those who continued to smoke.[69]

Other tobacco use, including vaping, water pipe smoking and smokeless tobacco

Electronic cigarettes (e-cigarettes) may be less lethal than conventional cigarettes, but they are still electronic nicotine delivery systems[70] and nicotine is not good for the vascular system.[71-77] Vaping is associated with increased cardiovascular events.[78]

Water pipe smoking is also extremely popular,[79] with the worldwide prevalence estimated to be 100 million - with an alarming increase in popularity among the youth.[80] Water pipe smoking leads to an increase in a multitude of health problems[81-84] and exhibits many detrimental effects on the vasculature.[85,86] Nicotine, along with other chemicals present in water pipe smoking contributes to an increase in cardiovascular events seen in these patients.[87-92]

Smokeless tobacco has been used for thousands of years and is still very popular.[93-98] Smokeless tobacco use is associated with several health problems.[99-102] There is damage to the vascular system,[103-106] with a higher risk of ischemic heart disease and stroke.[107,108]

Smoking/Tobacco use and Peripheral artery disease

Smoking is a major risk factor for Peripheral artery disease, both overt[109-116] and subclinical.[117] Diabetics with PAD who smoke have a worse survival and diminished event-free survival.[118]

Smoking/Tobacco use and Erectile dysfunction

Cigarette smoking is an independent risk factor for the development of erectile dysfunction.[119-121] It damages the endothelium and impairs eNOS mediated vasodilation – both important for erectile function.[122,123] Smoking is associated with a decrease the level of free nitric oxide in the corpora cavernosa.[124] Direct damage to the penile vasculature may also occur in these patients.[125]

Smoking/Tobacco use and venous disease

Smoking may also play an important role in venous thromboembolism.[126-128] Smoking may result in a procoagulant state, reduced fibrinolysis, inflammation, and increased blood viscosity – all raising VTE risk.[129-131] Smokers also have more cardiovascular diseases, diabetes, lung dysfunction and certain types of cancer – all of these further increase the risk of VTE.[132-135]

Yoga and smoking

Yoga is defined as *'Yogas Chitta Vritti Nirodhah'* or 'Yoga is the cessation of all modifications in consciousness'. In other words, yoga philosophy frowns upon all substances that alter consciousness (this would include smoking and nicotine). It is not surprising therefore that Ross and associates found that only 2% of yoga practitioners smoked - compared to a national average of 21% (4,307 randomly selected individuals from 15 US Iyengar yoga studios (n = 18,160), representing 41 states; 1087 individuals responded, with 1045 (24.3%) surveys completed.[136]

Most studies on yoga have focused on smoking cessation in smokers with encouraging results.

In a study of 20 nicotine addicted participants from a residential drug and alcohol rehabilitation center, simple yoga stretches with breath awareness for 60 minutes once a week for five weeks resulted in a statistically significant shift toward an intention to stop smoking (as assessed through the Stages of Change/Transtheoretical Model Questionnaire).[137] Similarly, in another controlled study, the rhythmic breathing processes of Sudarshan Kriya and *pranayama* were found effective in reducing tobacco consumption in cancer survivors at the end of 12 weeks of the practice. The effects were sustained at the end of a six-month follow-up.[138] Reduced craving for nicotine was also seen following hath yoga exercises.[139] In another study of fifty-five women, all exposed to an eight-week group-based cognitive–behavioral therapy for smoking cessation, patients in a Vinyasa yoga group when compared to general health wellness program group, showed improved abstinence from smoking at seven days and at six months. Yoga also helped reduce anxiety and improved perceived health and well-being when compared with controls.[140] Other studies have also shown that yoga helps patients to stop smoking.[141,142] In a review of four studies, Todd and associates found that the practice of yoga resulted in smokers to have increased desire and motivation to quit smoking. There are fewer urges to smoke and reduced temptations to smoke.[142] Yogic breathing has also shown to reduce the craving for cigarettes.[143] Chia-Liang and Sharma reviewed 10 studies published between 2004 and 2013 in English Language and reported: "Most studies indicated that yoga-based interventions were effective in reducing craving and number of cigarettes smoked during smoking cessation."[144] In a post intervention focus group study of 20 women who had participated in a 8-week vinyasa yoga intervention which included twice weekly 60-minute classes involving breathing exercises, yoga postures, and relaxation techniques, researchers concluded that yoga was viewed by the participants as positive and potentially helpful for quitting smoking.[145] In a review/meta-analysis of 19 randomized controlled trials, Klinsophon and group concluded that yoga when combined with cognitive-behavioral therapy had a positive effect on smoking cessation.[146]

There is no specific published data available on the benefits if any, of using yoga for preventing/deterring/stopping other forms of tobacco/nicotine use such as vaping, water pipe smoking or smokeless tobacco use.

30. Social Isolation/Loneliness

Human beings have "a need to belong".[1] Loneliness – an emotional state, arises from the subjective experience of suffering from social isolation.[2] It is a major social and public health problem, all over the world.[3] It is estimated that 1 in 3 adults age 45 and older, in the USA, feel lonely.[4-6]

The feeling of loneliness is associated with many negative physical and mental health outcomes.[7-11] Loneliness is strongly associated with depression[12-14] and suicidal behavior.[15] It is associated with greater cognitive decline[16,17] and doubles the risk of Alzheimer's disease.[18] It also decreases functionality with a decline in activities of daily living, and a decline in mobility, including difficulty in climbing.[19] A decrease in the quality of life also occurs in these patients.[20]

Loneliness or social isolation plays an important role in premature death and decreased longevity. In a meta-analytic review of 70 independent prospective studies conducted between 1980 and 2014 – featuring a total of 3,407,134 participants – researches found an increased likelihood of premature mortality of 26% for reported loneliness, 29% of social isolation, and 32% for living alone.[21] Increased mortality in those socially isolated has also been reported by others.[22,23]

Loneliness also deleteriously affects the heart and circulation,[24] increasing several risk factors associated with vascular diseases.[25-42] Social isolation or loneliness is related to an increased vascular resistance[25] and increased blood pressure.[26,27] Socially isolated elderly are also more likely to be distressed.[28] They are less physically active[29] and experience less restorative sleep.[30] Social interactions and loneliness also impact obesity.[31] Lonely people are less likely to walk for leisure or transportation, which would increase activity and help them lose weight.[32] Loneliness may be associated with diabetes and higher risks of metabolic syndrome.[33,34] Loneliness increases systemic[35,36] and vascular inflammation.[37] Lonely people are also more likely to smoke.[38] They are also more likely to abuse alcohol.[39] They have autonomic dysfunction - in animal studies involving prairie voles, animals that have similar social interactions as humans, social isolation produced increased heart rate, heart rhythm abnormalities, and autonomic imbalance due to increased sympathetic and decreased parasympathetic drive to the heart.[40] Lonely people also suffer from more depression[41] and anxiety.[42]

Loneliness is associated with an increase in cardiovascular diseases,[43] especially in women.[44,45] Loneliness also impacts health care utilization in patients with heart failure.[46] A large study (meta-analysis of 23 scientific papers) found that lack of socialization and social relationships increased the risk of stroke and coronary heart disease by about 30%.[47] Loneliness increases the prevalence of stroke, with increased mortality and disability.[48,49] Social isolation results in poor post-stroke outcomes.[50] It is also associated with premature cardiovascular mortality.[51]

There was no published association of perceived or real level of social support with the occurrence of PAD.[52]

Socially active (less lonely) people thrive better.[53-55] However, social isolation and loneliness is often difficult to resolve,[56] but remains beneficial - randomized controlled trials of modification of social supports after myocardial infarction show a decrease in cardiac death or reinfarction rates.[57]

Yoga and social isolation

Yoga may help reduce social isolation, especially in the elderly, bereaved, and depressed, as well as individuals undergoing interpersonal crises.[58,59]

Yoga improved social relationships (67%) in an anonymous online survey.[60] Mindfulness based stress reduction has also shown to be useful for reducing loneliness.[61]

31. Spirituality

Spirituality has been defined by many[1,2] and refers to an individual's search for ultimate meaning of life through participation in various modalities, including religion. It's connection with physical health is well established.[3] Prayer can be considered a spiritual practice and is commonly used by most people, especially as a CAM modality.[4-7]

Higher levels of spirituality are also strongly associated with lower levels of depressive symptoms, less anxiety, and less anger.[8] Increasing spirituality helps cope with a chronic or life-threatening diseases[9] and can lead to significant symptomatic improvements in psychiatric disorders.[10]

Spiritual people have a significantly decreased risk of CHD.[11] Spirituality is often used by cardiovascular disease patients to cope during hospitalization.[12] Patients with cardiovascular disease have a better quality of life, if they are spiritual.[13]

Yoga and spirituality

Yoga practitioners are more spiritual.[14] Increase in spirituality is often given as the main reason for continuing the practice of yoga.[15] Studies suggest that more yoga one practices, the more spiritual the practitioner gets.[16]

Beneficial effects of yoga practice related to spirituality have been seen in psychiatric disorders[17] as well as in coping with life threatening illnesses.[18,19]

32. Stroke

Stroke is a common disorder,[1] affecting about 15 million people worldwide each year.[2] It is responsible not only for a large number of deaths,[3] but a major percentage of survivors (80%-90%) are left with some type of disability.[4,5] It is the third major cause of loss of disability-adjusted life years among 291 adverse health conditions worldwide.[6] These patients are also burdened with a significant decrease in their quality of life.[7,8]

Stroke has several modifiable risk factors,[9] which include atrial fibrillation,[10] diabetes mellitus,[11] unhealthy diet,[12] dyslipidemia,[13] hypertension,[14] obesity,[15] physical inactivity,[16] and smoking.[17]

Yoga and stroke

Yoga practice helps ameliorate several of the risk factors responsible for an increased risk of stroke.[18-26] Several studies demonstrate yoga related benefits in atrial fibrillation,[18] diabetes mellitus,[19] hypertension,[20] diet,[21] physical inactivity/exercise,[22,23] dyslipidemia,[24] obesity,[25] and smoking.[26] These improvements in risk factors should have a beneficial effect in decreasing strokes.

The benefits of yoga, as a modality for stroke rehabilitation, have been documented in several studies.[27-29]

33. Stroke Rehabilitation

As discussed in the previous chapter, stroke is a common disorder, affecting about 15 million people worldwide each year.[1] A major percentage of stroke survivors (80%-90%) are left with some type of disability.[2,3] It is the third major cause of loss of disability-adjusted life years among 291 adverse health conditions worldwide.[4] These patients are also burdened with a significant decrease in their quality of life.[5] Post stroke rehabilitation helps improved functionality and reduces long-term disability.[6] Co-morbidities are common in stroke patients, the top three being hypertension, cardiovascular diseases and diabetes mellitus.[7,8] Post-stroke depression is also a common emotional disorder in these patients.[9] Post-stroke rehabilitation is continued following hospital discharge.[10]

Rehabilitation is aimed at recovery of function and cognition to the maximum level achievable, allowing stroke survivors to engage in meaningful life activities. Post-stroke rehabilitation involves many different techniques, mostly based on motor learning to induce neural plasticiticity.[11] Complementary and alternative medicine therapies have also been used in stroke rehabilitation.[12]

Yoga and stroke rehabilitation

Yoga practice has also been tried in this physical and mental rehabilitation process.[13] In a study involving eight female participants, with a mean age of 84 years, and 8 control participants, 5 women and 3 men, average age 81.3 years, an 8-week, 80-minute biweekly Kripalu yoga class was noted to improve postural control, mobility, and gait speed. The researchers suggested that these benefits should also be possible in post-stroke patients with the practice of yoga.[14]

In another study by Garrett and group, nine post-stroke patients underwent a 10-week yoga training program. The patients reported improved sensation, feeling calmer and becoming connected to a new body. Yoga practice also resulted in improvement in strength, range of motion, walking ability[15] and balance.[16]

In a small study involving four post-stroke patients, functionality was monitored using the Berg Balance Scale and the Timed Movement Battery. The patients underwent yoga practice for 1.5-hour sessions, 2 times per week, for 8 weeks, in their home. Improvements in mobility and balance were noted.[17] Improved balance with yoga was also reported in another study.[18]

Schmid and associates[19] recruited 47 patients with chronic stroke and randomized them to a therapeutic-yoga group (n=37) or a wait-list control group (n=10). After 16 sessions of therapeutic yoga (twice a week/8 weeks) they reported that the yoga group had significant improvements in pain, neck range of motion (ROM), hip passive ROM, upper extremity strength, and 6-minute walk scores.

Quality of life, related to motor functions and memory/emotions, also improved in the yoga group, in a randomized controlled trial after a 10-week yoga intervention (n = 11) compared to the group with no treatment (n = 11).[20]

A meta-analysis (five randomized controlled clinical trials, four single case studies and one qualitative research study) documented an overall improvement in cognition, mood, and balance and reductions in stress in post-stroke patients practicing yoga.[21] Improvements in depression and anxiety with yoga were also noticed in another meta-analysis.[2]. Yoga remains a viable modality for patient-centered stroke rehabilitation.[23]

34. Vascular dementia

Vascular dementia is the second most common cause of dementia after Alzheimer's disease,[1,2] and often coexists with the latter.[3] It results from vascular brain injury in regions important for memory and cognition.[4]

Vascular dementia may result from strokes involving the middle size arteries in the brain.[5] Dementia occurring with multi-infarcts account for about 15% of vascular dementia.[6] A major cause of vascular dementia, however, is cerebral small vessel disease.[7,8] This presents as white matter hyperintensities, lacunar infarcts, cerebral microbleeds, and/or brain atrophy on the MRI.[9] Small vessel disease has been linked with hypertension.[10,11] and diabetes.[12] Rarely, cerebral amyloid angiopathy with the deposition of the amyloid β-protein in the wall of leptomeningeal and cerebral blood vessels can result in vascular dementia.[13]

Vascular dementia commonly manifests with a decline in cognitive function, apathy and depression, and can eventually result in death.[14,15] Depression appears to play a significant role in aggravating cognitive decline in patients with dementia.[16,17]

Yoga and vascular dementia

The beneficial effects of yoga on reducing blood pressure[18] and diabetes[19] have been discussed in detail before. Reduction of depression with yoga[20] may also help reduce cognitive decline in these patients.

35. Vascular Elasticity

Reduction in the arterial wall elasticity occurs with aging,[1,2] and in patient with diabetes mellitus,[3] obesity,[4] smoking,[5] and sleep disturbances.[6]

Stiffening of the arteries is suspected if there is an increase in pulse pressure – systolic arterial pressure minus diastolic arterial pressure equals pulse pressure (in mmHg). Normal pulse pressure is between 30 and 50. Arterial stiffness ultimately leads to increased systolic arterial pressure and decreased diastolic arterial pressure – a condition often called 'isolated systolic hypertension'[7] – with an increase in pulse pressure.[8]

Stiffening of the arteries can be recorded by two methods. Carotid intima-media thickness measures the thickness of the inner two layers of the carotid artery—the intima and media – and its increased thickness (indicative of atherosclerosis) is sometimes used as a marker of arterial stiffening (loss of elasticity),[9] while the gold standard is the aortic pulse wave velocity (PWV).[10]

Arterial stiffening promotes left ventricular hypertrophy, left ventricular dysfunction, enhanced atherosclerosis[11] and impairs coronary blood flow.[7,12] Clinical sequelae include heart attacks,[13] heart failure[14] and stroke.[15,16] It is also associated with higher cardiovascular morbidity and mortality.[17-20]

Arterial stiffening documented by aortic pulse wave velocity independently prognosticates cardiovascular risk factors - as was concluded in a recent meta-analysis involving 17,635 subjects.[21] In a meta-analysis of 17 longitudinal studies (15,877 subjects followed for a mean of 7.7 years) Vlachopoulos and group noted that an increase in aortic PWV by 1 m/s corresponded to a risk increase of 14% in total cardiovascular events, 15% in cardiovascular mortality and 15% in all-cause mortality.[22]

Elasticity of the blood vessels can be improved therapeutically by drugs.[23] but also by following many healthy lifestyles, especially regular exercise.[24]

Yoga and arterial elasticity

In a study, 30 elderly patients with increased pulse pressure were assigned for yoga training (one hour in the morning for 6 days in a week for 3 months) and their cardiovascular profile compared with another 30 individuals that were assigned to brisk-walking. The researchers noted that that the yoga program was more effective than brisk-walk in reducing arterial stiffness in these individuals.[25]

In a more recent study of twenty hypertensive individuals (7 females), age range 30 to 60 years, a comprehensive residential yoga therapy program for one week resulted in an improvement in the pulse pressure, mainly due to a reduction of the systolic blood pressure, suggesting improved arterial elasticity.[26]

Another study on 24 young (mean age 30±1 years) and 18 middle-aged and older (mean age 53±2 years) adults was done using an 8 week Bikram yoga (90 minutes of yoga per session, three times per week, in a room heated to 40.5°C with 40%--60% relative humidity.) intervention. At the end of the study, there was a reduction in arterial stiffness (as measured by carotid artery compliance), in the young but not in the elderly.[27]

36. Vascular Inflammation

Inflammation ("to set on fire") acts as both a 'friend and foe': although it our immune-surveillance and host defense, a chronic low-grade inflammatory state becomes pathological and has been linked with several diseases.[1,2] These include obesity,[3] metabolic syndrome,[4] depression,[5] anxiety,[6] schizophrenia,[7] Alzheimer's disease,[8] rheumatoid arthritis,[9] osteoporosis,[10] periodontal disease,[11] type 2 diabetes mellitus[12,13] and cancer.[14,15] Inflammation is also a robust and reliable predictor of all-cause mortality.[16,17]

Vascular inflammation plays an important role in all aspects of atherosclerosis - initiation, progression and complications.[18] Patients with atherosclerosis have higher levels of serum inflammatory biomarkers, such as C-reactive protein, (CRP)[19] cell adhesion molecules, fibrinogen and various inflammatory cytokines.[20] The three commonly associated inflammatory biomarkers with the greatest risk of cardiovascular events are IL-6, TNF-α, and CRP.[21-24]

In clinical practice vascular inflammation is commonly assessed by measuring high-sensitivity C-reactive protein (hs-CRP) levels.[25] Baseline levels of CRP are considered an independent predictor of future cardiovascular events[26,27] and patients with elevated CRP have more cardiovascular events.[28] These include a wide range of cardiovascular, neurovascular and peripheral vascular diseases[29-31] - coronary artery disease,[32] myocardial infarction,[33,34] stroke,[35-37] and peripheral arterial disease.[38,39] The increased risk in one study was 23% more for myocardial infarction, 32% for ischemic stroke and 34% more for vascular death in a meta-analysis. This study evaluated the results of 160,309 people without a history of vascular disease (1.31 million person-years at risk, 27 769 fatal or non-fatal disease outcomes) from 54 long-term prospective studies.[40]

A large-scale prospective study among women without a history of cardiovascular disease, markers of systemic inflammation were also significantly related to atrial fibrillation.[41] The risk also increases for peripheral artery disease.[42] Several studies have also documented increased vascular mortality with increased inflammation.[43]

Reducing low grade inflammation helps reduce vascular disease. Low dose aspirin has some anti-inflammatory effects,[44,45] but its use in cardiovascular event protection is mainly based on its anti-platelet effects.[46] Statins, on the other hand, not only help lower LDL cholesterol, but they also have potent anti-inflammatory effects.[47-49] Mediterranean diet[50,51] and exercise[52] are associated with a reduction in vascular events. Lowering vascular inflammation with these lifestyles is an important factor in conferring this benefit.[53,54]

Yoga and inflammation

Regular practice of yoga reduces the resting levels of inflammatory cytokines like TNF-α and IL-6 and hsCRP.[55] Vascular inflammation was reduced as evidenced by a reduction in fibrinogen, hsCRP and ESR in 7 elderly women following hath yoga for 10 weeks, as compared to the levels before the intervention. The control group of 7 did not show any change.[56] The beneficial effects of yoga on reduction of vascular inflammation has been documented by several other studies, including those in healthy[57,58] and diseased individuals.[59-63]

In a study of 50 healthy women (mean age=41.32), 25 novices and 25 experts, were exposed to yoga, movement control, and passive-video control during three separate visits. Researchers found that novices' serum IL-6 levels were 41% higher and they were more than 4.75 times likely to have abnormal levels of CRP when compared to experts – indicating yoga's protection against inflammation in the experts.[57]

Regular practice of yoga also stunts the extent of increase of TNF-α and IL-6 following a challenge of moderate exercise and strenuous exercise – this was recorded in a study of 109 yoga practitioners (5 years of yoga experience) and 109 controls – both were exposed to a bout of moderate exercise and a bout of strenuous exercise.[58]

Heart failure patients (n=9) randomized to a two-month hatha yoga intervention showed a 22% reduction in IL-6 and a 20% reduction in CRP - the changes in 10 control patients who received standard medical care were minimal.[59] Another study of yoga intervention in breast cancer survivors reported decreases in IL-6, TNF-α, and IL-1β.[60] Yogic practice has also reduced inflammation in obese[61,62] and stressed individuals.[63]

Diet is also strongly related to increased inflammation, especially intake of red meat[64] while intake of fruits, vegetables, whole grains, nuts, seeds, and legumes is associated with lower inflammation.[65] Plant based diets are cardio-protective.[66] Yoga practitioners are more likely to eat more plant-based diet.[67]

37.   Venous Diseases

Venous insufficiency

Chronic venous insufficiency is a common disease, affecting about 15% of the total adult population, with a significant increase in elderly people.[1,2] In the United States, it is estimated that approximately 2.5 million people have chronic venous insufficiency.[3,4]

Contraction of the muscles of the feet and the legs actively compress the lower limb veins and help the normal venous return (against gravity) during standing and other dependency states.[5] The main muscles responsible for this 'deep vein muscle pump action' are the calf muscles – the soleus and to a lesser extent, the gastronemius.[6,7] This muscle pump is therefore sometimes called the 'peripheral heart'.[8]

Venous return of the leg is dependent on two systems: deep and superficial (either deep or superficial to the muscular fascia), connected by innumerable perforator veins between ankle and groin. The deep system also includes the venous sinuses within, mainly, the soleus and, to a lesser extent, the gastrocnemii muscles. The deep venous systems empty due to muscular actions in feet, calf and thigh, and the blood from the superficial system passes on to them guided by perforators and unidirectional intact valves. This action guides the blood towards the heart. Incompetence at the saphenofemoral junction in the groin is the commonest cause of reflux from the deep to superficial systems – resulting in retrograde flow.[9,10] Extended periods of sitting or standing lead to increased venous pressure in the legs and to stretched vein walls and damaged venous valves, ultimately leading to chronic venous insufficiency[11,12] Risk factors include age, gender, tall stature, pregnancy, history of leg injury, family history, prolonged standing at work as experienced by bus conductors, teachers and policeman on duty, and iatrogenic.[13,14] Patients may experience a vague feeling of heaviness in lower extremities, swelling of the legs, aching, itching due to eczema, and skin pigmentation and venous ulceration, particularly of the medial ankle.[15]

Chronic venous insufficiency can lead to telangiectasia, varicose veins, deep vein thrombosis, post-thrombotic syndrome and venous ulcers.[16-18]

Telangiectasia

Telangiectasia and/or reticular veins are the earliest indication that chronic venous insufficiency is present.[19]

Varicose Veins

Varicose veins in the legs is a common venous disease[20] with an incidence of 10% to 30% in the general population.[21] They result from dilatation of the branches of the great saphenous vein and small saphenous veins.[22] Major risk factors include family history, age, and pregnancy (especially women with two or more pregnancies).[22-25]

Patients with varicose veins may be asymptomatic or experience significant symptoms, including discomfort, cosmetic disfigurement, aching, throbbing pain, itching or eczema, and ankle/leg swelling.[26,27] Clinical manifestation and duplex ultrasound usually provide the diagnosis.[28] The CEAP (clinical, etiology, anatomy, pathophysiology) is an useful classification describing the degree of varicose veins.[29] Complications of varicose veins may lead to disability, and a decreased quality of life.[30]

Treatment options include conservative treatment with lifestyle changes, including exercise, proper diet, loss of weight, leg elevation, and compression stockings. Surgical options include open venous surgery, endo-venous thermal ablation with laser or radiofrequency energy, and sclerotherapy.[31-36]

Venous Thrombosis (Deep Vein Thrombosis -DVT)

Deep vein thrombosis occurs with the formation of a blood clot in the deep venous system, most commonly in the lower limbs (i.e. superficial femoral and popliteal veins in the thighs and the posterior tibial and peroneal veins in the calves)[37] It is a common disease.[38-40] DVT and pulmonary embolism has an estimated incidence rate of 1-2 per 1000 persons every year, and DVT is responsible for substantial short- and long-term morbidity and mortality.[41-43]

Morbidity is associated with long term complications in about one-half of the affected people (post-thrombotic syndrome) such as swelling, pain, discoloration, and scaling in the affected limb.[44,45] and a poor quality of life.[46]

If part of the venous thrombus dislodges and deposits occluding the vessels of the lung – it results in pulmonary embolism (occurs in approximately one-third of the patients with DVT).[47] Pulmonary embolism is immediately fatal in about 20% of patients - they die before diagnosis or on the 1st day of diagnosis.[48] It is estimated that 10 to 30% of people will die within one month of diagnosis.[49] The incidence of pulmonary embolism appears to be increasing.[50]

Risk factors for venous thromboembolism include advancing age, obesity, recent surgery (including hip or knee replacement), major trauma (including fracture), active cancer, acute medical illnesses (e.g. heart failure, respiratory failure), paralytic stroke or immobilization, antiphospholipid syndrome, inherited thrombophilia, previous venous thromboembolism, congenital venous malformation, varicose veins, central venous catheter or vena cava filter, long-distance travel, pregnancy/antepartum and oral contraceptives or hormone replacement therapy.[51]

Contrast venography is the gold standard for diagnosing DVT.[52] Besides clinical examination, other diagnostic tools include compression ultrasound,[53] D-dimer levels.[54] and CT scan and MRI scans.[55]

Since DVT is a chronic disease and carries a high risk for recurrence, treatment in usually long term and comprises of oral anticoagulants.[56,57]

Post-thrombotic Syndrome

The main complications after venous thrombosis is development of the post-thrombotic syndrome, which occurs in about 50% of patients with deep vein thrombosis.[58] Another complication, chronic thromboembolic pulmonary hypertension,[59] occurs in about 3.4% of those with pulmonary embolism.[60]

Symptoms of the post-thrombotic syndrome include swelling, pain and skin problems ranging from dryness to discoloration and venous ulcers. Risk factors of post-thrombotic syndrome at the time of or after DVT, include older age, male sex, recurrent ipsilateral DVT, obesity, distal or more extensive DVT, poor quality of initial anticoagulation, ongoing symptoms or signs of DVT 1 month after diagnosis, and elevated D-dimer at 1 month.[61-63]

Use of elastic compression stockings helps prevent post-thrombotic syndrome in those with DVT.[64,65] but no placebo-controlled trials are available.

Venous Ulcers

Venous ulcers result from chronic venous insufficiency and venous hypertension – the latter leads to dilated/tortuous capillaries and compromises the blood irrigation/tissue oxygenation of the tissues in the affected limb.[66-70]

In one study, an ambulatory foot vein pressure of 30 mm Hg or less was not associated with leg ulceration, while patients with a pressure greater than 90 mm Hg experienced consistent ulceration.[71] Venous ulcers account for 75% of all chronic leg ulcers.[72] Other non-venous causes of leg ulcers include arterial insufficiency, diabetes, rheumatoid arthritis, autoimmune disease, cancer, and tropical diseases.[73] The estimated prevalence of venous leg ulcers in adults is about 0.3%, and incidence is about 20% of those with chronic venous insufficiency. The prevalence of venous ulceration increases with age[74] – it is estimated that 1–3% of the population aged over 60 years is affected[75] and affect almost 600,000 Americans aged 65 years or older.[76]

Lifestyle factors, including proper nutrition, and cessation of smoking, are useful in the management of venous ulceration.[77] Lower limb exercise is also beneficial.[78] Compression therapy, delivered using compression hosiery[79] or multi-layer bandaging, is the mainstay of treatments for venous leg ulcers.[80] The objective is to provide graded external compression to the leg and oppose the hydrostatic forces of venous hypertension.[81] Compression (bandages and stockings)heals more ulcers compared with no compression. Therapeutic interventions also include vascular reconstruction, shaving surgery with graft coverage, ulcer excision with fasciectomy with graft coverage and other advanced treatment modalities.[82]

Clinical outcomes in these patients are poor with many patients experiencing delayed healing and recurrent ulcerations.[83,84] Many patients become disabled[85] and experience a poor quality of life.[86,87]

Yoga and venous disease

Several yoga poses involve activating the muscle pump in the legs and stimulating venous return. However, no published studies were found linking yoga with prevention or improvement of venous diseases of the legs. However, leg up poses and social support as is provided by yoga, may be helpful in patients with chronic venous disease, especially venous ulceration.[88]

38. Other Cardio-vasculo-protective Lifestyles

Several lifestyles are associated with decreased heart and circulatory system disease and its related mortality.[1,2] It is my observational opinion that yoga practitioners are more likely to indulge in several vasculo-protective lifestyles.

Aromatherapy: Essential oils are obtained by steam distillation of aromatic plants. Controlled use of these essential oils is aromatherapy ("aroma" meaning a pleasant scent and "therapy" meaning healing). These fragrant essential oils are absorbed into the human body through the airway or the skin.[3] Vascular benefits of aromatherapy (using specific oils) include reduction in blood pressure,[4,5] better sleep[6-8] and decreased anxiety in sick cardiac patients.[9,10]

Yoga and aromatherapy: Most yoga practitioners will use some 'incense/aromatic oil' in the room during yoga practice.

Dental/Oral health: Tooth brushing suppresses halitosis and may help prevent tooth decay and gum disease by delivering active ingredients such as fluoride. Regular brushing of the teeth also helps prevent periodontal disease. Periodontal disease, a chronic infection of the tissues surrounding the teeth, results in increased inflammation.[11-13] Inflammation is a major player in the pathogenesis of atherosclerosis.[14] Periodontal disease also raises several cardiovascular risk factors such as diabetes mellitus and dyslipidemia.[15] An association with an increased risk of cardiovascular diseases,[16] including non-fatal and fatal coronary artery disease events[17,18] with periodontal disease has been well established.

Yoga and dental health: *Niyama* or personal observances in Pantajali's eight-fold yoga sutras includes *sauca*: outer and inner cleanliness.

Gardening: Gardening is a common leisure-time physical activity among older adults[19] It helps improve nutrition,[20] decreases obesity and diastolic blood pressure,[21] improves mood,[22,23] mental health,[24] decreases social isolation[25] and increases physical activity[26] – all factors that help improve the vascular health. Habitual gardeners have decreased acute coronary events.[27] Gardening also improves the quality of life post stroke.[28] It is good for general health[29] and helps increase longevity.[30]

Yoga and gardening: Many yoga retreats encourage '*karma* yoga' - to give selflessly for the good of others without thought of one's self or attachment to the results of one's actions.[31] This is practiced in many forms at the yoga retreats and often includes working in their gardens, cooking and serving food.

Hobbies: Hobbies are leisure time activities that one enjoys doing alone. They can include stamp collecting, photography, knitting, doing crossword puzzles etc. They act as mental tonics, and often keep one physically active. They also help one relax. Hobbies can thus help reduce cardiovascular disease by inducing relaxation, generating happiness, improving social interaction and increasing leisure time exercise. In a study of 121 men and women, those with hobbies showed better coronary vasculature reactivity and had lower incidence of major adverse cardiovascular events during several months of observation (average follow-up period was 916 +/- 515 days).[32] Hobbies help modify several emotional risk factors - they reduce stress and increase happiness.[33] Leisure time hobbies help improve social interaction.[34] And these people, especially the elderly, become more active, which is cardioprotective.[35]

Yoga and hobbies: I could not find any published data in the English literature that substantiates my opinion that yoga practitioners are more likely to have hobbies. Interestingly, in a survey by Telles and group, 5.5% of the males and 5.9% of the females (especially the young) considered doing yoga itself a hobby.[36]

Marriage: Marriage is a legally or a formally recognized union of two people as partners in a personal relationship. According to the United States Census in 2014, there were 39,833,000 single adults, 50 years of age and older, living in the United States.[37] The majority of these older singles do not date and continue to remain single. This group is at an increased risk of poor health, including cardiovascular disease and early death. Married people have better general health than the unmarried.[38] In one study, married people had 5% less vascular disease, 8% less abdominal aortic aneurysm, 9% less cerebrovascular disease and 19% less peripheral arterial disease.[39] They also tend to live longer.[40,41]

Yoga and marriage: Yoga practitioners are less likely to be divorced/widowed/separated – only 18.1% according to one study.[42]

Mindfulness: Mindfulness is defined as "paying attention in a particular way: on purpose, in the present moment, and non-judgmentally".[43] Many individuals practice mindfulness in their daily life and many yoga teachers will teach mindfulness meditation as part of the multi-modal yoga routine. Mindfulness based stress reduction programs are also popular.[44] Mindfulness meditation has been practiced and prescribed successfully for a reduction of anxiety, depression and stress.[45,46] Besides neuro-psychological benefits,[47] mindfulness also positively affects many physical ailments, including cardiovascular diseases.[48] It helps reduce inflammation,[49] and blood pressure,[50] better control blood glucose.[51] improve lipid profiles,[52] reduce anxiety,[53] depression[54] and encourages healthy lifestyles.

Yoga and mindfulness: Mindfulness living is taught as a part of multi-modal yoga.

Music: Music is considered an art form and is deeply ingrained in many people's way of life.[1] Music is often used as a complimentary therapy to promote health in several health ailments,[55-60] such as reducing agitation in psychiatry patients,[55] relaxing patients in stressful situations,[56] and reducing pain, anxiety and distress in hospitalized[57-59] and post-operative patients.[60]

Music is also good for the cardiovascular system.[61-65] It is helpful in reducing stress in patients with coronary heart disease,[62] as well as thrombotic activity and inflammatory cytokines.[63] In a study of 60 patients undergoing open heart surgery, relaxing music helped reduce postoperative pain.[64] In cardiac rehabilitation, music increases the time of physical activity undertaken and helps in exercise adherence.[65]

In a study of 60 stroke patients recruited between March 2004 and May 2006 at the Department of Neurology of the Helsinki University Central Hospital, cognitive recovery and prevention of negative mood was enhanced in the early post-stroke phase with music.[66]

Yoga and music: Literally every yoga class in the West has soothing background music. 'Yoga music' may include drums, harmonicas, and many other instruments that are immediately familiar and many other Indian instruments such as esraj or bansuri. The difference from other music is that yoga music often makes use of *mantras* from the Sanskrit and Gurbani traditions. These mantras are often hundreds, if not thousands of years old. Yoga music is also designed to complement and facilitate the yoga practice. The music can set the appropriate mood and even have specific tempos or lengths of time coinciding with the duration of certain *asanas*, *kriyas* or meditations.

A study on yoga music and anxiety was recently (2018) presented at the European Society of Cardiology (ESC) Congress in Munich, Germany.[67] One hundred and forty-nine healthy people participated in three sessions on separate nights. The first was yoga (soothing or meditative) music before sleep at night, the second pop music with steady beats, and the third no music or silence before sleep. This study assessed anxiety levels before and after each session using the Goldberg Anxiety Scale. The study that found anxiety levels fell significantly after participants listened to yoga music and rose after pop music or no music. People felt significantly more positive after the yoga music than after the pop music.

Pets: Pet ownership is popular.[68] Pet owners have reduced cardiovascular disease risk factors.[69,70] and having pets is therefore cardioprotective.[71] Pet owners are more active[72,73] and experience more positive emotions.[74] Pets help lower blood pressure.[75] They experience less coronary artery disease[76,77] and live longer following a heart attack.[78,79]

Yoga and pet ownership: I could not find any published data in the English literature that substantiates my opinion that yoga practitioners are more likely to be pet owners.

Pollution (both air and noise): Air pollution is detrimental for our health, and is a major preventable environmental risk.[80] In 2012, the World Health Organization (WHO) recorded an increase to nearly seven million deaths from combined ambient and household air pollution.[81] Besides exerting a major negative impact on the pulmonary and digestive system, it is also responsible for a significant number of cardiovascular events and deaths.[82] Most studies show that PM2.5 particles (particulate matter in the environment is primarily divided into three categories according to their aerodynamic diameter: coarse: PM10 – PM2.5; fine: PM2.5 to PM1 and ultrafine: <PM1.) play a major role in cardiovascular morbidity and mortality.[83] Particulate air pollutants affect the cardiovascular

system in many ways. They cause endothelial dysfunction and vasoconstriction, increase blood pressure and heart rate, increase prothrombotic and coagulant activity, increase systemic inflammation, and raise oxidative stress responses. They decrease heart rate variability, increase autonomic imbalance, induce arrhythmias, raise insulin resistance, and lead to the progression of atherosclerosis. Besides an increase in coronary disease events[84] air pollution also increases the incidence of ischemic strokes[85] and stroke related hospitalizations and deaths.[86] There is worsening of heart failure in patients, resulting in an increase in heart failure hospitalizations and an increase in heart failure mortality.[87] Patients dying of sudden cardiac death appear to do so more when ambient air pollution is high.[88] There is an increase in deaths related to coronary artery disease, with an increase in air pollution.[89] Overall, increasing air pollution results in increased cardiovascular morbidity and mortality.[90]

Transportation generated noise - road traffic, railways and aircraft, are common causes of outdoor noise. Indoor noise pollution may occur at work dur to machines or at home from listening to loud music. Noise pollution is detrimental to general[91] and cardiovascular health[92,93] High noise exposure may alter glucose control[94] and increase depression,[95] annoyance[96] and vascular dysfunction, oxidative stress and inflammation[97] – all risk factors for cardiovascular diseases. Blood pressure is increases[98] and there is an increase in risk for myocardial infarction.[99] The rates of heart failure also go up with increasing noise exposure. This association was confirmed in a study involving 104,145 cases of heart failure and/or hypertensive heart disease patients, followed during the years 2006-10 and compared with 654,172 control subjects in Germany.[100] There is also an increase in the rates of stroke with exposure to noise from different sources.[101] Chronic exposure to excessive noise at workplace has also been noted to increase cardiovascular mortality. In a study done on a group of 27,464 blue-collar workers who worked for at least one year, at 14 lumber mills in British Columbia, and followed between 1950 and 1995, researchers found that the group with the highest exposure to noise, ended up having 50% higher heart attack related deaths.[102]

Yoga and pollution: Yoga stresses breathing exercises and meditation – both against air and noise pollution. Yoga retreats are also usually held in places with natural surroundings, usually with clean air and a quiet environment. However, no published data could be found on yoga and pollution.

Sports: Evidence based data from several scientific studies and meta-analyses persuasively confirm a positive association between increased athletic activity (both recreational and competitive) and better general[103] and cardiovascular health.[104] It also improves longevity.[105]

Sports-persons practicing yoga derive many vascular health benefits, which include a reduction in blood pressure,[106] improvement in the lipid profile,[107] reduction of abdominal adiposity,[108] improved insulin sensitivity,[109] better glucose metabolism,[110] reduced systemic inflammation,[111] and improvement in overall cardio-vascular function.[112] They also have a more positive attitude, with less depression and anxiety.[113]

Yoga and sports: Yoga practice leads to improved functional fitness.[114,115] In a study of Bikram yoga in healthy young individuals, researchers found that practicing subjects exhibited increased deadlift strength, substantially increased lower back/hamstring flexibility, increased shoulder flexibility, and modestly decreased body fat compared with control group.[116] Yoga also improves balance and produces modest improvements in leg strength and leg muscle control.[117] Athletes also develop better flexibility and balance[118,119] and benefit from improved motivation for the activity.[120] They have improved aerobic cardio-respiratory functions[121-123] and improved anaerobic capacity functions.[124] There is also improvement in relaxation.[125] All these make yoga a common modality in exercise routine of many atheletes.[126] Whether normal people are more sports active due to yoga practice is not known.

Tea drinking: Tea is one of the most consumed beverages in the world.[127] Health benefits of tea have been noted in several diseases, including cancer,[128] cognitive dysfunction[129] and osteoporosis.[130]

The phenolic compounds present in black tea[131,132] help reduce several cardiovascular disease risk factors such as hypertension,[133] diabetes mellitus,[134] dyslipidemia,[135] obesity,[136] stress, and depression.[137] Tea drinking is also associated with reduced inflammation[138] and reduces platelet activation.[139] Drinking 3 cups of tea per day decreases the risk of myocardial infarction by 11%.[140] Tea drinking also reduces strokes by 10%–20%.[141,142] Tea drinking also helps reduce cardiovascular mortality.[143-145]

Yoga and tea drinking: Tea is often a part of yoga class and is preferred over coffee. Yogi Tea is a type of masala (spiced) chai (tea) and is, traditionally made of black tea and aromatic Indian spices such as cloves, cardamom, ginger, black pepper and cinnamon. It is usually sweetened with honey and milk.

Many yoga teachers will suggest an invigorating tea after the morning yoga sessions - green, ginger, chai or yogi tea. A calming tea such as chamomile, lavender, mint or jasmine is often imbibed after an evening session.

Vacation: Vacationing is associated with a litany of healthy outcomes.[146-153] These include psychological well-being,[146,147] and an improved physical status.[148,149] Vacations lead to less severe disease outcomes,[150] and increased longevity.[151,152] Vacations also enhances positivity.[153]

Cardiovascular benefits have been noted in vacationers.[154-156] In a 20-year study, researchers found that women who took vacation once every six years or less were almost eight times more likely to develop coronary heart disease or have a heart attack than women who took at least two vacations per year.[154] In a study of middle aged men at risk of developing coronary heart disease, taking vacations resulted in several health benefits: a 17% reduction in all-cause mortality, a 29% reduction in cardiovascular mortality, and a 32% reduction in coronary heart disease and heart attacks.[155,156]

Yoga and vacations: Many yoga sessions are provided in yoga retreats – these are vacations that include yoga with exposure to often exotic destinations.

Vitamin D: Vitamin D (sunlight related synthesis in the human epidermis is responsible for almost 80% of the human vitamin D supply) levels should be >30 ng/mL.[157] Vitamin D deficiency is responsible for rickets in children and osteomalacia in adults.[158] Together with calcium, vitamin D also helps protect older adults from osteoporosis. Vitamin D has other roles in the body, including modulation of cell growth, neuromuscular and immune function, and reduction of inflammation.[159,160]

Its deficiency has also been associated with increased risk for many chronic diseases,[161] including autoimmune diseases,[162] some cancers,[163] infectious disease,[164] schizophrenia,[165] type 2 diabetes,[166] and also results in increased mortality.[167]

Low vitamin D levels appear to increase cardiovascular risk.[168] Low vitamin D levels have been associated with several cardiovascular risk factors. A connection between low vitamin D levels with obesity,[169] and lower high-density lipoprotein cholesterol and higher triglycerides, as well as higher apolipoprotein E levels, has been noted.[170] A meta-analysis of 11 prospective studies involving 3,612 cases and 55,713 non-case participants provided evidence for a strong inverse association between vitamin D levels and incidence of type 2 diabetes.[171] Some studies have suggested that vitamin D deficiency is associated with higher blood pressure levels, while others find this association not consistent.[172]

In a study of 1,739 participants from the Framingham Offspring cohort, researchers found that a vitamin D concentration below 15 ng/mL was consistently associated with an increased risk of cardiovascular events. They estimated that patients with vitamin D deficiency had a 5-year rate of developing a cardiovascular event two times higher than in those with adequate vitamin D stores.[173] A clear association between vitamin D status and the occurrence of acute myocardial infarction and coronary heart disease has however not been firmly established. Low levels have also been associated with heart failure.[174]

In a meta-analysis of seven studies, involving 47,809 individuals and 926 cerebrovascular events, the risk for cerebrovascular disease was significantly lower in subjects with high vitamin D levels compared to those with low levels.[175] Low vitamin D levels are also linked with excess peripheral arterial disease.[176] Low vitamin D levels are also associated with an increase in cardiovascular mortality and overall mortality.[177,178]

However, most vitamin D supplementation trials have not demonstrated improvement in CVD.[179,180] This suggests that naturally obtained vitamin D (for a light skinned person, 10-15 minutes of sun exposure) is cardioprotective and this protection cannot be obtained by oral supplementation.

Yoga and vitamin D: Yoga is preferentially done outdoors in nature. *Surya namaskars* are encouraged to be done facing the rising run in the early morning hours on grass – exposing the human body to natural vitamin D (and low exposure to the harmful UVA radiation). In the early morning, average person of median skin complexion, 30 minutes to an hour in the sun without sunscreen will create adequate amounts of vitamin D. Morning exposure might have to be a little longer than this due to less sunlight intensity than midday sun (10 AM to 3 PM), as recommended by the National Institutes of Health.[181]

Work and long work hours: Working regular hours is often associated with stress – chronic work-related stress is detrimental to the physical and mental health of humans.[182] It can also increase the risk of cardiometabolic diseases by as much as 50%.[183]

Working long hours also brings in emotional burnout[184] and physical exhaustion.[185] Besides poor job performance, there is an associated negative impact on social and family life. The quality of life is obviously affected.[186]

An increase in working hours is associated with an increase in hypertension. A study looked at 1,079 subjects, with average working time of 47.68 hours per week. The proportion of overtime workers was 61.0% (cutoff of 40 hours per week). In this study, as the number of overtime hours increased, so did the diagnosis of hypertension.[187] A study of 2,194 workers indicate that those working more than 50 hours overtime per month in Japan, had a 3.7 times higher risk of non-insulin dependent diabetes mellitus after controlling for known risk factors.[188] Another study found that working more than 10 hours/day resulted in an increased risk of metabolic syndrome among Japanese male workers.[189] Long working hours are also related to an increase in several other cardiovascular risk factors, including decreased physical activity, increased smoking, increased stress and depression.[190]

A meta-analysis of 11 studies have confirmed that long working hours were associated with an increased risk of cardiovascular disease.[191-193] A retrospective cohort study of 1,926 individuals from the Panel Study of Income Dynamics, revealed that increasing work week was associated with a dose-related increased risk of cardiovascular disease. These employees were employed for at least 10 years and were studied from 1986 to 2011.[194]

Regular work stress is associated with an increased incidence of coronary heart disease and stroke.[195-197] Evaluation of Karoshi or deaths attributed to overwork in Japan revealed that over 70% of the sudden deaths were due to a sudden stroke or a fatal cardiac event.[198]

Yoga and work: Yoga has shown in several studies to reduce work related stress, exhaustion and burnout.[199-202] A Swedish study involving 33 workers showed positive effects of yoga on psychological and physiological stress outcomes with yoga intervention.[203] The relationship between stress with increased cardiovascular diseases is well known.[204,205] This link between stress and disease is influenced to a large extent by autonomic imbalance implicating an overactive or dysregulated sympathetic nervous system and an up-regulated hypothalamus-pituitary-adrenal (HPA) axis. Yoga practice decreases sympathetic activity[206] and downregulates the HPA axis.[207]

YOGA PROGRAM FOR THE HEART AND CIRCULATORY SYSTEM

A regular lifelong practice of multimodal yoga – a combination of *asanas* (poses), *pranayamas* (breathing exercises), *dhyana* (meditation) and *yoga nidra* (relaxation) with an understanding of the yogic philosophy – will greatly help one achieve a healthy, happier, longer and more spiritual life. A sample program is presented here (heart and circulation friendly):

Timings:

    Opening prayer 1-2 minutes

    Warming Exercises 5 minutes

    Surya Namaskar 5 minutes

    20 slow yoga poses 20 minutes

    Breathing exercises 10 minutes

    Meditation 10 minutes

    Yoga *Nidra* 5 minutes

    Closing prayer 1-2 minutes

Total session: approximately 60 minutes (the duration may be cut down to 30 minutes per session, if needed – most clinical studies have used 45-60 minutes of yoga)

Frequency: 3 times per week

Duration: no stop date – continue for the rest of your life

    Yoga and props: Yoga props are commonly used in yoga studios all over the world. They not only help you deepen your pose but also help improve your alignment. The difficult, awkward and uncomfortable poses become easier to do, and this not only increases your self-confidence but also improves your ability to them in the future without the help of props. A yoga mat is almost a necessity for performing the exercises. Commonly used props are towels and blankets. Commercially available props are numerous and include pillows/belt/strap/wheel/bolster/cushion/blocks and other contraptions. These may be used as and when needed.[1]

    Yoga music may help set the mood or otherwise help during this practice.

1. Opening Prayer

"Prayer is the key of the morning and the bolt of the evening."

Mahatma Gandhi

Traditionally, most 'gurus' in India will prefer reciting a mantra/prayer or two before the start of the yoga session. This helps set the mood for the practice – which is 'holistic' in nature and prayers also remind us that we are a part of the universal consciousness. Sample opening prayers:

Om bhur bhuvah svah
tat savitur varenyam
bhargo devasya dhimahi
dhiyo yo nah prachodayat

The divine light that pervades the earth,
heavens, and the in-between –
may this protect us,
sustain us
and illuminate our consciousness.

•

Om saha nav avatu
saha nau bhunaktu
saha viryam karavavahai
tejasvi navadhitam astu ma vidvishavahai
Om shanti

May god protect us both
May god nourish us both
May we work together with energy and vigor,
May our study be enlightening.
Om, peace, peace, peace!!
Or you can use any of your own prayers.

2. Loosening (Warm-up) Exercises

Yogic literature describes warm up exercises as loosening exercises (*Sukṣma vyayāma* and *Sithilikarana vyayama*) which should be done before proceeding to the *asanas*. These should ideally be done five times each, but you can vary this to your liking and timing.

Neck:

1. Chin to chest and back bend: exhale and bring chin to chest; inhale and bring it back to center
2. Chin to shoulder and back: exhale and turn chin to right shoulder; inhale and bring it back to center. Repeat left side.
3. Ear to shoulder and back: exhale and bend neck to bring right ear to right shoulder, inhale and come back to center. Repeat on left side.
4. Neck rotation; looking forward, do a clockwise neck rotation and then one counter-clockwise.

Shoulders:

1. Shoulder shrugs – inhale while shrugging them and exhale while returning to baseline.
2. Bring the arms up over your head with inhalation and interlace the fingers and try to push up and press the palms to the ceiling, without losing your flat footing. Exhale and arch the interlaced hands over to the right side. Return to the ceiling pose with inhalation. Now exhale and arch over to the left side. Return to normal standing pose.
3. Bring the arms up over your head with inhalation and interlace the fingers and try to push up and press the palms to the ceiling, without losing your flat footing. Now bring and extend the hands forward, while your upper/middle spine gets rounded. Inhale and bring the palms back towards the ceiling. Now exhale and push the hands backwards behind the head – limited but do the best you can. Inhale and bring the palms back to the ceiling.
4. Bring the arms up over your head with inhalation and interlace the fingers and try to push up and press the palms to the ceiling, without losing your flat footing. Exhale and bend the right elbow downwards and behind the head on the right side. Inhale and bring the palms back towards the ceiling. Exhale and bend the left elbow behind and below the head on the left side. Inhale the palms to back the ceiling. Relax in the standing pose.
5. Shoulder roll: Making slow big circles, roll the shoulders up, down and back. Then reverse direction of the circles.

Spine:

1. Backward arch to forward bend – standing with feet somewhat apart, raise both arms above your head and then exhaling, bend your spine backwards so that your face looks at the ceiling and your arms are stretched back. Inhaling bend forwards till arms are above the head and now exhaling, bend further forwards as if trying to touch your feet. Return to the rest pose.
2. Stretched arm twists – inhale and spread your arms on each side outwards so that they are parallel to the ground and both form a straight line together. Now exhale and twist first right side and then left side.
3. Side bends – from the same stretched out arms, exhale and bend right so that your right hand is trying to touch your right foot. Inhale and return to normal. Now repeat on the left side and return to baseline.

Hips

Wide legged squat:

1. Stand with your feet slightly more than hip distance apart.
2. Maintaining your balance, lower your hips into a squat till your thighs are parallel to the ground.
3. The weight should be equally borne by both feet.
4. The arms can be stretched out in front or on the sides.
5. After a pause, raise your body to the resting pose again.

Lateral stretch (for hips and inner thighs)

1. Stand erect with feet wider than shoulder-width apart.
2. Keep your toes pointing forward, hands on your hips and back straight.
3. Now take a step toward the left with your left foot. Keep your right leg straight, bend your left knee slightly and lower your body towards your left leg – till you feel a stretch in the right leg.
4. Hold the position and then pushing with your left leg, return to an upright position.
5. Repeat the exercise to the right.

Legs

Quad stretches:

1. Lift your right foot so that you are standing on your left foot. Grab the right shin while bending the right leg behind you.
2. Pull your shin and right heel towards your glutes. The pull should not be sideways.

3. Bring the foot back to the floor.
4. Repeat with the other foot.

Hamstring stretch:

1. Stand up straight with the right leg straight forward and on its heel. Make sure both knees are not bent.
2. Now with your arms up in the air, slowly bend forward towards the right foot. You will feel the stretch in the hamstrings. Come back to the standing position.
3. Repeat on the other side.

Calf Stretch

Lunge

1. Stand with your hands on your hips.
2. Step one foot back into a mini lunge, bending your front leg and keeping your back leg straight. The further apart the feet, the deeper the stretch.
3. Press your back heel down and make sure it is flat on the ground.
4. Return to the standing position.
5. Repeat on the other side.

Heel raise

1. From a standing position, slowly raise up on the balls of your feet, lifting your heels in the air.
2. Go as high as possible without losing your balance.
3. Hold for few seconds.
4. Slowly lower your heels as you return to your starting position.

Deep breath:

1. Stand with your feet hip-width apart, spine tall and arms along your sides.
2. Take a deep breath in and lift your arms straight up into the air above your head as you breathe in.
3. Pause at the top. As you breathe out, lower your arms back down by your sides.

Meditation:

A minute of internal meditation with eyes closed and standing still.

3. *Asanas* (Physical Postures)

Physical postures form the core of yoga practice. I have described one *surya namaskar* (sun salutation) and twenty slow *asanas* in this book. There are many more *surya namaskars* and *asanas* and many of these can be found in my book, 'Yoga for Life'.

Precautions:

Although yoga *asanas* are safe, some precautions are needed:

- Yoga should be practiced in a place that is spacious, clean, airy, bright and away from disturbances. A carpet or mat will help prevent slipping and potential injuries. Outdoors on the grass (and immersed in nature) is also suitable.
- Wear loose comfortable and clean clothes.
- Use the restroom prior to the practice.
- Although yoga can be done anytime, early morning is preferable.
- Yoga should be practiced at least 2 times a week and preferably every day.
- Movement during each pose and during transition should be slow and smooth. Remember – there should be no stress.
- Timed inhalation, timed exhalation and normal breathing during hold or transitions should remain smooth and even. However, the breathing advice and timings are just a rough guidance. Adjust breathing patterns and timings according to your convenience.
- You will be able to do yoga better on an empty stomach. Ideally solid food should have been consumed 3-5 hours before practicing and liquids 1 hour before practicing.
- Try to shut off your awareness of all external stimuli during the practice – your ears are open, but you do not hear anything, your eyes are open, but you do not notice anything – and so on.
- Do not exceed your current ability, even if otherwise healthy. You will find that your ability will gradually increase with continuing practice.
- Limit your stretch or hold if suffering from restrictive joint diseases like arthritis.
- Limit your postures and timings if you have high blood pressure or heart disease – get clearance from your health care provider first.
- If you feel dizzy, pain, or any other uncomfortable sensation, come out of the pose, rest and get some medical advice before continuing again.
- If you have a medical problem requiring medications, you may want to get an approval from your private physician or health care professional.
- Do not stop taking any medications.
- Always have a bottle of water or athletic drink with you during practice. You do not want to get dehydrated.
- Carry a spare towel – for sweating and also to use as a seat/eye cover in the *savasana* pose or as a prop.
- Women may want to avoid practice during menstruation and pregnancy.

(special postures are described that may be done during menstruation and pregnancy by several authors)
- Have faith and become fully immersed in the practice – yogic literature states you should have "*Tatodwanabhighatah*" - the practice should lead to disappearance of duality of cold-hot, happiness-sorrow, stress-satisfaction and so on.
- And finally, do not break any local rules - whenever you are performing yoga on the go.

Surya Namaskar (Sun Salutation)

Sun salutations are usually done facing the rising sun - and ideally on the morning grass. The following sequence provides a good workout:

1. Start: Mountain pose *(Tadasana)* – normal breathing
2. Inhalation: Upward salute pose *(Urdhva Hastasana)*
3. Exhalation: Deep forward fold *(Uttanasana)*
4. Inhalation: Standing half forward bend *(Ardha Uttanasana)*
5. Exhalation: Four limbed staff pose *(Chaturanga andasana)*
6. Inhalation: Upward facing dog *(Urdhva Mukha Svanasana)*
7. Exhalation: Downward facing dog *(Adho Mukha Svanasana)*
8. Inhalation: Standing half forward bend *(Ardha Uttanasana)*
9. Exhalation: Deep forward fold *(Uttanasana)*
10. Inhalation: Upward salute *(Urdhva Hastasana)*
11. Exhalation: Back to Mountain pose *(Tadasana)*

Sun salutations can be done at home or in yoga studios. Move through this sequence relatively quickly – one pose during inhalation (2-5 seconds) and one pose during exhalation (2-5 seconds). A complete *surya-namaskar* will take anywhere from approximately 15 seconds to one minute. Do five-ten repetitions. This sequence is stimulating and will warm you up quickly. Start at a slow pace – maybe do five slowly. Sun salutations can be done faster as you get more accustomed to the routine – to get maximum benefits of moderate intensity exercise.

Sun Salutation
(Clockwise from the top)

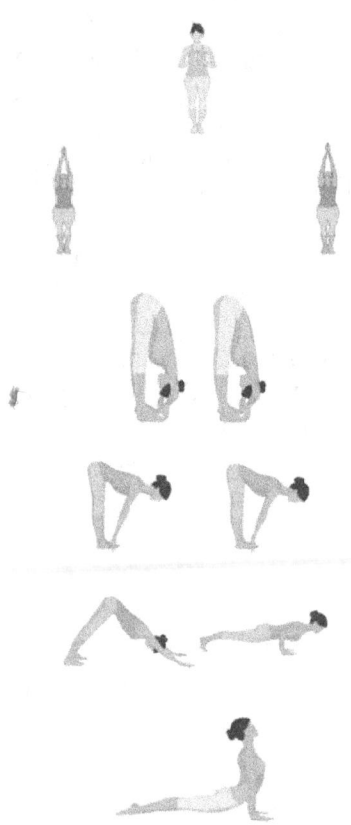

Sun Salutation

1. **Mountain Pose** — *Tadasana*
Stand with your feet slightly apart. Press your palms together in prayer position (*Anjali* mudra). Your thumbs should be touching your sternum and fingers pointing up. You should be relaxed.

2. **Upward Salute** — *Urdhva Hastasana*
Inhale as you lift your arms out to the side and overhead. Press the palms against each other. Arch your back gently and look upwards.

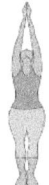

3. **Standing Forward Fold** — *Uttanasana*
Exhale as you fold forward from the hips. Try to reach the toes with your hands and touch the knees with your nose. Go only as far as you can go comfortably.

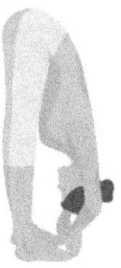

4. **Half Standing Forward Fold** — *Ardha Uttanasana*
Inhale as you lift your torso halfway and parallel to the floor. Your hands should be touching your feet or your shins.

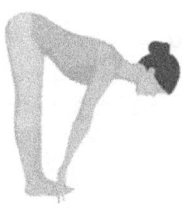

5. Four-Limbed Staff Pose — *Chaturanga Dandasana*

Exhaling lower your body towards the floor. Stretch yourself so that you are body is parallel to the floor and you are resting on your toes and palms. The palms should be flat on the floor and you are looking at the floor in front of you. Your wrists and elbows are in one line.

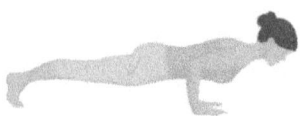

6. Upward-Facing Dog Pose — *Urdhva Mukha Svanasana*

Inhaling lift your upper chest towards the sky. Your arms will become straight and the wrists, elbows and shoulder are now in one line. Your thighs should be off the floor. The elbows are touching the sides of the body. The upper side of the feet are flush with the floor.

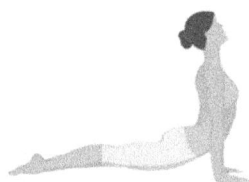

7. Downward-Facing Dog Pose — *Adho Mukha Svanasana*

Exhaling lift your hips and move the soles of the feet on the floor. As you get into the pose, the heels may move off the floor. Stretch your arms forwards, with the palms on the floor, as you arch the back upwards. Your sitting end should be the highest point and facing the ceiling/sky.

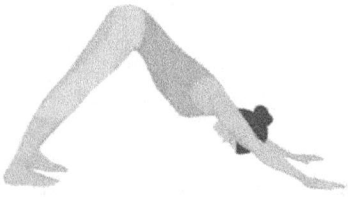

8. Half Standing Forward Fold — *Ardha Uttanasana*

Inhale as you lift your torso halfway, so that it becomes parallel to the floor. Bring your fingertips to your feet or your shins. You are looking at your feet.

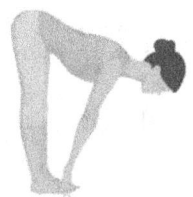

9. Standing Forward Fold — *Uttanasana*
Exhale as you go into a deep fold, bringing your nose if possible, to your knees. You may try to hold the toes with your fingers. Go only as far as you can without discomfort.

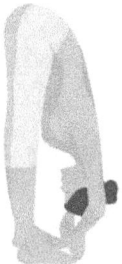

10. Upward Salute — *Urdhva Hastasana*
Inhaling straighten your back while your feet are firmly on the ground. Raise your arms from the side and extend the upwards. Let the palms of both hands touch each other while you arch your back and look upwards.

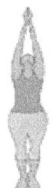

11. Back to Mountain Pose — *Tadasana*
Exhale as you come back into Mountain Pose. Bring your hands into prayer position (*Anjali* mudra). Rest your thumbs on your sternum with the fingers pointing up.

Move through this sequence rather quickly – one pose during inhalation and one pose during exhalation. This sequence is stimulating and will warm you up quickly. Do 5 repetitions (5 minutes). These can be done at the start of the slow yoga sequence or independently anytime during the day – especially in the morning.

Stay within your comfort zone and do not painfully force a shape onto the body. Yoga means 'gain with no pain'. Be careful if you have bad knees or bad back.

There are several variations of sun salutation but the above is easy to follow with alternating inhalations and exhalations.

Slow Yoga Poses

Getting into the pose should be smooth and gentle and take about 5-10 seconds. Each pose is held for approximately 30 seconds or to a slow count of 30 (one-Mississippi, two-Mississippi onwards). This will also mean approximately 7 complete breaths - each inspiration being about two seconds and each exhalation being about two seconds – or as you become better trained at taking lesser breaths per minute, your respiratory rhythm may become slower. If unable to hold for 30 seconds, do less but with practice you will be able to hold the pose longer. Getting out of pose should again be smooth and gentle (no jerking movements) and last for 5-10 seconds.

These timings are approximate. You have 20 minutes for 20 poses – or approximately one minute per pose. Once you get comfortable in the poses, you may want to hold them for about 40 seconds each.

Become completely immersed in the poses. There should be no distractions. Pantanjali describes yogasana as "*Sthir Sukham Asanam*" - the poses should be stable, stress free and enjoyable.

After finishing the '*surya-namaskar*' you should already be in the mountain pose, which is the first 'slow asana' pose. I will describe it in a little more detail here.

1. Mountain Pose

Tadasana

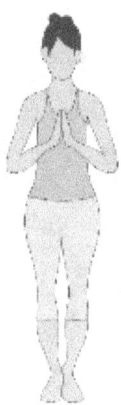

1. Stand upright on your feet. Both feet are close together, with the big toes touching or slightly apart. The feet are pointing straight forward. The weight is equally spread on either side and between the front and the back of the feet. The torso/trunk of the body is upright with the head and neck resting erect on the main body. The arms are on the side with the palms facing the thighs.

2. Now raise both arms and bring your hands forward, opposing palms firmly but gently pressing against each other, with the thumbs resting against the breast bone and fingers pointing up - the prayer position. This is our basic mountain pose with the hands in the prayer pose (*anjali* mudra) – with this mudra it is sometimes called the *prarthanasana (prathana* = prayer, *asana* = pose).

3. This is the starting point. Stay grounded, look forward at the infinite and breathe peacefully in and out with ease.

Drishti (Gaze): front - infinity

2. Crescent Moon in Mountain Pose

Ardha Chandrasana

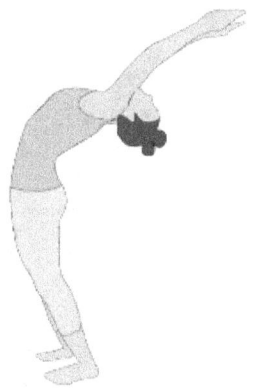

1. Inhaling from the mountain pose, stretch your arms upwards while keeping the palms pressed together.

2. As you continue inhaling, bend your torso backwards and turn your head upwards, facing the sky above.

3. The whole body should be firmly grounded on both feet and arched back like a crescent moon.

4. The knees are not bent.

5. Hold the pose. Breathe normally.

6. Exhaling slowly move to the next pose – deep forward bend pose.

Drishti: upwards sky - infinity

3. Deep Forward Bend Pose

Uttanasana

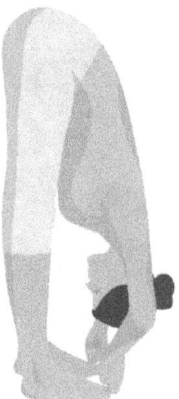

1. From the crescent moon, instead of stopping at mountain pose, keep bending forward till your fingers touch your feet.

2. This is done during exhalation in one fluid motion.

3. The feet are firmly on the ground and the knees are kept straight.

4. The body is bent from the hip upwards and folded like a pancake.

5. After the pose is reached, the Drishti is tip of the nose.

6. Hold pose. Breathe normally.

7. Inhaling raise the head and upper trunk to an upright position and exhaling bring the hands into the prayer position.

Drishti: toes

4. Revolved Triangle Pose

Parivrtta Trikonasana

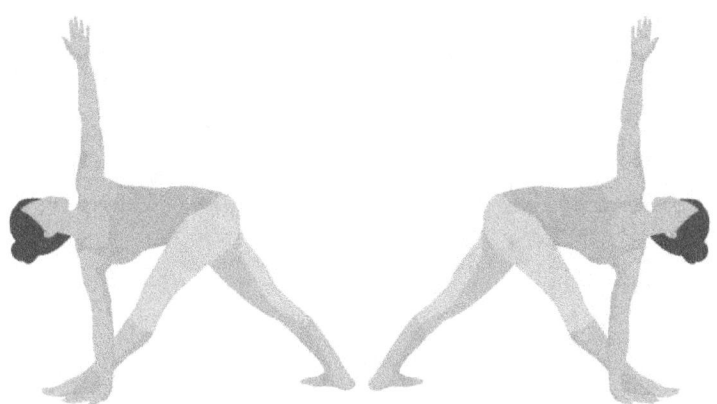

1. From the mountain pose, spread your legs and arms on the sides. This is the five-pointed star position.

2. Turn the toes of the right foot towards the right about 90 degrees.

3. Turn the left toes slightly inwards – about 45 degrees.

4. Now rotating, bring the right hand downwards against the right leg with the palm facing downwards/forward.

5. The left arm is raised upwards with the fingers pointing to the ceiling.

6. The arms are stretched and stay in one line with the shoulders.

7. Hold pose. Breathe normally. Come back to the mountain pose.

8. Repeat on the other side.

Drishti: upper hand

5. Warrior I Pose

Virabhadrasana I

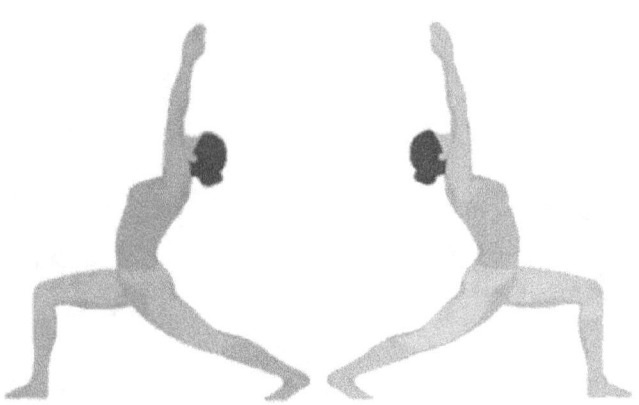

1. Start from the mountain pose.

2. Now step your left leg and foot back, behind you, about 1-2 feet. The left foot will be rotated outwards (towards the left front end of the mat) about 30-45 degrees or more. The right foot stays firmly grounded with the toes pointing forward.

3. Now bend the front knee to a 90 degree, with the knee (right knee) directly over the right ankle. You may stretch the left leg further backwards if needed. Both hips stay aligned with the front edge of the mat.

4. From here, reach up with both arms, stretching your belly chest upwards. Reach out as high as you can. The arms can be parallel to each other or the palms can be flat against each other. The biceps are touching the ears.

5. Lift your head back and Drishti at the thumbs. You should feel your shoulder blades pressing inwards. Breathe normal while holding this pose.

6. Come back to the mountain pose. Repeat on the other side.

Drishti: upwards/hands

6. Hero Pose

Veerasana

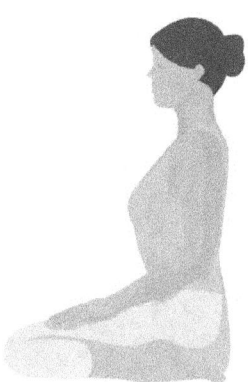

1. Kneel with the knees together and thighs perpendicular to the floor.

2. The toes point backwards and touch the floor.

3. The calves are pushed outside the thighs – do not sit on them or on the heels.

4. The hands are on top of thighs just near to knees, with the palms facing down.

5. The spine is straight and tall. The head is held proudly with the crown pointing to the ceiling.

6. Hold pose. Breathe normally.

Drishti: tip of the nose or straight ahead/infinity

7. Child Pose

Balasana

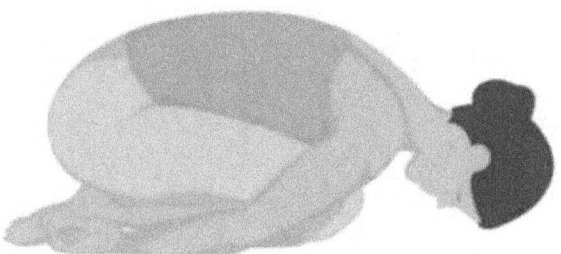

1. You are in the hero pose. Push your calves under your thighs so that you are now sitting on them. The buttocks rest on the heels.

2. Exhaling bend your torso forward, with your chest resting on your thighs and your forehead touching the floor.

3. Your arms at the same time move backwards with the palms facing up. The arms should be straight and extended with the palms resting on the floor or clasped behind your buttocks.

4. The buttocks should continue to rest on your heels.

5. The forehead continues to touch the floor.

6. Hold this position. Breathe normally.

7. Inhaling straighten the body from waist up.

Drishti: knees or eyes closed

8. Cat Pose

Marjaiasana

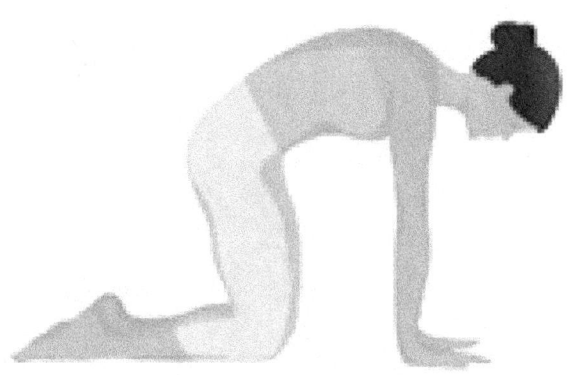

1. From the previous pose, raise your thighs so that your lower legs are on the floor and your body is upright and perpendicular to the floor.

2. The hips directly above the bent knees.

3. Slowly bend forward at the waist till your hands rest on the floor in front of your knees and the trunk of the body is parallel to the floor.

4. Straighten your arms so that they are perpendicular to the floor and the shoulders are directly above the bent wrists.

5. Exhaling draw your belly to your spine and round your back toward the ceiling.

6. You are now looking like a cat stretching its back.

7. You can let the head drop forward gently.

8. Hold the pose. Breathe normally.

Drishti: floor/hands

9. Cow Pose

Bitilasana

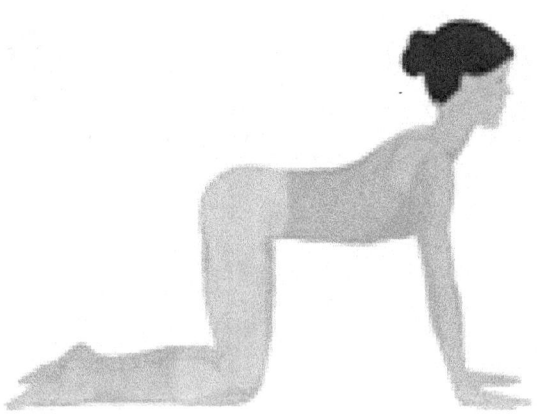

1. From the cat pose, inhaling, drop your belly towards the floor so that your back is concave upwards.

2. The head moves upwards, and you are now seeing up and front.

3. This is the cow pose

4. Hold the pose (a few cow and cat poses can be done back to back)

Drishti: upwards - front

10. Downward Facing Dog Pose

Adho Mukha Svanasana

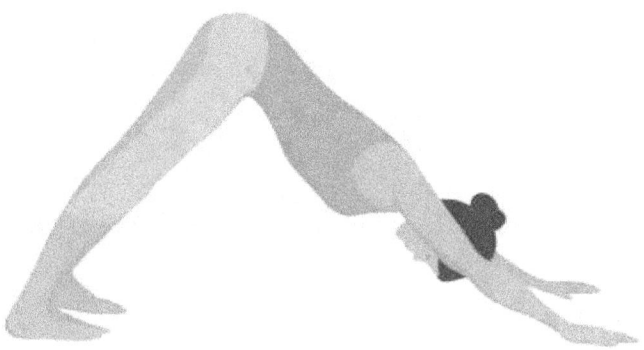

1. From the previous pose, your palms should be shoulder length apart and on the floor in front of you.

2. Spread the fingers and have the weight of the front body rest on the palm and fingers.

3. Now gradually lift your knees off the floor, straightening your legs and having the soles of the feet flat on the ground.

4. The pelvis is now raised, and you are in an inverted 'V' shape.

5. The face is looking down.

6. The muscles in the arms and legs should be tight and firm.

7. Hold this pose. Breathe normally.

Drishti: forward hands/floor/back legs

11. Sphynx Pose

Salamba Bhujangasana

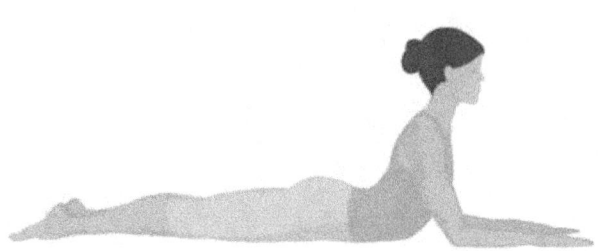

1. From the downward facing dog position, slowly glide down on the floor.

2. The belly is on the floor and the legs are brought together.

3. Now raise your upper torso, bring your elbows under your shoulders and your forearms on the floor parallel to each other. The hands stay flat on the floor.

4. Inhale and lift your upper torso and head away from the floor into a mild backbend.

5. Hold this pose. Breathe normally.

Drishti: front - infinity

12. Cobra Pose

Bhujangasana

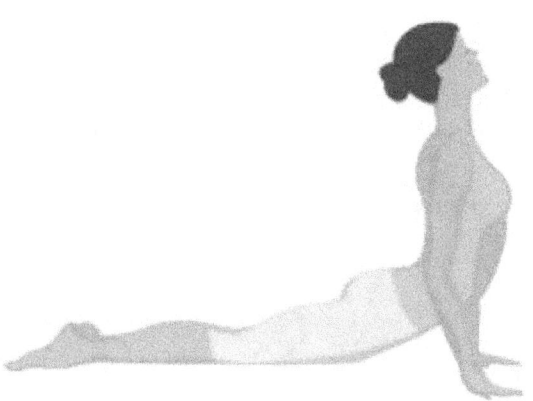

1. You are in the sphinx pose.

2. Exhaling press the tops of the feet and thighs and the pubis firmly into the floor.

3. Inhaling gradually lift the chest and elbows off the floor. The groin should be touching the floor.

4. Raise your upper body to a comfortable height. The head and neck should be perpendicular to the floor.

5. Pull the shoulder blades backwards and towards each other while opening the chest in the front.

6. Hold the pose. Breathe normally.

7. Gradually lower yourself back to the sphinx pose.

Drishti: front - infinity

13. Four Limbed Staff Pose

Chaturanga Dandasana

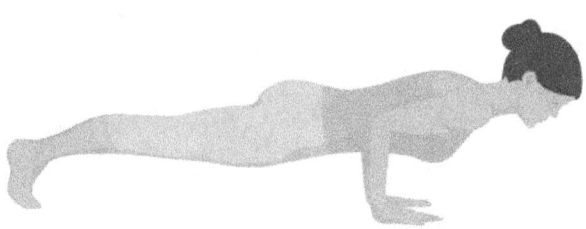

1. From the sphynx pose, slowly raise your entire body to become parallel with the floor.

2. The body rests on the toes and the flat of the hands.

3. The elbows will bend to 90 degrees and will come to be at the same level as the shoulders. The spine stays straight and firm.

4. Hold the pose. Breathe normally.

5. Finally, slowly lower your body back to the sphynx pose.

Drishti: floor in front

14. Locust Pose

Salabhasana

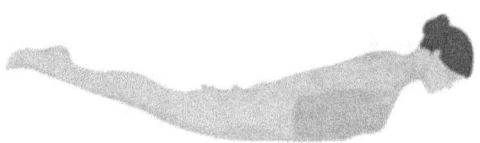

1. From the sphinx position, raise your head and upper torso to bring your arms by your side going backwards, and the palms resting besides your body on the floor.

2. Continue lifting your head and upper torso away from the floor. The upper body is now resting on your lower ribs and the belly.

3. Raise the legs away from the floor so the lower torso is resting on the lower pelvis and the feet, which are pointing back with the upper part of the feet against the floor. (soles facing up)

4. Hold pose and breathe normally.

5. Gradually lower yourself back to the sphynx pose.

Drishti: floor/front

15. Crocodile Pose

Makrasana

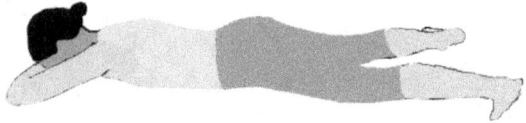

1. Bringing your arms forward and downwards, slowly lower your torso and move your legs backwards.

2. Lie down on the belly.

3. Move both arms forward and fold them with the hands placed on opposite elbows.

4. The forehead rests on the forearms. The face can also be turned on either side.

5. The legs should be extended and stretched back.

6. The legs are now spread about shoulder-width apart with the toes turned out and heels turned in.

7. Relax and breathe normally.

Drishti: floor/side infinity/eyes closed

16. Corpse Pose

Savasana

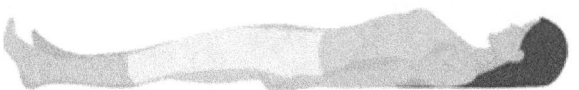

1. From the crocodile pose, flip over so that you are now lying face up. Ensure that your body is stretched, and your arms are by your side. Your entire body is resting against the ground.

2. The palms are facing up.

3. The legs which are on the floor, will rotate out with the toes facing up and away from each other.

4. Make sure you are in a 'neutral' position with no tension.

5. Hold this pose. Breathe nice and easy through the nostrils.

Drishti: upwards/infinity or eyes gently closed

17. Boat Pose

Navasana

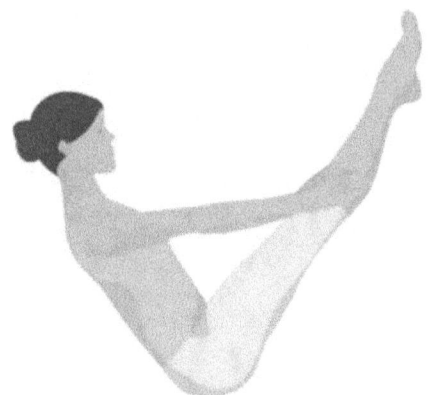

1. From the corpse pose (face up), sit up, pushing with the hands and arms. The palms are flat on the floor. Now bend your knees 90 degrees and perpendicular to the floor. Bring your feet, with the soles against the floor and with the palms flat on the ground, as close to the buttocks as possible.

2. Now, slowly lean back slightly, keeping your spine straight. Lift your feet off the ground and bring your shins parallel to the floor.

3. Sitting on the back bone, lift your hands off the floor and bring the arms parallel to the floor, on either side of the legs, with the palms facing towards each other.

4. The spine should remain straight. This is half boat.

5. Now straighten your legs so the that feet are now pointing up and the legs are at an angle of 45 degree from the ground. The body now assumes a 'V' shape.

6. This is the full boat pose. Hold this pose. Breathe normally.

7. Gradually bring your arms and legs down and assume the corpse pose.

Drishti: legs/feet

18. Bridge Pose

Setubandha

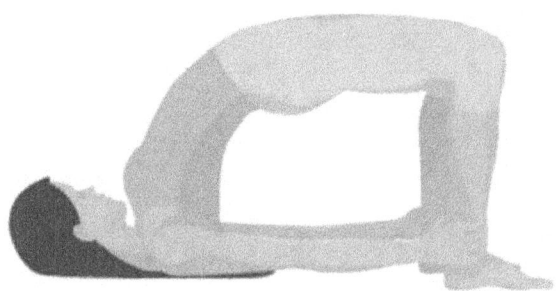

1. From the corpse pose, bend your knees and bring them as close to the buttocks as possible.

2. Press on your palms and feet downwards and inhaling lift your buttocks in the air towards the pubic bone.

3. The lower legs should be perpendicular to the floor now and the thighs and feet aligned in a straight line.

4. The knees should be above the ankles.

5. Lift your shoulder blades pushing your sternum upwards.

6. Bring your hands under your torso and clasp them together.

7. The head and feet stay flat on the floor.

8. Drishti is upwards infinity. Hold pose. Breathe normally.

9. Return to the corpse pose

Drishti: ceiling/upwards infinity

19. Legs Up Pose

Viparita Karani

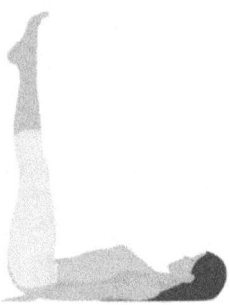

1. From the corpse pose, slide close to a wall.

2. Sit alongside a wall with the feet on the floor in front.

3. The left side of the body is touching the wall.

4. Lie backwards while wiggling around so that the legs are now up against the wall.

5. The backs of the legs press against the wall and the soles of the feet are facing up.

6. Your body is flat on the floor and it forms a 90-degree angle at the waist/hips.

7. The arms are by your side with the palms facing downwards

8. Move away from the wall and come back to the corpse pose.

Drishti: feet

20. Supine Spinal Twist Pose

Jathara Parivartanasana

1. From the corpse pose, draw your knees with the back of the feet touching your bottom and the knees bent.

2. The soles are flat on the ground. Extend arms to a T position.

3. Lower both legs down towards the left, with the left knee touching the ground. Hold this pose. Breathe normally.

4. Bring knees to center. Extend knees to return to the corpse pose.

5. Repeat on the other side. Come back to the corpse pose.

Drishti: thumb on the side of the face

Rest in the corpse pose (with your eyes closed) and gentle breathing till you are ready to move on to the breathing exercises.

"This thing called 'corpse' we dread so much is living with us here and now."

Milarepa, The Tibetan book of living and dying

4. *Pranayama* (Breathing Exercises)

Yoga says that breath contains more than air/oxygen - you breathe *'prana'* (good energy) on inhalation (*puraka*) and you discard *'apana'* (bad energy) on exhalation (*rechaka*).

Most people in the modern world breathe improperly and inefficiently. We subconsciously train ourselves to perform chest breathing- a breathing pattern associated with prolonged sitting - in car, sofa or at work. This breathing is restricted, usually limited to the middle chest. There is hardly any abdominal movement during such breathing. It is often associated with stress and anxiety and results in a faster shallower breathing and a fast heart rate. Besides the vascular benefits, yogic breathing will help lower your breathing rate, improve your breathing capacity and exercise all the numerous muscles, ligaments and bones involved with respiration (besides the diaphragm – the main muscle of respiration). For more breathing techniques, see my book, 'Yoga for Life'.

1. **Complete breath:**

Savasana or Corpse Pose

You are already in the *savasana* pose. Place both hands palm down on either side of the belly button with the tips of the middle fingers touching gently. The entire inhalation and the entire exhalation is divided into three sections - without a specific demarcation. We inhale first into the lower lungs (diaphragm), then into the middle lungs (intercostal muscles) and finally into the upper lung (clavicular muscles) in one smooth continuous action. After a normal pause. we exhale in the reverse direction - first start exhaling from the upper lung, then the middle lung and finally the lower lung. This is the complete breath.

While in the corpse pose, inhale and fill your lower lung first - the belly should move up and the tips of the fingers should separate. The continuing inhalation into the middle lung will result in an expansion of the chest cavity while the final segment - inhalation into the upper lobes will make the collar bone and shoulders rise. After a normal pause. exhalation is done in a controlled but reverse manner - first exhale from the top, then the middle and finally the lower part of the lung. The latter will result in the stomach being sucked in and the middle fingers coming in opposition again. Breathing is done through both nostrils only and the smooth process is not accompanied by any sounds or other bodily movements. Inspiration is 5 seconds and expiration is slightly longer - maybe 7-10 seconds. There is a normal pause both at the end of inspiration and the end of expiration. Remember, during complete breathing, we are executing only 6 or so breaths per minute. Practice complete breaths for 5 minutes (approximately 30 complete breaths). You can vary the timings according to your ability.

The other two breathing exercises are best done in *sukhasana*. Although other poses like *veerasana* can be used, I recommend *sukhasana* as you can then go on to the meditation phase without changing position.

Sukhasana or Easy Pose

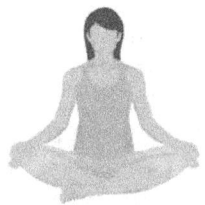

1. Breathing normally, lower your torso, place both hands on the floor, sit down on your buttocks and straighten out the legs in front of you. The arms are resting along your sides.
2. Sit up straight. (this is the *dandasana* pose)
3. Cross your legs in front of you and fold them near your torso.
4. With the knees wide apart, tuck your feet beneath the opposite knee. Either shin can be on top – it is good to alternate on different days. The position should be easy and relaxed.
5. Place your palms on the knees, facing down or up, and without any tension. Adopt a *pranayama* mudra as described under each technique.

2. Alternate nostril breathing:

The yogis believe that breathing through the right nostril (sun energy) heats the body and increases catabolism while breathing from the left nostril (moon energy) cools the body and increases anabolism. The aim is to balance the two.

Use the **Vishnu Mudra:** In this mudra, the forefinger and middle finger are curled in toward the palm, while the thumb and the other two fingers remain extended.

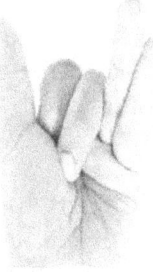

First close the right nostril with the fleshy tip of the right thumb. Breathe in gently from the left nostril for five seconds. Now with the thumb still on the right nostril, using the same hand, close the left nostril with the ring and little finger. Now let go the thumb while keeping the left nostril closed. Breathe out smoothly over five seconds. Close both nostrils again. Now open the right nostril and breathe in from the right nostril for 5 seconds. Close the right nostril again with the right thumb and letting go the little and ring finger, open the left nostril and breathe out for 5 seconds. This is one breath cycle (20 seconds). Restart breathing in from the left nostril to continue the next cycle. Do this for 12 cycles (4 minutes). Remember the ratios starting with left nostril inspiration are as follows 1: 1: 1: 1 for the one complete cycle. You can vary the ratio (especially expiration may require more time) according to your convenience. Always initiate this breathing from the left nostril – this will potentiate the good parasympathetic activity and decrease the troublesome increased sympathetic activity - in most people, the sympathetic activity is very high.

3. *Bhastrika*

Bhastrikā, is also known as bellows breath. Sit comfortably, with the spine straight (upright) and both hands on the knees with the palms down. Start with a few normal breaths. Follow this with breathing characterized by forceful inhalation and then forceful exhalation through nostrils at a rate of about 20–30 respirations/minute (about 2 seconds per cycle) while using strong abdominal muscle contractions. Perform bhastrika for 30 seconds.

Relax for 30 seconds after this exercise with eyes closed before proceeding to meditation.

Brahmari *(Bumblebee Breath): This also improves the autonomic tone. Slow breathing is done while eyes and ears are covered with placement of hands over face and external ear flaps. There is long slow inhalation and then a gentle humming sound is made with exhalation. Breathing occurs at a rate of about 6 respirations/minute. If you have time, do this breathing also for a few minutes.*

5. Dhyana (Meditation)

"Meditation is listening to the Divine within."

Edgar Cayce

Meditation is popular in the in the United States. According to published data, the 12-month prevalence for meditation practice was 3.1% for spiritual meditation, 1.9% for mindfulness meditation, and 1.6% for mantra meditation. This represents approximately 7.0, 4.3, and 3.6 million adults respectively.[2]

Meditation brings about a host of general health benefits. In the brain it enhances cortical thickening and neuroplasticity. It increases the levels of GABA and serotonin while reducing the sympathetic activity. Brain waves show higher levels of alpha activity – indicative of increased calmness.

"... a timeless state where there is no death or birth or growth, where there is no pain or sorrow, where there is no day or night, nor any distance........such a state can be achieved by meditating upon the self within, and realizing that I am everywhere and in everything."

Swami Vishnu-Devananda

After finishing Bhastrika breathing exercise, stay in the *sukhasana* pose. Take a few calm breaths by noticing the silky caress of your breaths on the nostrils. Calm your mind and clear it of all clutter. You should be relaxed and can now proceed to meditation. Continue in the *sukhasana* pose. Close your eyes and concentrate on the third eye (area around the middle of the forehead, slightly above the junction of the eyebrows - brow (*ajna*) chakra) Choose either the *gyana* or the *dhyana* mudra.

Other poses often used for meditation are *Padmasana* (Lotus pose) *Siddhasana* (Perfect pose) and *Svastikasana* (Prosperous or Auspicious Pose) – see appendix.

Gyana Mudra: In this mudra the tips of the thumb and index fingers are brought to touch each other at the tips, and they form a circle. The remaining three fingers are stretched, and the palm is facing upward (in chin mudra the palm is facing downwards). It is commonly done with both hands resting on the knees and with the elbows straight.

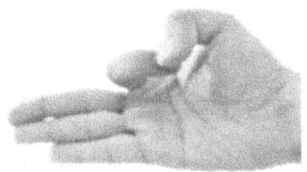

Dhyana Mudra: The right-hand rests on top of your left palm. The hands are resting at the level of the navel, facing up. The right hand represents enlightenment and higher spiritual faculties, and rests over the left hand, representing the world of *maya*, or illusion.

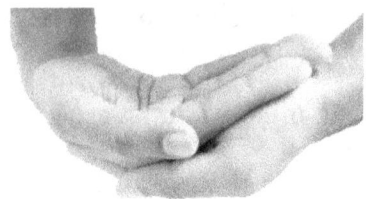

Meditation can be done in several ways. For the purpose of this book, I will only delve into 'mantra' meditation. In this, repeat a *mantra*, ideally as a whisper or if not possible - in the mind. The East Indians like to use '*Aum*'. Several other mantras can be used – there are millions of them, and they can be used 'generically', without any religious favoritism. A phrase can be picked up from the bible or other religious texts and repeated. Verbalization appears to benefit partially from the resultant vibrations produced.

Chanting mantras calms the mind, brings focus and is great for controlling the breath. Repetition of the mantras (*jap*) is a means to get closer to the divinity within, and it creates positive vibrations that benefit both the one who chants and the one who listens. The Sanskrit word is derived from the root, *jap/japa*, meaning "to repeat quietly and internally."

It is believed that there are about 70 million mantras. Each mantra has its own sound and vibration, so when you chant it, you begin to vibrate within the same frequency – with healing effects. Most commonly used 'short jap mantras':

- *Aum/Om*

Aum is an ancient Sanskrit "word" that represents the sound of immortality. It represents everything - the beginning, middle and the end of it all or the past, present and future. The word/sound is multifaceted. '*Aum*' has four parts:

The A (aahhh) sound represents the creation aspect of the universe; the U signifies the inherent energy of the universe; the M (mmmm) sound characterizes the transformative energy of the universe while the fourth sound – or the silence or anagata, represents the pure consciousness of the Self or the *Atman*.

OM is said to vibrate at 432 Hertz, which is the natural musical pitch of the Universe. It is considered a primordial sound – with its origins at the time of the creation of the cosmos ('Big Bang').

- *Om śāntiḥ*

Om Peace

- *So Hum*

So-hum reflects the sound of the breath – so is inhalation and hum is exhalation. It also means: "I am that" (so = "I am" and hum = "that") – 'that' is the breathing of the whole creation or I am with the breathing of the whole creation.

- *Om Namo Bhagavate Vasudevaya*

It means abandon all varieties of religion and just surrender unto me – your Lord, that dwells in all.

- *Hari Om*

Hari' means 'the remover'. Chanting this mantra helps remove all obstacles.

- *Om mani padme hum*

"The jewel is in the lotus." We all have a lotus inside us, but it is covered up by a lot of mud and muck. By cleaning this 'dirt' with repetition of the mantra, we unveil the sparkling, pure, compassionate and wise self. The Buddhists use prayer wheels of various sizes and spin them while meditating upon or chanting the mantra, to cleanse themselves.

Or use any positive/spiritual/religious word or phrase of your liking.

You can recite these mantras without the beads, with the palms in either the *gyana* mudra or the *dhyana* mudra described before.

Meditation should last 10 minutes.

More meditations are described in my book, 'Yoga for Life'.

6. Yoga *Nidra*

Following meditation, move to the corpse pose.

- Lie on your back (on a comfortable yoga mat or blanket) with legs extended straight, feet rolling slightly apart from each other.

- Lay your arms alongside your body, without the upper arms touching the sides of the chest.

- The hands should be a slight distance away from the hips with palms facing up, fingers curved upwards and inwards and relaxed (not clenched).

- Head, neck and spine should all be in line with each other. The thighs are positioned slightly apart (the legs may be spread out to about 45 degrees).

- The feet may flop outwards completely relaxed.

- The eyes are gently closed.

- Cover yourself with a blanket if needed (will keep you warm).

- Soft and gentle, slow beat instrumental music may help – suggestion: Yoga *Nidra* by Max Gandossi.

- If you go to actual sleep during the practice – it is fine.

- Suggested time frame: 5 minutes

Process:

- Feel your soft silky breath touching your nostrils both during inhalation and exhalation.

- Make a positive intention to yourself. (see intentions below) and repeat it to yourself three times.

- Start whole body relaxation process by consciously focusing and relaxing different parts of your body – start with the left toes and move up to the whole left foot, then the ankle, to the left lower leg, the left knee and the left upper leg, Move up to the left hip, left side of the pelvis, left abdomen, left side of the chest, left shoulder, left upper arm, left elbow, left forearm and left hand and fingers. Relax each section as you move on. Now come back up to the left side of the neck, left side of the face and left side of the head and start heading down the right side of the head to the right face and reversing the entire sequence from the right arm, right side of the torso, right leg and finally to the right toes. The whole body should be now completely relaxed, and it should feel like a log on the ground.

- Breathe quietly through your nostrils, feeling the air on the nostril tips, and try to keep your mind thought free. You will have now blocked all sensory inputs except for hearing – to receive instructions from a yogi or recording. Or you may proceed to positive affirmations/positive visualizations/gratitude recitations (see appendix) – one or all.

- Stay in this pose and mental state for about 5 minutes. When done, wake up slowly.

- Gently roll over to the right side before sitting up.

- Smile.

"No thought, no reflection, no analysis, no cultivation, no intention; let 'It' settle Itself."

Zen Saying

Intentions for Yoga *Nidra*

Yoga *nidra* provides sensory deprivation (a hypnagogic state) and you should lose your duality during this process (the identification between *purusha* and *pakriti* should dissolve) – this prevents the ego and/or doubts to block or prevent your intention/affirmations/positive visualizations from coming true. During yoga *nidra* you transcend above any self-imposed conscious/subconscious limitations. The scientific literature has extensively documented the benefits of yoga *nidra*.[1-5]

"Our intention creates our reality."

Wayne Dyer

Setting an intention, unlike setting a goal, requires no plans. Your intention is based on "being" in the present moment – with the process and result surrendered to the universe. Examples of intentions:

- I intend to stay healthy and happy.

- I intend to stay positive and smile more.
- I intend to simplify my life and lead by example.
- I intend to be real and authentic in everything in my life.
- I intend to forgive others and myself.
- I intend to follow my heart and set a course of its vision.
- I intend to be non-judgmental.
- I intend to help and serve others.
- I intend to respect nature and everything in it.
- I intend to use my journey through this life creating good Karma – to radiate light.
- I intend to deepen and strengthen my loving relationship with my creator and caretaker.

Specific intentions are also available on liveandlifeyoulove.com - for a good collection of intentions written by Boni Lonnsburry[6]. You can also write and recite your own specific intentions. Yoga *nidra* is also an excellent yoga pose to rewrite your mind's software (neuroplasticity) with positive affirmations, happy visualizations, gratitude recitations and prayers (see appendix).

"It is intent which establishes one's consequential outcomes.

T.F. Hodge

7. Closing prayers

"I believe that prayer is our powerful contact with the greatest force in the universe."

Loretta Young

Following yoga *nidra*, roll over to your right/left side and slowly sit up and stay in this position for a minute or so. Now gradually stand up in the *tadasana* pose with the *anjali* mudra (prayer mudra) and recite a closing prayer.

The closing prayer brings the practice to a peaceful end, sealing in the work done and offering the efforts of our practice to improve the state of the world.

Om Sarvesām Svastir Bhavatu
Sarvesām Śāntir Bhavatu
Sarvesām Pūrnam Bhavatu
Sarvesām Mangalam Bhavatu
Om Shanti Shanti Shanti

May there be happiness in all.
May there be peace in all.
May there be completeness in all.
May everything prosper.
Om, peace, peace, peace

The prayer pose (*Anjali mudra*) – is also called '*namaste*'.

"Namaste means that whatever is precious and beautiful in me honors whatever is precious and beautiful in you."

Debasish Mridha

In yoga, there's a belief that there is a divine spark in everyone, located in the heart chakra. This chakra — one of seven — affects the ability to love and is located just above your heart in the center of your chest. By gesturing *namaste*, you acknowledge that spark and the soul in another person. Literally translated, *nama* means "bow," *as* means "I" and *te* means "you" — "Bow I you," or "I bow to you." Some instructors consider namaste to mean, "the light in me honors the light in you".

YOGIC LIFESTYLE

Besides the practice of yoga described above, for good health, especially good vascular health, try to incorporate yogic philosophy into your life. These are described in the eightfold path of yoga by Pantajali:

Yama – morality. *Yamas* are further classified into five limbs:

Ahimsa: nonviolence toward all living things. Kindness and compassion to all. During your daily life, you will come across many occasions where you can practice 'non-violence' – even thinking negative of others, creating judgment, criticism, and anger is violence – so practice 'non-violence' both physically and mentally. Accept everything – good and bad with compassion.

Satya: being truthful – being always transparent. Dishonesty will not only harm others but will foster negativity in you. Being honest in life will help you reach the true spirituality that yoga teaches and inspires.

Asteya: non-stealing. You do not mentally or physically take something that is not yours. Not only do not 'steal' but also become more generous – this way you overcome greed. Yoga teaches that when you are devoid of greed, you get what you would have coveted.

Brahmacharya: celibacy – or proper use of sexual energy. By being moderate and not harming others with our sexual energy, we become stronger – and the extra energy can be used to make us more spiritual.

Aparigraha: the virtue of non-possessiveness, non-grasping or non-greediness. It also encompasses non-attachment. Everything you own today belonged to someone else before and everything you own today will belong to someone else when you leave this earth – you cannot take those 'coveted' items with you. So, enjoy a clean and good life – rather than acquiring material things. Remember, memories count – you keep and take memories with you and not materialistic things.

Niyama – personal observances –also five in number:

Sauca: outer and inner cleanliness. This includes physical as well as mental cleanliness. There should be simplicity in our lives. External cleanliness also counts - wherever you are - help keep the place clean.

Santosa: contentment – finding happiness in whatever we have. Not longing for what we do not have. Contentment must be both internal and external – one must be content with oneself and with others (accepting them as they are without judgement and not coveting what they have). Yoga tells us that by being truly content - we attain true joy and happiness. Travel often exposes us to spiritual riches of others (and poverty) – you won't feel frustrated or egoistic if you are internally content.

Tapas: discipline – in life, and in everything we do. Creating an internal flame that burns up our internal fears and procrastinations and keeps us aligned to the path devoid of impure impulses and 'negative behavior'. Life will often present us with immoral and illegal baits – stay steadfast on your honest and honorable path.

Svadhyaya: self-inquiry, self-realization. Becoming aware of one's limitations. By looking objectively at the mirror that reflects our life's flaws and weaknesses, we can, improve our future behaviors - and with the help of spiritual knowledge from texts and *gurus*, realign our lives with the 'truth' – our oneness with the universal spirit.

Isvarapranidhana: establishing spirituality – a connection with a higher power. Our lives should be spent in 'purity' with the realization that everything we do is for the higher power – and anything otherwise will create bad '*karma*' which will at some stage of our lives (in this life or in our future life) we will have to rectify.

Pratyahara – sense control. We are constantly being bombarded by sensory stimulants – to our five senses (seeing, hearing, touching, tasting and smelling). By *pratyahara* we mean selectively using these sensations to establish positive impressions in our minds (positive experiences such as gazing at the ocean, the mountains or the blue sky.) and avoiding negative ones (news/politics on television/newspapers). *Pratyahara* does not means physically withdrawing or 'hiding' from the world – it means that in the midst of sensory overstimulation, we seek, accept and respond to the ones (positive) we want to and ignore the ones that are negatively poised for us. It also means practicing a positive life – thinking positively, being mindful of speech and action, practicing good eating and entertainment habits and going to bed on time. Yogic practice of *asanas*, *pranayamas* and *dhyana* also help in developing *pratyahara*.

Three forms of *pratyahara* that you can practice:

- Silence (*maun*)– no speaking (and preferably no hearing)

- Intermittent fasting – maybe once a week (with the approval of your personal health care provider) – drink only water and/or fruit juices or eat fresh fruit. Remember – fasting is not for everyone.

- Practicing periods of voluntary celibacy – both mental and physical.

The *savasana* pose in yoga – described earlier, is a great pose for achieving sensory *pratyahara* and looking inwards for peace and relaxation. Paying attention to your breath in the corpse pose and focusing on the third eye (between the eyebrows) during meditation will help develop the ability to block out external and internal stimuli. Establishing a good practice of *pratyahara* will help achieve the next stage somewhat more easily – Dharana.

Dharana – concentration. *Dharna* prepares you for *dhyana* (meditation) – in *dhyana* the mind eventually becomes so absorbed in that one entity that it enters a thoughtless state—completely aware but unengaged with itself.

Samadhi – union with the Almighty. *Samadhi* has been described by Pantajali as being of two kinds - *Samprajnata* samadhi (*savikalpa* samadhi) and *Asamprajnata* samadhi (*nirvikalpa* samadhi). During *samprajnata* samadhi, the meditator's soul merges with the infinite consciousness but limited to the period of meditation. The body is still controlled by the ego-consciousness – *'I' am the one with infinite power*. During *asamprajnata* samadhi, the ego bondage is removed, the karmic bonds are broken and there is a state of unconditioned oneness with the Almighty.

The last three limbs of yoga – *dharana* (concentration), *dhyana* (meditation) and *samadhi* (enlightenment) -- are collectively referred to as *sanyam*, which means "control." Pantajali states that the last three limbs should be considered together, as they are progressive stages of concentration.

According to yoga, we are spiritual beings, or souls (causal body/spirit), who spend time on earth in a physical body. We have a spirit that relates to the Universal Source. Samadhi is a state where material possessions lose their meaning; where we can come to realize that we don't own anything, not even our bodies. Everything physical will dissolve, everything in our physical world will eventually disappear - at the very end we will lose them when we leave this physical world. But the spirit is eternal, and *it* knows this. We just need to reconnect with this inner knowledge and reach a state of consciousness where individual awareness dissolves into the great Whole.

आप खाली हाथ आए, और आप खाली हाथ छोड़ देंगे।

You came empty handed, and you will leave empty handed

Bhagwad Gita

YOGA AND SAFETY

'Primum non nocere' – 'first, to do no harm'

Yoga is mostly practiced by Americans for health and fitness – and more and more as an adjunct therapeutic modality[1]. Yoga has become one of the top 10 complementary and integrative health interventions and is being increasingly used as an adjunct therapeutic modality for medical diseases[2-4]. Worldwide, it is estimated that more than 30 million people practice yoga[5]. It is therefore important to review any possible dangers associated with this practice.

Poses:

In an Australian study[6], yoga-related injuries occurring under supervision in the previous 12 months were low - 2.4% of respondents of the 3,892 respondents reported injuries in this national survey. Most of these yoga practitioners were interested in yoga for health, fitness and stress management. About one in five practiced yoga for its medical benefits[6].

In a review of yoga related injuries published in the scientific media through February 15, 2013, Cramer and associates[7] found 76 cases of injuries – the main ones being associated with head stand, shoulder stand, lotus position and forceful breathing. Other causes of injuries were voluntary vomiting and postures that included putting 1 or 2 feet behind the head, kneeling posture (*Vajrasana*), locust pose (*Salabhasana*), bridge pose (*Setu bandha*), seated forward bend (*Paschimottasana*), and downward-facing dog (*Adho mukha savasana*).

Swain and McGwin reviewed the data from the National Electronic Injury Surveillance System from 2001 to 2014 for yoga related injuries. They found that of the 29,590 yoga-related injuries seen in hospital emergency departments during this period, the most frequent area injured was the trunk (46.6%), and the most common diagnosis was sprain/strain (45.0%). The injury rate was higher in those aged 65 years or more (57.9/100,000) compared with those aged 18 to 44 years (11.9/100,000) and 45 to 64 years (17.7/100,000)[8].

Fishman and group surveyed more than 1,300 yoga teachers worldwide. They found that yoga injuries usually involved the neck, lower back, knee, shoulder, and wrist. According to them, the most common causes were poor technique, poor instruction, previous injury, and excess effort[9]. They reported that some injuries were linked with certain asanas. According to them, neck injuries were commonly attributed to *sarvangasana* (shoulder stand) while lower-back injuries were associated with forward bends, twists, and backbends. Shoulder and wrist injuries were usually due to *adho mukha svanasana* (downward-facing dog) and different plank poses (e.g., *chaturanga dandasana* - four-limbed staff pose and *vasisthasana* - side plank pose). The knees were more likely to be injured in *virabhadrasana* (warrior pose I and II), and *virasana* (hero's pose).

While most injuries are minor[10], serious injuries such as bone fractures[11] and tendon/ligament injuries[12] may occur. Non-musculoskeletal injuries have also been reported[13,14]. However, according to one study, injuries led to stoppage of yoga practice in less than 1% of the participants[15].

Another study of 2,508 people taking yoga classes (271 yoga therapists) demonstrated that 27% of the yoga class attendees experienced some type of adverse event during class. The most common were simple musculoskeletal - muscular pain, joint pain, and muscle cramps. They were often seen in students who were "overexerting and overdoing" and were in "poor physical condition".[16]

Mace and Eggleston reported that practitioners performing hot yoga reported dizziness (60%), feeling light headed (61%), nausea (35%), and dehydration (34%), amongst other symptoms.[17]

In general, adverse effects with *asana* practice are uncommon in healthy people. Advanced postures such as headstand or lotus position (not part of the yoga routine suggested in this book) should be avoided by beginners. Fast aggressive breathing techniques, likewise, should be learnt and practiced gradually. Advance cleansing techniques, including voluntary vomiting, esophagus and stomach cleaning, or enemas should also be avoided.

Breathing

Yogic breathing exercises are essentially safe.[18] There is an isolated report of a complication (pneumothorax) with *kapalbhati pranayama* in the published literature.[19]

Meditation

Side effects with meditation are not common[20] and most are deemed minor in character and usually do not require discontinuation of yoga practice or medical attention.[21] Some studies have indicated that long meditation periods can be contraindicated for people with psychiatric problems[22] as they may result in the precipitation of mental illness, such as psychosis,[23-25] posttraumatic stress disorder,[26,27] and epileptic attacks.[28] In general, if you have significant neurological or psychiatric problems, discuss the yoga prescription with your physician before starting.

The National Institute of Health in the US recommends that yoga should be practiced with a well-educated instructor (or 'guru'). *Guru* means 'teacher'. In Sanskrit, the word '*Guru*' has two roots – 'Gu' which means darkness and 'Ru' which means light or the remover of darkness. Yoga modalities can also be learnt from a book or video - but having a guru or teacher is still essential. A guru will teach you to do the physical practice (besides instilling spirituality) the correct way – this will help prevent injuries.

Poses with injury potential:

1. Shoulder stand

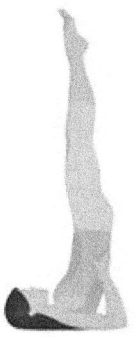

2. Downward facing dog

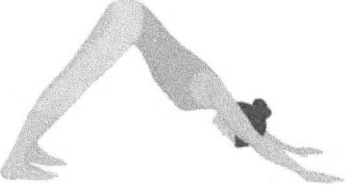

3. Four-limbed staff pose

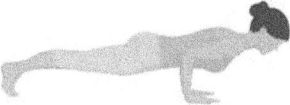

4. Side plank pose

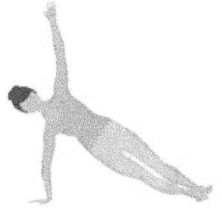

5. Warrior poses I and II

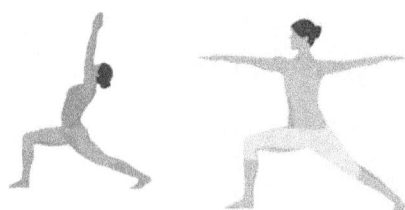

6. Hero pose

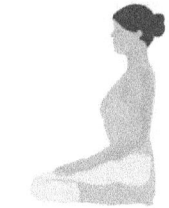

7. Lotus pose

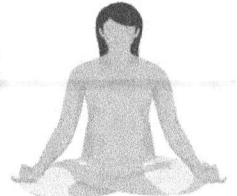

8. Bridge pose

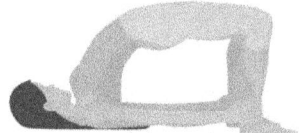

9. Locust pose

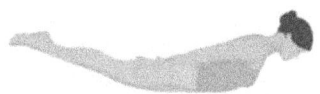

10. Head Stand

Elderly people and those with limitations need to practice extra caution with yoga practice.

"Safety is as simple as ABC - Always Be Careful."

Unknown

CLOSING REMARKS

The health benefits of yoga are tremendous – and these are especially evident in the research data supporting its complementary use in the prevention and management of diseases of the heart and circulation.

Yoga has survived through several millennia – mainly because the practitioners felt better and lived healthier.

> *"Yoga teaches us to cure what need not be endured and endure what cannot be cured."*

B.K.S. Iyengar

Yoga posture (*asana*) practice bring strength, flexibility and improved coordination.

> *"We do not stop exercising because we grow old - we grow old because we stop exercising"*

Kenneth Cooper

Breathing exercises (*pranayama*) bring clean fresh energy (*prana*) into the body and get rid of the toxic energy (*apana*).

> *"God is the breath inside the breath"*

Kabir

Meditation (*dhyana*) helps remove or restrain unnecessary and damaging brain activity – often constantly running in the brain's 'unconscious' background.

> *"Quiet the mind, and the soul will speak."*

Ma Jaya Sati Bhagavati

Along with these modalities, incorporation of *yamas* and *niyamas* in life and the practice of *pratyahara* and *dharna*, one will become more peaceful in this 'tumultuous' physical and emotional life.

> *"The mountains, I become part of it*
> *The herb, the fir tree, I become a part of it*
> *The morning mist, the clouds, the gathering waters*
> *I become part of it*
> *The wilderness, the dew drop, the pollen...*
> *I become a part of it."*

Navajo Chant

Yoga practice also induces subtle yet profound transformations in the non-physical (spiritual) 'atoms' – a beneficial metamorphosis, that significantly alters the course of one's karmic journey, both in time and quality - and profoundly enhances one's ability to achieve the ultimate goal – 'nirvana".

> *"Every human being's essential nature is perfect and faultless, but after years of immersion in the world, we easily forget our roots and take on a counterfeit nature."*

Lao- Tzu

Make yoga practice a lifelong habit. Do not expect immediate changes – but with time, you will not only live healthier, happier and longer, but also change into someone you (and the Universal Spirit) will like.

> *"Your Life Only Gets Better When You Get Better."*

Brian Tracy

Wish you a happy and healthy heart and a robust circulation.

Namaste.

Shashi K. Agarwal, MD

APPENDIX

Meditation poses

Besides *sukhasana,* which is commonly used, meditation can also be done in the following poses:

Lotus Pose (*Padmasana*)

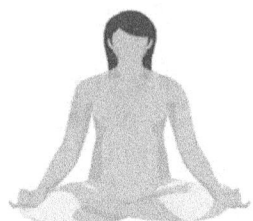

- Breathing normally, lower your torso, place both hands on the floor, sit down on your buttocks and straighten out the legs in front of you.
- Sit up straight. (*dandasana* pose).
- Bending the right knee with both hands, bring the right ankle to the groin.
- Now raise the foot to rest on the left thigh with the heel touching the lower belly/hip area.
- The left knee is now bent, and the left heel is brought towards the navel, (with the help of both hands) over the right shin, with the left foot resting now on the right thigh and the left heel gently touching the lower belly/right hip.
- The outer edges of your feet will be pressing down onto your thighs.
- Straighten your arms and with them partially resting on the knees, join the hands together in a meditation mudra.
- The back is straight, and you are calm and breathing normally.

Although the above instructions bring the left leg on top, the sequence can start with the left leg first to bring the right leg on top. Do them alternatively to open both hips.

This pose may be initially difficult, but your hips/knees will gradually open and you will find this 'classic yoga pose' not only easy to do but comfortably maintainable for hours.

Perfect pose (Siddhasana)

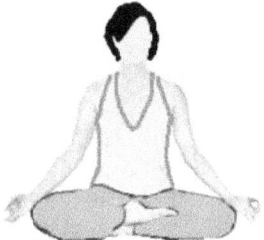

- Breathing normally, lower your torso, place both hands on the floor, sit down on your buttocks and straighten out the legs in front of you.
- Sit up straight. (*dandasana* pose)
- Now bending your left knee slide the left heel towards the groin. Leave the heel in this position touching your groin.
- Bend the right knee and bring the right ankle over the left ankle, resting it near your pubic bone (the central bone above your groin)
- Rest your hand on the knees and adopt a meditation mudra.

Prosperous or Auspicious Pose (Svastikasana)

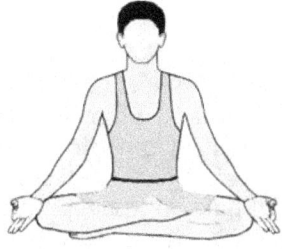

In India, 'Swastika' – the name being the name *svastikasana*, is a symbol of happiness, good luck or auspiciousness.

- Breathing normally, lower your torso, place both hands on the floor, sit down on your buttocks and straighten out the legs in front of you. Sit up straight. (*dandasana* pose)
- Fold your left leg; keep the sole of your left leg against the inner thigh of your right leg.
- Now bend your right leg and keep your right foot in the space between left thigh and calf muscles.
- Catch your left foot by the toes and try to pull it up and place it between the right calf and thigh. Your knees must firmly touch the floor. Maintain the pose so that you feel relax.
- Your body and trunk should erect. Place your hands on your knees in any mudra.

Again, either leg can be on the top and practice both so that you become comfortable in both poses.

Yoga and laughter

Lion posture (*Simhasana* pose) is commonly used for simulated laughter in yoga.

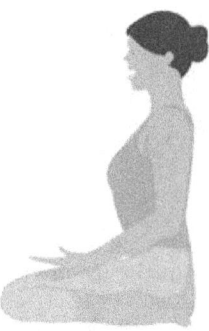

- Sit in virasana.
- Place your palms on your thighs/knees and spread out the fingers like the claws of a feline.
- You can even bend forward and put the palms in front of the knees on the floor. The focus of the eyesight (*drishti*) is on the tip of the nose.
- Take a deep breath, stick your tongue out.
- The tongue is stretched out with its tip curled towards the chin.
- Now exhaling, roar like a lion (Haaa) followed by a good belly laugh.

Laughter clubs:

Laughter at these clubs is usually done standing up. The initial action is clapping – it helps you warm up and stimulate beneficial pressure points. Clap with a 1-2-3 rhythm – move your hands up and down and swing them from side to side during the clapping process. Loudly chant "ho ho, ha-ha-ha", while clapping, with fast deep breaths from your belling and exhaling in co-ordination. You may move in the room during this process.

Some benefits of asanas:

General health benefits of doing sun salutations, especially with bare feet on grass facing the rising sun include:

2. It is an exercise – tones muscles and ligaments, strengthens bones, makes joints more flexible, improves posture and balance and provides mild to moderate intensity aerobic workout.
3. Induces production of vitamin D
4. Protects against melanoma – the morning sun is less damaging to the skin
5. Stabilizes the circadian rhythm – better sleep
6. Provides earthing – anti-oxidants improve
7. Foot health is better
8. Improves mental health – endorphins are released
9. Individual asanas have specific health benefits
10. Provides exposure to nature
11. Allows better and cleaner air to be breathed – non-polluted.

12. Increases positivity

Slow *asanas* provide low intensity exercise and work on your body's framework, strengthening it and making it more flexible.

1. **Standing Poses**: These are grounding postures. While standing on your feet, your spine and body is aligned, and the center of gravity is in the middle. These poses create strength in your legs, allow spinal movements in all directions including twisting, while anchoring your hips. They help create stability and improve coordination. Most standing poses work on lower body toning (muscles, bones, ligaments and other joint structures), spine range of motion, posture and balance. They help tone the shoulders and arms.

2. **Kneeling/Seated Poses**: These are sitting poses and often involve kneeling – with a heavy emphasis on the hip and knee joints. Most seated poses work on the spine – twists and flexion and extension. Some hip (adductor muscles) and knee stretches also occur. These muscles and bones get stretched, toned and relaxed.

3. **Prone Poses**: These are done lying face down, on your stomach. Mostly work on the spine range of motion. Some strengthening of the wrists, shoulder joints, back muscles and ankles also occurs.

4. **Supine Poses**: These poses are done with face up and lying on the back. These help you work on your upper front chest and abdominals, shoulders and back muscles. They specifically work on the spine and core abdominal muscles. The supine pose is also conducive to total body relaxation, natural breathing and meditation.

Mantra Meditation

Mantra yoga can be practiced in at least six ways.

The first way is called *baikhari*, wherein the mantra is chanted in a loud manner. This type of chanting is advantageous for removing unwanted thoughts from the mind in order to make the meditation process easier.

The second method of chanting is called *upanshu*, in which the mantra is chanted in a very low voice that only the practitioner can hear.

The third method is chanting the mantra silently to one's self. This is called *manasic* and it is used by advanced practitioners.

A fourth method is *kirtan* meditation – in this the mantra is musically chanted.

Likhita japa, the fifth method, which refers to the writing of a mantra again and again.

The sixth method is by using a *mala* (yoga beads). *Japa* engages the mind spiritually and leads the practitioner to a deep meditative state. Malas can be made of many materials — including gemstones, rudraksha seeds and sandalwood. They are tied together with overhand knotting which provides the perfect space for japa meditation. Jap meditation uses each bead to recite the mantra. Rudraksha beads are commonly used for the mantra '*Om Namah Shivaya*' as Lord Shiva wears these beads. Rudraksha beads are the seeds of several species of large evergreen broad-leaved tree in the genus Elaeocarpus, especially the species *Elaeocarpus ganitrus*. Because of their 'coarse' feel and comfortable size, I prefer these for jap meditation.

There are 108 beads on a *mala* (plus a *guru* beat, the 109th bead – also known as the '*meru*' or '*bindu*' bead). A different size or shaped bead may be placed at every 27th bead to make it easier to keep track of the count. Most religions use some similar '*mala*' devices for spirituality/prayers.

Japa meditation session with beads: Do this in the *sukhasana* pose. Hold your mala in your right hand, draped between your middle and index fingers. Start at the '*guru*' bead, use your thumb to count each smaller bead, pulling it toward you – each bead movement is associated with a recitation of a mantra. After 108 times, you will reach the '*guru*' bead and instead of pass

Yoga *Nidra*

Yoga literature also describes a pose that is named after yoga *nidra*:

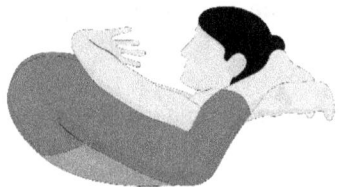

This pose is an expert pose and I recommend that you do yoga *nidra* in the corpse pose.

Yoga *Nidra* with Positive Affirmations

"Once you replace negative thoughts with positive ones, you'll start having positive results."

Willie Nelson

Some positive affirmations (a quality or virtue you wish to achieve and reinforce)

- "I am at peace."
- "I am compassionate and kind."
- "I forgive myself. "
- "I am balanced in mind and body."
- "I have an open heart."
- "I am a good person."
- "I am a healthy person."
- "I am a strong person."
- "I am a loving person."
- "I am a caring person."
- "I am a capable person."
- "I am loved person."
- "I am an honest person."
- "I am non-judgmental."

- "I am full of vitality."
- "I am a happy person."
- "I am a unique person."
- "I am perfect."
- "I am one with the Source."

Positivity and happiness centers in the brain are spread all over, with extensive connections. They include the anterior cingulate cortex, the ventral striatum, the ventral pallidum, and the midbrain dopamine neurons.[1] Repeating positive affirmations over a period of time, will rewire the brain and change the electrical routes to the more positive centers in the brain – a positive neuroplasticity. Positivity results in the brain directed increase in the production of serotonin and a decrease in cortisol – changes that produce feelings of happiness. Other beneficial hormones released with positivity - and happiness include dopamine, oxytocin, and endorphins.[2]

"You can search throughout the entire universe for someone who is more deserving of your love and affection than you are yourself, and that person is not to be found anywhere. You yourself, as much as anybody in the entire universe deserve your love and affection."

Buddha

Yoga *Nidra* with Happy Visualization

"An attitude that creates joy is one in which you interpret what happens to you through the filter of joy. Your attitude and outlook act like a filter. When you have a positive, optimistic outlook, it filters out the negative and denser perspectives and leads to joy. Bring joy into your life today."

Sanaya Roman

Positive visualizations can help achieve several goals. Achieving desires and fulfilling dreams. It helps your brain generate creative ideas to achieve your goal. It helps your brain to perceive and recognize resources in order to achieve these goals. It attracts people, resources, and circumstances that will help you achieve your goals. It helps develop motivation and perseverance to reach your goals.

Calming down: Happy memories help buffer stress.[1] Closing your eyes and imagining yourself in your favorite experienced place, position or among your favorite people or things is extremely beneficial to your underlying brain wiring especially during the event, during rumination or when faced with anxiety about future events. Develop a mental bank of happy 'visual' memories – your favorite beach, your enjoyable hike, your memorable party etc. – events and places that you can automatically retrieve during troubled times and then relive those moments. Remember, on a spiritual scale, everything happens for the good.

जो भी हुआ, अच्छे के लिए हुआ जो भी हो रहा है, अच्छे के लिए हो रहा है जो भी हो, वह भी अच्छे के लिए होगा

Whatever happened, happened for the good. Whatever is happening, is happening for the good. Whatever will happen, will also happen for the good

Bhagvad Gita

Positive visualizations prevent negative thoughts from occurring, thereby un-strengthening those neurons and its negative connections/pathways – for example, your connections between the amygdala and the prefrontal cortex and insula.[2,3] On the flip side, it helps fortify the positive stores in the brain and their favorable connections - thereby raising baseline hope and happiness, though at a subconscious level. It also helps you bounce back faster from negative situations.[4]

Mental vacation: dip into your bank of stored good and happy memories – travel, awards, birthdays, children's achievements – whatever you find uplifting. This way you can float away on a happy visual break – even when not under stress. Memories that you cherish are encoded via the midbrain and ventral striatum[5,6] and stored in the hippocampus and you can recall them and relive them vividly – be rich with 'happiness'.[7]

Better health: visualizing one being active and youthful, say gardening, fishing, running etc. – you guessed it – you will probably stay healthier. Data suggests that even visualizing exercising makes the muscles subjected to 'mental gymnastics' bigger and stronger.[8]

Competitions – especially sports. Visualizing repeatedly hitting a homerun or making a birdie etc., during yoga nidra, will help you improve your sports ability. You can also visualize a presentation or speech... and so on. Your results will be better.

Better habits: visualizing not smoking and having whiter teeth and fresh breath – will help you break a bad habit and achieve those goals – other habits improve if similarly visualized.

Better dreams: positive visualization during yoga nidra of one being able to overcome negative psychological challenges in life, real or imagined, should help turn your negative dreams into positive ones. You will sleep better and wake up happier. Negative dreams may be result from experiencing these threatening or painful experiences[9,10] during waking times and visualization of our mastery over these will make your rapid eye movement sleep much more enjoyable.

It is therefore important to establish a bank of rich rewarding happy memories – your exercises will help trigger and recall them rapidly – consciously or unconsciously. These happy memories should be 'visually' revisited often ('visual gymnastics') – the storage in the brain becomes vivid, the neuronal connections become stronger and the recall is easier. Examples include: a childhood camping trip, picking sea-shells by the ocean, a first kiss, graduation, first pay check, birth of a child, a memorable vacation ... and so on.

"Memories are the treasures that we keep locked deep within the storehouse of our souls, to keep our hearts warm when we are lonely."

Becky Aligada

Yoga Nidra with Gratitude Recitations

"Those who have the ability to be grateful are the ones who have the ability to achieve greatness."

Steve Maraboli

Also, be thankful, during certain yoga nidra practices:

- I am thankful for continuing my soul's journey in this body – allowing me to experience being a human.
- I am thankful for being able to live this experience and learn from it.
- I am thankful for everything I have received during this journey.
- I am thankful for happiness experienced during good times and the lessons learnt from adversity.
- I am thankful for mastering the ability to live in the present - not regretting the past and not fretting about the future.
- I am at thankful for being at peace - accepting serenely what I cannot change.
- I am thankful to my spirit for keeping me energized.
- I am thankful to the Universal Creator/Source for providing me with this energy and keeping my soul's journey on its course.

Everything that we get, everything that we have and everything that we consider ours – is all a gift.

आप खाली हाथ आए, और आप खाली हाथ छोड़ देंगे।

You came empty handed, and you will leave empty handed

Bhagvad Gita

So be grateful. Gratitude confers health benefits – both mental[1] and physical[2] Neuroimaging studies confirm stronger neuronal changes in the brain's reward system regions with gratitude behaviours.[3]

"I would maintain that thanks are the highest form of thought; and that gratitude is happiness doubled by wonder."

G.K. Chesterton

Yoga Nidra with Prayers

While in yoga nidra, concentrate on the third eye – this incorporates dharna and will help prevent your 'monkey brain' from wandering. Repeat any or all of these prayers in your mind (or even audibly) again and again. Or recite gratitude and sing to the glory of the Supreme.

Prayer is man's greatest power!

W. Clement Stone

Prayer in any form —petition, praise, and confession, can be practiced during meditation. It will bring stillness in your chaotic brain and connect you with the Creator.

God grant me the serenity
to accept the things, I cannot change;
courage to change the things I can;
and wisdom to know the difference.

Reinhold Niebuhr (1892-1971)

A few prayers from different major religions:

Jewish Prayer

Modeh Ani Lefanecha
Melech Chai Vekayom
Shehechezarta Bi Nishmati
Bechemla
Raba Emunatecha

I offer thanks to You,
living and eternal King,
for You have mercifully restored my soul within me;
Your faithfulness is great.

Islamic Prayers

Subhaan Allah: Glory to Allah.

Alhamdo lillah: All praise belongs to Allah

Subhaan Allah, Alhamdo lillah, Allaho Akbar: Glory to Allah, all praise belongs to Allah, Allah is the Greatest.

Budhhist Prayer

May you be at peace
May your heart remain open
May you awaken to the light of your own true nature
May you be healed
May you be a source of healing for all beings

Christianity prayer

Our Father, which art in heaven,
Hallowed be thy Name.
Thy Kingdom come.
Thy will be done in earth,
As it is in heaven.
Give us this day our daily bread.
And forgive us our trespasses,
As we forgive them that trespass against us.
And lead us not into temptation,
But deliver us from evil.
For thine is the kingdom,
The power, and the glory,
For ever and ever.
Amen.

Hindu prayer

Om Bhur Bhuvaḥ Swaḥ
Tat-savitur Vareñyaṃ
Bhargo Devasya Dhīmahi
Dhiyo Yonaḥ Prachodayāt

We meditate on that most adored Supreme Lord,
the creator,
whose effulgence (divine light) illumines
all realms (physical, mental and spiritual)
May this divine light illumine our intellect

Follow the yoga nidra with preparations to wake up with silk breath rejuvenation. Feel your breath coming in and out of your nostrils and gently caressing them. Your thoughts should be completely devoted to following the breath at the tips of the nostrils. Gradually wake up to reality – you should feel repaired and revitalized.

General health benefits of yoga

Yoga plays an important prophylactic role in modern medicine. The overall health benefits experienced by otherwise healthy people with yoga are numerous[1]. These include:

1. Improved academic performance[2]
2. Aerobic exercise[3]
3. Addiction is decreased[4]
4. Aging is slowed[5]
5. Anger/Aggressiveness/Hostility is diminished[6]
6. Anxiety is less[7]
7. Arthritis is reduced[8]
8. Atherosclerosis is retarded[9]
9. Athletic activity improves[10]
10. Balance improves[11]
11. Blood count improves[12]
12. Blood is thinner[13]
13. Blood pressure is reduced[14]
14. Blood sugar is better[15]
15. Bones get stronger[16]
16. Bowels function improves[17]
17. Brain blood flow is increased[18]
18. Brain waves are better[19]
19. Breathing is improved[20]
20. Cholesterol levels improve[21]
21. Circulation (blood) is improved[22]
22. Circulation (lymph) is facilitated[23]
23. Cleansing is enhanced[24]
24. Cognition is better[25]
25. Common cold (rhinitis) is less[26]
26. Connective tissue is better[27]
27. Coordination is better[28]
28. Creativity improves[29]
29. Death fear lessens[30]

30. Decision making improves, problem solving improves[31]
31. Dementia is prevented[32]
32. Dental health improves[33]
33. Depression is reduced[34]
34. Detoxification via increased sweating occurs[35]
35. Discipline occurs in life[36]
36. Eating quality improved[37]
37. Efficiency increases[38]
38. Energy levels rise[39]
39. Empathy/compassion gets better[40]
40. Endurance increases[41]
41. Exercise desire and ability increases[42]
42. Fertility increases[43]
43. Fitness is improved[44]
44. Flexibility/ROM improves[45]
45. Focus improves, attention improves, ability to work under distractions/stress improves[46]
46. Gastrointestinal function improves[47]
47. Gene expression improves[48]
48. Grief is better handled[49]
49. Grey matter increases[50]
50. Happiness is enhanced[51]
51. Headaches are decreased[52]
52. Healing improves[53]
53. Heart Attacks are prevented[54]
54. Heart pumps better[55]
55. Immunity increases[56]
56. Incontinence is prevented[57]
57. Inflammation is decreased[58]
58. Injury protection is increased[59]
59. Joint health improves[60]
60. Lifestyle improves[61]
61. Loneliness is decreased[62]
62. Longevity increases[63]
63. Lung parameters improve[64]
64. Memory improves, memory recall improves[65]
65. Menopause is easier[66]
66. Menstrual disorders are less[67]
67. Muscles are stronger[68]
68. Neuroplasticity (positive) is enhanced – white matter is increased[69]
69. Nostril breathing is encouraged with beneficial effects[70]
70. Organs (internal) are massaged[71]
71. Pain is reduced[72]
72. Parasympathetic tone is improved[73]
73. Performance improves[74]
74. Positivity rises[75]
75. Posture improves[76]
76. Pregnancy results are better[77]
77. Prevents several diseases – helps diseases[78]
78. Pulse rate goes down[79]
79. Quality of life improves[80]
80. Relationships improve[81]
81. Relaxation occurs[82]

82. Respiratory muscles are strengthened[83]
83. Self-awareness improves (better body image)[84]
84. Self-esteem is enhanced[85]
85. Self-confidence improves[86]
86. Sexuality improves[87]
87. Sinuses are cleaner[88]
88. Sleep is better[89]
89. Smoking cessation is enhanced[90]
90. Social Support improves[91]
91. Spine health improves[92]
92. Spirituality increases[93]
93. Stress is reduced[94]
94. Sympathetic activity goes down[95]
95. Urination is improved[96]
96. Vascular health improves[97]
97. Venous return improves[98]
98. Vision Improves[99]
99. Weight is better managed[100]

Medical benefits of yoga

Yoga as an adjunct therapeutic (complimentary) therapy may play a role in the following conditions[1] (and more are being added as new research continues to emerge)

1. ADHD[2]
2. Alcohol Use Disorder[3]
3. Alzheimer's Disease[4]
4. Anxiety[5]
5. Asthma[6]
6. Autism[7]
7. Back Pain[8]
8. Cancer[9]
9. Cardiac Rehabilitation[10]
10. Carpel Tunnel Syndrome[11]
11. Chronic Fatigue Syndrome[12]
12. Chronic Kidney Disease[13]
13. Chronic Obstructive Pulmonary Disease[14]
14. Coronary Artery Disease[15]
15. Congestive Heart Failure[16]
16. Depression[17]
17. Diabetes Mellitus[18]
18. Drug addiction/withdrawal[19]
19. Eating disorders[20]
20. Epilepsy[21]
21. Firbromyalgia[22]
22. Hypertension[23]
23. HIV/AIDS[24]
24. Infertility[25]
25. Insomnia[26]
26. Irritable Bowel Syndrome[27]
27. Menopausal Disorders[28]
28. Menstrual Disorders[29]

29. Metabolic Syndrome[30]
30. Migraine[31]
31. Multiple Sclerosis[32]
32. Neuro-degenerative disorders[33]
33. Neurosis[34]
34. Obesity[35]
35. Obsessive compulsive disorder[36]
36. Osteoarthritis[37]
37. Osteoporosis[38]
38. Pancreatitis[39]
39. Parkinson's disease[40]
40. Periodontal disease[41]
41. Pleural effusion[42]
42. Polycystic Ovaries[43]
43. Post-op recovery[44]
44. Post stroke rehabilitation[45]
45. Pregnancy/Perinatal Disorders[46]
46. Psoriasis[47]
47. Psychosis[48]
48. PTSD[49]
49. Restless leg syndrome[50]
50. Rheumatoid arthritis[51]
51. Rhinitis/Sinusitis[52]
52. Schizophrenia[53]
53. Scoliosis[54]
54. Smoking cessation[55]
55. Tuberculosis[56]
56. Urinary Incontinence[57]

The benefit of multi-modal yoga is being studied in many other conditions.

GLOSSARY

ACE: angiotensin converting enzyme – their inhibitors are common drugs that relax arteries and promote renal excretion of salt and water and help reduce blood pressure.
Adenopectin: a protein made by fat cells that plays a role in the development of insulin resistance and atherosclerosis.
Adipocyte: also known as lipocytes and fat cells that are specialized in storing energy as fat
Adrenal: glands found above the kidneys – they secrete a variety of hormones including adrenaline and the steroids aldosterone and cortisol
Adrenaline: hormone secreted by the adrenal glands in response to stress - increases heart rate, pulse rate, and blood pressure, and raises the blood levels of glucose and lipids.
Aerobic: occurring only in the presence of oxygen
Aggregability/ aggregation: the tendency or the process whereby the platelets clump together and form a clot
Algae: chlorophyll containing unicellular or multicellular organisms, present in fresh or salt water or moist ground
Angiogenesis: the growth of new blood vessels
Anthocyanins: red, purple, or blue pigment found in blueberries, cherries and plums and other colored vegetables and fruits – they are powerful antioxidants
Anthropometric: relating to measurements used to assess the size, shape and composition of the human body.
Antibodies: a blood protein produced by B cells as a primary immune defense. It is a response to and counteracting a specific antigen – usually an alien such as a virus or bacteria
Anticoagulants: substances that hinder coagulation of blood – could be a drug
Antioxidant: a substance that inhibits oxidation such as beta-carotene, vitamin C, and alpha-tocopherol
Anti-proliferative: retarding cell growth or spread
Aortic: relating to the aorta – the largest artery in the body arising from the top of the left ventricle which is the main pumping chamber of the heart
Apolipoprotein: proteins that bind lipids to form lipoproteins (and help transport the lipids)
Arrhythmia: an irregular or abnormal heart rhythm
Arterial: relating to an artery
Atherosclerosis: a silent process leading to the buildup of plaque inside the arteries and leading to narrowing and blockages – the usual cause of heart attacks, strokes, and peripheral vascular disease
Atherothrombotic: the formation of a blood clot within an artery, usually as a result of atherosclerotic lesion disruption
Atrial fibrillation: a fast and irregular heartbeat - may lead to blood clots, stroke, heart failure and other heart-related complications
Autoimmune: usually referred to an autoimmune disorder where the immune system attacks healthy cells in its own body by mistake
Autonomic nervous system: the nervous system that regulates the functions of the internal organs such as the heart, stomach and intestines
Bariatric surgery: weight loss surgery. The most common bariatric surgery procedures are gastric bypass, sleeve gastrectomy and adjustable gastric band
Baroreflex: feedback loop that plays an important role in short term blood pressure regulation
Bioactive: having an effect on a living tissue
Bioavailability: the degree and rate a substance is available for physiological activity –

usually referred to an absorbed drug and the amount available in the body for bioactivity

Biomarker: a distinct biochemical, genetic, or molecular characteristic or substance that is an indicator of a particular biological condition or process

Bipolar: bipolar disease is a serious manic-depressive illness

Body Mass Index (BMI): a weight-to-height ratio - defines normal weight, overweight, and obesity in adults

Caffeine: a central nervous system stimulant found in coffee – it is the world's most widely consumed psychoactive drug

Calorie: the energy needed to raise the temperature of 1 gram of water through 1 °C – commonly used as a measurement of the amount of energy that food provides

Carbohydrates: substances such as sugar and starches that are major sources of energy for the human body

Carcinogens: a substance or agent capable of causing cancer

Cardiac rehabilitation: an outpatient medically supervised program of exercise and education for people following a heart attack, heart failure, heart valve surgery, coronary artery bypass grafting, or percutaneous coronary intervention

Cardiogenic: relating to the heart

Cardiomyopathy: a disease affecting the heart muscle – it causes the heart to become enlarged, thick, or stiff.

Cardiotoxicity: toxicity that affects the heart – may occur with cancer therapy

Cardiovascular: relating to the heart and blood vessels

Carotenoids: a group of pigments that are responsible for the bright red, yellow and orange colors of many fruits and vegetables

Cataracts: progressive opaqueness of the lens of the eyes – resulting in blurry or cloudy vision

Catecholamines: a group of sympathomimetic amines (including dopamine, epinephrine, and norepinephrine) that act as hormones and/or neurotransmitters

Cerebrovascular: relating to the brain and its blood vessels

Cholesterol: a steroid that's found in all cells of the body – high levels are associated with an increased risk for heart and blood vessel disease.

Chylomicron: a small lipoprotein particle – they transport exogenous cholesterol and triglycerides from the small intestine to the liver and adipose tissues

Circadian rhythm: an internal body clock – it regulates many physiological processes including when to sleep and when to rise

Cognitive: concerning mental processes such as perception, thinking, learning, and memory

Cohort: a group of individuals with something in common

Co-morbidity: the presence of two disorders or illnesses simultaneously or sequentially in the same patient

Congestive heart failure: failure of the heart to pump blood

COPD: Chronic Obstructive Pulmonary Disease – chronic obstruction of lung airflow interfering with normal breathing and not fully reversible

Coronary Artery Disease: disease (usually atherosclerosis) of the arteries that supply blood to the heart – the result may be angina or a heart attack

Coronary Heart Disease: heart diseases resulting from coronary artery narrowing or blockage

Cortisol: a steroid based hormone produced by the adrenal glands – it is also known as hydrocortisone

CRP: C-reactive protein – is a marker for inflammation in the body

Cytokines: a group of proteins (such as interferon, interleukin) that trigger inflammation

Dementia: a progressive condition characterized by multiple cognitive deficits. Alzheimer's disease accounts for 60 to 80 percent of cases.

Deoxyribonucleic acid: DNA – carries the genetic information for the transmission of hereditary traits
Diabetes Mellitus Type 2: a long-term metabolic disorder characterized by high blood sugar, insulin resistance, and relative lack of insulin – causes damage to the heart, eyes, kidneys, nerves, and other parts of the body.
Diastolic blood pressure: it indicates the pressure the blood is exerting against the walls of the arteries while the heart is resting between beats. If the blood pressure is 120/80, the diastolic pressure is 80 mm Hg (millimeters of mercury).
Dopamine: neurotransmitter; essential to the normal functioning of the central nervous system
Eclampsia: a life-threatening high blood pressure complication during pregnancy – with one or more convulsions
Endogenous: produced internally
Endothelium: the single layer of cells lining the insides of the blood vessels, heart, and lymphatic vessels
Epidemiological: the incidence, distribution, and control of diseases in large populations
Epinephrine: also known as adrenaline – a hormone secreted by the adrenal gland. It is a stress hormone and causes increases in heart rate, pulse rate, and blood pressure, and raises the blood levels of glucose and lipids.
Ethanol: the intoxicating ingredient of alcoholic beverages – usually obtained from the fermentation of sugars and starches
Fibrinogen: a protein in the blood plasma that is changed into fibrin to form a blood clot
Flavanols/Flavanoid: plant-based nutrients that have major antioxidant activities
Foam cells: macrophages (phagocytic white cells) laden with lipids – accumulating in the walls of the arteries and a part of the process of developing atherosclerosis
Gestational: period of fetal development from conception until birth
Glycated hemoglobin: is a form of hemoglobin that when measured gives the three-month average plasma glucose concentration - hemoglobin A1c, HbA1c, A1C, or Hb1c
Glycemic Index: a relative ranking of carbohydrate in foods according to how they affect blood glucose levels. Carbohydrate-containing foods can be classified as high- (≥70), moderate- (56-69), or low-GI (≤55) relative to pure glucose (GI=100). A low GI indicates a slow absorption
Growth hormone: also known as somatotropin is secreted by the pituitary and helps children grow and helps adults maintain tissues and organs
HDL: high density lipoprotein – the 'good cholesterol'. It carries the 'bad' LDL cholesterol away from the arteries and back to the liver
Hemodialysis: kidney dialysis – the process of purifying the blood, by removing fluid and waste products, from a person whose kidneys are not working normally
Hemorrhagic stroke: brain damage caused by a rupture of a weakened blood vessel – it is responsible for about 15% of all strokes
Hydrogenation: the process of converting liquid vegetable oils into solid or semi-solid fats, such as those present in margarine.
Hypercholesterolemia: high cholesterol levels in the blood
Hyperglycemia: excess of glucose in the blood – as seen in diabetes mellitus
Hyperlipidemia: increased levels of fats or lipids in the blood – increasing the risk of disease of the blood vessels leading to stroke and heart disease
Hypertension: blood pressure is higher than 140 over 90 mmHg
Hypertrophy: enlargement resulting from an increase in the size of cells
Hypotensive: abnormally low blood pressure
Hypothalamic: relating to the hypothalamus – the hypothalamus controls the pituitary gland and regulates many body functions

Incident: An incident is an occurrence of something that is often unpleasant
Inflammation: a complex biological response of body tissues to harmful stimuli
Inotropic: increasing or decreasing the force of muscular contractions – a positive heart inotropic agent increases the force of contraction; a negative ionotropic agent, the reverse
Insomnia: difficulty in falling or staying asleep
Insulin resistance: inability of the body cells to respond to insulin effectively, often leading to high blood sugar.
Interleukin-6: an endogenous chemical which is active in inflammation
Intima: the innermost layer of a blood vessel
Intracranial: within the skull
Intravenous: situated within, performed within, occurring within, or administered by entering a vein (intravenously)
Immune function: the response of the immune system to protect the body – when threatened by foreign substances, cells, and tissue
Ischemia: in cardiology usually referred to a shortage of blood and oxygen to the heart muscle – often resulting from a narrowing or blockage of the coronary arteries
Ischemic heart disease: heart disease due to ischemia – usually due to atherosclerosis
Lactose: a disaccharide (sugar) present in milk – some people are lactose intolerant and develop symptoms such as bloating and diarrhea on drinking milk
Lipid: fatty acids, oils, waxes, sterols, and triglycerides – they are insoluble in water
Lipoprotein: a particle that is the primary mean of transport of cholesterol and triglycerides in the blood
LDL: low density lipoprotein – the 'bad' cholesterol
Macrophages: large white blood cells in the tissues or blood – they engulf foreign substances or invaders such as cellular debris, foreign substances, microbes, cancer cells
Macular degeneration: deterioration of the small central area of the retina of the eye that controls visual acuity
Marfan's syndrome: a genetic disorder affecting the body's connective tissue
Mediterranean: referring to the Mediterranean Sea or the lands surrounding it
METs: A metabolic unit used to quantify the intensity of physical activity - commonly used in stress testing of the heart
Meta-analysis: a quantitative statistical analysis of several separate but similar experiments or studies – the pooled data usually provides more precise conclusions
Metabolic Syndrome: the co-occurrence of several known cardiovascular risk factors, including insulin resistance, obesity, atherogenic dyslipidemia and hypertension
Minerals: naturally occurring inorganic compounds
Mitral valve prolapse: a condition in which the leaflets of the mitral valve bulge (prolapse) into the heart's left upper chamber (left atrium) when the heart contracts
Monosaccharides: a class of sugars that cannot be broken down to simpler sugars
Monounsaturated: A fatty acid chain is monounsaturated if it contains one double bond
Myocardial Infarction: a heart attack – resulting from an abrupt stoppage of blood flow to the heart and causing heart muscle damage
NEPA: non-exercise physical activity
Neuro-hormonal: a hormone produced by or acting on nervous tissue – examples: acetylcholine or norepinephrine
Nicotine: the chief active constituent of tobacco – an addictive alkaloid
Nitric oxide: a major vasodilator
Noradrenaline: norepinephrine – a neurotransmitter that constricts blood vessels, raising blood pressure and heart rate and dilates bronchi of the lungs
Nor-epinephrine: noradrenaline - a neurotransmitter that constricts blood vessels,

raising blood pressure and heart rate and dilates bronchi of the lungs
Obstructive sleep apnea: a serious breathing disorder – the throat muscles intermittently relax and block the airway during sleep
Oligosaccharides: a saccharide containing a small number (typically two to ten) of simple sugars (monosaccharides).
Omega 3: essential fatty acids found in fish oils, that help to lower the levels of cholesterol and LDL (low-density lipoproteins) in the blood.
Omega 6: long-chain polyunsaturated fatty acids, such as linoleic acid and arachidonic acid
Orthostatic: relating to or caused by erect posture
Osteoporosis: increased bone weakness from loss of bone mineral density increasing the risk of fractures
Oxidation: the process or result of oxidizing
Oxidative stress: imbalance between the production of free radicals and the ability of the body to counteract or detoxify their harmful effects
Parasympathetic: part of the autonomic nervous system that controls equilibrium of the physiological processes of the body at rest - the "rest and digest" function.
Pathogenesis: the biological mechanism that leads to the development of a disease
Percutaneous coronary intervention
Periodontal: supporting structures of the teeth including the gums, cementum, periodontal membranes, and alveolar bone.
Peripheral: situated away from the center
Peripheral artery disease: narrowing of the peripheral arteries, usually the leg arteries - due to atherosclerosis
Peroxidation: rancidity from oxidative deterioration of lipids
Phenols: A simple cyclic compound in fruits and green tea which is cardioprotective
Phobia: a persistent, abnormal, or irrational fear of a specific thing or situation
Phytochemicals: naturally occurring, plant-based chemicals, that are biologically active and beneficial to our health.
Phytonutrients: plant-based compounds that have health-protecting qualities
Phytosterols: sterols derived from plants. When consumed, they help block cholesterol absorption, resulting in a reduction of the blood cholesterol levels
Pituitary: a pea sized endocrine gland attached to the brain – it produces hormones that control other *glands*
Placebo: a harmless pill, medicine, or procedure
Plaque: atherosclerotic lesion within the wall of an artery that causes its inner lining to bulge into the lumen
Plaque vulnerability: the vulnerability of an atherosclerotic vessel plaque to rupture or cause the formation of a blood clot in the vessel – may lead to a myocardial infarction or sudden death.
Platelets: a small, round, thin blood cells that circulate through our bloodstream. Their role is to help stop bleeding
Polyphenols: naturally occurring plant compounds with antioxidant activity that prevents or neutralizes the damaging effects of free radicals.
Polysaccharides: long chains of monosaccharide units bound together by glycosidic linkages – examples are starch, glycogen, and cellulose
Polycystic ovary syndrome: a hormonal disorder in women that can affect their periods, ovulation, fertility and pregnancy.
Polyunsaturated: A fatty acid chain is *polyunsaturated* if it contains more than one double bond.
Postmenopausal: after menopause
Postprandial glucose: blood sugar after eating a meal, usually after 1 and 2 hours
Prehypertension: blood pressure between 120/80 mmHg and 139/89 mmHg

Premature: occurring before the expected time
Premenstrual syndrome: a wide variety of complex symptoms experienced by some women prior to *menstruation*
Prevalence: proportion of a population that is affected with a particular disease at a given time.
Primary prevention: to prevent disease or injury before it occurs
Prophylactic: preventive – more details in the appendix section of this book
Prothrombotic: increasing the risk of thrombosis (developing a blood clot in a blood vessel)
PTSD: Post Traumatic Stress Disorder
Pulmonary: relating to the lungs
Quintile: used in statistics - where the sample or population is divided into fifths
Randomized: make unpredictable; in a clinical trial, people are allocated by chance to receive one of several clinical interventions
Revascularization: to restore blood flow – usually by vascular bypass and angioplasty
Ribonucleic acid: RNA - acts as a messenger between DNA and the protein synthesis complexes, called ribosomes
Saturated fats: saturated fats have no double bonds because they are saturated with hydrogen molecules. Saturated fats are typically solid at room temperature.
Schizophrenia: a chronic and severe mental disorder which affects how a person thinks, feels and acts.
Secondary prevention: to stop or slow the progression of a disease or injury already established
Snuff: smokeless tobacco made from ground or pulverized tobacco leaves
Statins: a group of cholesterol lowering drugs
Stroke: cutting off blood flow to a part of the brain resulting in permanent damage
Supplement: a product taken orally that contains one or more ingredients, such as vitamins or amino acids to add further nutritional value
Sympathetic nervous system: A part of the autonomic nervous system that accelerates the heart rate, constricts blood vessels, and raises blood pressure – the fight or flight response.
Systolic blood pressure: pressure your blood is exerting against your artery walls when the heart beats. If the blood pressure is 120/80, the systolic pressure is 120 mm Hg (millimeters of mercury).
Therapeutic: healing/curing; relating to the treatment of disease
Thermogenesis: heat production by metabolic processes; the process of energy production in the body
Thrombosis: the formation of a blood clot inside a blood vessel
Thrombotic: pertaining to thrombosis
Thrombus: a blood clot within a blood vessel
Tobacco: dried leaves of this plant - smoked in cigarettes, pipes, or cigars, or chewed
Tocopherols: organic chemical compounds with vitamin E antioxidant activity
Transcendental meditation: silent *meditation using a mantra* and other yogic practices
Transient ischemic attack: a mini-stroke, usually lasting only a few minutes and causing no permanent damage
Trans-fat: artificially created by adding hydrogen to liquid vegetable oils to make them more solid
Triglycerides: lipids that are esters formed from one molecule of glycerol and three molecules of one or more fatty acids They are stored in the fat cells and are a major source of energy in the body.
Unsaturated fats: a *fat* or fatty acid in which there is at least one double bond within the fatty acid chain – these are healthier than saturated fats

Unstable angina: angina due to inadequate blood flow to the heart that may lead to a myocardial infarction
Vasoconstriction: the narrowing/constriction of the blood vessels
Vasomotor: relating to the caliber of the blood vessels (constriction or dilatation)
Vasospasm: spasm of a blood vessel – constriction which may lead to the restriction of blood flow
Ventricular arrhythmias: Abnormal rapid heart rhythms originating in the ventricles of the heart
Visceral: relating to the inner organs of the body
Vitamin: group of organic compounds required by the body in small amounts for proper functioning and growth

REFERENCES

Introduction

1. Heart Disease and Stroke Statistics—2018 Update: A Report From the American Heart Association. Circulation 2018;Jan 31: From: https://www.acc.org/latest-in-cardiology/ten-points-to-remember/2018/02/09/11/59/heart-disease-and-stroke-statistics-2018-update.
2. Ziglio E, Currie C, Rasmussen VB. (2004). The WHO cross-national study of health behavior in school aged children from 35 countries: findings from 2001–2002. J School Health, 74 (6): 204– 206.

What is Yoga?

1. Strauss S. The master's narrative: swami sivananda and the transnational production of yoga. Journal of Folklore Research 39 2002;2:217.
2. Hammond H. Yoga pioneers: how yoga came to America. Yoga Journal 2007. https://www.yogajournal.com/yoga-101/yogas-trip-america (accessed July 16, 2017).
3. https://en.wikipedia.org/wiki/Richard_Hittleman.
4. McDermott RA. Indian spirituality in the west: a bibliographical mapping. Philosophy East and West 1975;25:213–39. 10.2307/1397942.
5. Schmidt T, Wijga A, Von ZurMuhlen A, Brabant G, Wagner TO (1997) Changes in cardiovascular risk factors and hormones during a comprehensive residential three month kriya yoga training and vegetarian nutrition. Acta Physiol Scand Suppl 640: 158-162.
6. https://nccih.nih.gov/health/yoga.
7. Barnes P, Bloom B, Nahin R. Complementary and alternative medicine use among adults and children: United States, 2007. Natl Health Stat Report. 2008. December 10;(12):1–23.
8. Larson-Meyer DE. A Systematic Review of the Energy Cost and Metabolic Intensity of Yoga. Med Sci Sports Exerc. 2016 Aug;48(8):1558-69. doi: 10.1249/MSS.0000000000000922.
9. NHS . Your health, your choices. A guide to yoga. 2013.
10. https://www.usatoday.com/story/opinion/2013/05/18/yoga-religion-column/2158377/ (accessed 1/2/18).
11. Keosaian JE, Lemaster CM, Dresner D, et al. "We're All in This Together": A Qualitative Study of Predominantly Low Income Minority Participants in a Yoga Trial for Chronic Low Back Pain. Complementary therapies in medicine. 2016;24:34-39. doi:10.1016/j.ctim.2015.11.007.
12. Firestone KA, Carson JW, Mist SD, Carson KM, Jones KD. Interest In Yoga Among Fibromyalgia Patients: An International Internet Survey. International journal of yoga therapy. 2014;24:117-124.
13. Berger DL, Silver EJ, Stein REK. Effects of yoga on inner-city children's well-being: a pilot study. Alternative Therapies in Health and Medicine. 2009;15(5):36–42.
14. Curtis K, Hitzig SL, Bechsgaard G, et al. Evaluation of a specialized yoga program for persons with a spinal cord injury: a pilot randomized controlled trial. Journal of Pain Research. 2017;10:999-1017. doi:10.2147/JPR.S130530.
15. Balasubramaniam M., Telles S., Doraiswamy P. M. (2012). Yoga on our minds: a systematic review of yoga for neuropsychiatric disorders. Front. Psychiatry 3:117. 10.3389/fpsyt.2012.00117.
16. Rector K, Vilardaga R, Lansky L, et al. Design and Real-World Evaluation of Eyes-Free Yoga: An Exergame for Blind and Low-Vision Exercise. ACM transactions on accessible computing. 2017;9(4):12. doi:10.1145/3022729.
17. https://www.livestrong.com/article/394069-do-you-need-to-use-a-yoga-mat - accessed 12/5/17.
18. Tew GA, Howsam J, Hardy M, Bissell L. Adapted yoga to improve physical function and health-related quality of life in physically-inactive older adults: a randomised controlled pilot trial. BMC Geriatrics. 2017;17:131.
19. Cramer H, Krucoff C, Dobos G. Adverse events associated with yoga: a systematic review

of published case reports and case series. PLoS One. 2013;8(10):e75515. doi: 10.1371/journal.pone.0075515.
20. Cheema BS, Marshall PW, Chang D, Colagiuri B, Machliss B. Effect of an office worksite-based yoga program on heart rate variability: A randomized controlled trial. BMC Public Health. 2011;11:578. doi:10.1186/1471-2458-11-578.
21. Berger DL, Silver EJ, Stein RE. Effects of yoga on inner-city children's well-being: a pilot study. Altern Ther Health Med. 2009 Sep-Oct;15(5):36-42.
22. Chen KM, Fan JT, Wang HH, Wu SJ, Li CH, Lin HS. Silver yoga exercises improved physical fitness of transitional frail elders. Nurs Res. 2010 Sep-Oct;59(5):364-70. doi: 10.1097/NNR.0b013e3181ef37d5.
23. Flegal K, Kishiyama S, Zajdel D, Haas M, Oken B. Adherence to yoga and exercise interventions in a 6-month clinical trial. BMC Complementary and Alternative Medicine. 2007;7:37. doi:10.1186/1472-6882-7-37.
24. Tew GA, Howsam J, Hardy M, Bissell L. Adapted yoga to improve physical function and health-related quality of life in physically-inactive older adults: a randomised controlled pilot trial. BMC Geriatrics. 2017;17:131. doi:10.1186/s12877-017-0520-6.
25. Findorff MJ, Wyman JF, Gross CR. Predictors of Long-term Exercise Adherence in a Community-Based Sample of Older Women. Journal of Women's Health. 2009;18(11):1769-1776. doi:10.1089/jwh.2008.1265.
26. Mishra SK, Singh P, Bunch SJ, Zhang R. The therapeutic value of yoga in neurological disorders. Annals of Indian Academy of Neurology. 2012;15(4):247-254. doi:10.4103/0972-2327.104328.
27. Findorff MJ, Wyman JF, Gross CR. Predictors of Long-term Exercise Adherence in a Community-Based Sample of Older Women. Journal of Women's Health. 2009;18(11):1769-1776. doi:10.1089/jwh.2008.1265.
28. Agarwal SK. Evidence Based Therapeutic Effects of Yoga. 2017.Available at: https://www.amazon.com/Evidence-Based-Therapeutic-Effects-Yoga/dp/1983936367/ref=sr_1_3?s=books&ie=UTF8&qid=1517713441&sr=1-3&keywords=agarwal+shashi+k
29. National Center for Complementary and Alternative Medicine. Yoga for Health: Side Effects and Risks. Online document at: http://nccam.nih.gov/health/yoga/introduction.htm#hed3 Accessed January30, 2014.
30. https://www.yogajournal.com/lifestyle/8-travel-yoga-poses-work-small-spaces - accessed 12/15/17.
31. Vyavahare SV. Yoga for jail inmates. Proceedings of the 1st International Conference on Frontiers in Yoga Research and Applications; December 1991; Bangalore, India. VKYRF.
32. Ross A, Friedmann E, Bevans M, Thomas S. National Survey of Yoga Practitioners: Mental and Physical Health Benefits. Complementary therapies in medicine. 13;21(4):313-323. doi:10.1016/j.ctim.2013.04.001.
33. Birdee GS, Ayala SG, Wallston KA. Cross-sectional analysis of health-related quality of life and elements of yoga practice. BMC Complementary and Alternative Medicine. 2017;17:83. doi:10.1186/s12906-017-1599-1.
34. Yanping Li, An Pan, Dong D. Wang et al. Impact of Healthy Lifestyle Factors on Life Expectancies in the US Population. Circulation. 2018; CIRCULATIONAHA. 117.032047.

Prophylactic and therapeutic benefits of yoga on the heart and circulation

1. Haidich AB. Meta-analysis in medical research. Hippokratia. 2010;14(Suppl 1):29-37.
2. Gülpınar Ö, Güçlü AG. How to write a review article?. Turk J Urol. 2013;39(Suppl 1):44-8.
3. Kabisch M, Ruckes C, Seibert-Grafe M, Blettner M. Randomized controlled trials: part 17 of a series on evaluation of scientific publications. Dtsch Arztebl Int. 2011;108(39):663-8.
4. Song JW, Chung KC. Observational studies: cohort and case-control studies. Plast Reconstr Surg. 2010;126(6):2234-42.

Alcohol

1. Ferreira MP, Willoughby D. Alcohol consumption: the good, the bad, and the indifferent. Appl Physiol Nutr Metab. 2008 Feb;33(1):12-20. doi: 10.1139/H07-175.

2. Takkouche B, Regueira-Mendez C, Garcia-Closas R, Figueiras A, Gestal-Otero JJ, Hernan MA. Intake of wine, beer, and spirits and the risk of clinical common cold. Am J Epidemiol. 2002;155(9):853–858. doi: 10.1093/aje/155.9.853.
3. Ouchi E, Niu K, Kobayashi Y, et al. Frequent alcohol drinking is associated with lower prevalence of self-reported common cold: a retrospective study. BMC Public Health. 2012;12:987. Published 2012 Nov 16. doi:10.1186/1471-2458-12-987.
4. Scragg RK, McMichael AJ, Baghurst PA. Diet, alcohol, and relative weight in gall stone disease: a case-control study. Br Med J (Clin Res Ed). 1984;288(6424):1113-9.
5. Wang J, Duan X, Li B, Jiang X. Alcohol consumption and risk of gallstone disease: a meta-analysis. Eur J Gastroenterol Hepatol. 2017 Apr;29(4):e19-e28. doi: 10.1097/MEG.0000000000000803.
6. Avogaro A, Watanabe RM, Gottardo L, et al. Glucose tolerance during moderate alcohol intake: Insights on insulin action from glucose/lactate dynamics. J Clin Endocrinol Metab. 2002;87:1233–8.
7. Furuya DT, Binsack R, Machado UF. Low ethanol consumption increases insulin sensitivity in Wistar rats. Braz J Med Biol Res. 2003;36:125–30.
8. Koppes LL, Dekker JM, Hendriks HF, Bouter LM, Heine RJ. Moderate alcohol consumption lowers the risk of type 2 diabetes: a meta-analysis of prospective observational studies. Diabetes Care. 2005 Mar 1;28(3):719-25.
9. Schrieks IC, Heil AL, Hendriks HF, Mukamal KJ, Beulens JW. The effect of alcohol consumption on insulin sensitivity and glycemic status: a systematic review and meta-analysis of intervention studies. Diabetes Care 2015;38:723–32.
10. De Oliveira e Silva ER, Foster D, McGee Harper M, et al. Alcohol consumption raises HDL cholesterol levels by increasing the transport rate of apolipoproteins A-I and A-II. Circulation. 2000;102:2347–52.
11. Hendriks HF, Veenstra J, van Tol A, Groener JE, Schaafsma G. Moderate doses of alcoholic beverages with dinner and postprandial high density lipoprotein composition. Alcohol Alcohol 1998;33:403–10.
12. Agarwal DP. Cardioprotective effects of light-moderate consumption of alcohol: a review of putative mechanisms. Alcohol Alcohol. 2002 Sep-Oct;37(5):409-15.
13. Ginter E, Simko V. Ethanol and cardiovascular diseases: epidemiological, biochemical and clinical aspects. Bratisl Lek Listy. 2008;109:590–594.
14. Collins MA, Neafsey EJ, Mukamal KJ, Gray MO, Parks DA, Das DK, Korthuis RJ. Alcohol in moderation, cardioprotection, and neuroprotection: epidemiological considerations and mechanistic studies. Alcohol Clin Exp Res. 2009;33:206–219.
15. Kiechl S, Willeit J, Poewe W, et al. Insulin sensitivity and regular alcohol consumption: large, prospective, cross sectional population study (Bruneck study). BMJ. 1996;313(7064):1040-4.
16. Huang P.H., Chen Y.H., Tsai H.Y., Chen J.S., Wu T.C., Lin F.Y., Sata M., Chen J.W., Lin S.J. Intake of red wine increases the number and functional capacity of circulating endothelial progenitor cells by enhancing nitric oxide bioavailability. Arterioscler. Thromb. Vasc. Biol. 2010;30:869–877.
17. Lefevre J., Michaud S.E., Haddad P., Dussault S., Menard C., Groleau J., Turgeon J., Rivard A. Moderate consumption of red wine (cabernet sauvignon) improves ischemia-induced neovascularization in ApoE-deficient mice: Effect on endothelial progenitor cells and nitric oxide. FASEB J. 2007;21:3845–3852.
18. Liu P., Zhou B., Gu D., Zhang L., Han Z. Endothelial progenitor cell therapy in atherosclerosis: A double-edged sword? Ageing Res. Rev. 2009;8:83–93. doi: 10.1016/j.arr.2008.11.002.
19. Krenz M., Korthuis R.J. Moderate ethanol ingestion and cardiovascular protection: From epidemiologic associations to cellular mechanisms. J. Mol. Cell. Cardiol. 2012;52:93–104.
20. Albert MA, Glynn RJ, Ridker PM. Alcohol consumption and plasma concentration of C-reactive protein. Circulation. 2003;107:443–7.
21. U.S. Department of Health and Human Services and U.S. Department of Agriculture. 2015-2020 Dietary Guidelines for Americans. 8th Edition, Washington, DC; 2015.

22. Colditz GA, Branch LG, Lipnick RJ, Willett WC, Rosner B, Posner B, et al. Moderate alcohol and decreased cardiovascular mortality in an elderly cohort. Am Heart J 1985;109:886-9.
23. Camargo CA, Hennekens CH, Gaziano JM, Glynn RJ, Manson JE, Stampfer MJ. Prospective study of moderate alcohol consumption and mortality in US male physicians. Arch Intern Med 1997;157:79-85.
24. Berger K, Ajani UA, Kase CS, Gaziano JM, Buring JE, Glynn RJ, et al. Light-to-moderate alcohol consumption and risk of stroke among US male physicians. N Engl J Med 1999;341:1557-64.
25. Djousse L, Lee IM, Buring JE, Gaziano JM. Alcohol consumption and risk of cardiovascular disease and death in women: potential mediating mechanisms. Circulation 2009;120:237-44.
26. U.S. Department of Health and Human Services and U.S. Department of Agriculture. 2015-2020 Dietary Guidelines for Americans. 8th Edition, Washington, DC; 2015.
27. Ronksley Paul E, Brien Susan E, Turner Barbara J, Mukamal Kenneth J, Ghali William A. Association of alcohol consumption with selected cardiovascular disease outcomes: a systematic review and meta-analysis BMJ 2011; 342: d671.
28. Zheng YL, Lian F, Shi Q, et al. Alcohol intake and associated risk of major cardiovascular outcomes in women compared with men: a systematic review and meta-analysis of prospective observational studies. BMC Public Health. 2015;15:773. Published 2015 Aug 12. doi:10.1186/s12889-015-2081-y.
29. Djousse L, Gaziano JM. Alcohol consumption and heart failure: a systematic review. Curr Atheroscler Rep. 2008;10:117–20.
30. Abramson JL, Williams SA, Krumholz HM, Vaccarino V. Moderate alcohol consumption and risk of heart failure among older persons. JAMA. 2001;285:1971–1977.
31. Walsh CR, Larson MG, Evans JC, et al. Alcohol consumption and risk for congestive heart failure in the Framingham Heart Study. Ann Intern Med. 2002;136:181–191.
32. Bryson CL, Mukamal KJ, Mittleman MA, et al. The association of alcohol consumption and incident heart failure: the Cardiovascular Health Study. J Am Coll Cardiol. 2006;48:305–311.
33. GBD 2016 Alcohol Collaborators. Alcohol use and burden for 195 countries and territories, 1990–2016: a systematic analysis for the Global Burden of Disease Study 2016. Lancet. 392, 10152, 1015-1035, 2018; doi:https://doi.org/10.1016/S0140-6736(18)31310-2.
34. Costanzo S, Di Castelnuovo A, Donati MB, Iacoviello L, de Gaetano G. Alcohol consumption and mortality in patients with cardiovascular disease: a meta-analysis. J Am Coll Cardiol. 2010;55:1339–47.
35. Rupp H, Brilla CG, Maisch B. Hypertension and alcohol: Central and peripheral mechanisms. Herz. 1996;21:258–264.
36. Corrao G, Rubbiati L, Bagnardi V, Zambon A, Poikolainen K. Alcohol and coronary heart disease: a meta-analysis. Addiction. 2000 Oct;95(10):1505-23.
37. Gonçalves A, Claggett B, Jhund PS, Rosamond W. Alcohol consumption and risk of heart failure: The Atherosclerosis Risk in Communities study. Eur Heart J. 2015;36:939–945. doi: 10.1093/eurheartj/ehu514.
38. Larsson SC, Wallin A, Wolk A, Markus HS. Differing association of alcohol consumption with different stroke types: a systematic review and meta-analysis. BMC Med. 2016;14(1):178. Published 2016 Nov 24. doi:10.1186/s12916-016-0721-4.
39. George A, Figueredo VM. Alcoholic cardiomyopathy: A review. J Cardiac Fail. 2011;17:844–849. doi: 10.1016/j.cardfail.2011.05.008.
40. Menz V, Grimm W, Hoffmann J, Maisch B. Alcohol and rhythm disturbance: The Holiday Heart syndrome. Herz. 1996;21:227–231.
41. Templeton AH, Carter KLT, Sheron N, Gallagher PJ, Verrill C. Sudden unexpected death in alcohol misuse—an unrecognized public health issue? Int J Environ Res Public Health. 2009;6:3070–3081. doi: 10.3390/ijerph6123070.
42. Mukamal KJ, Longstreth WT Jr, Mittleman MA, Crum RM, Siscovick DS. Alcohol consumption and subclinical findings on magnetic resonance imaging of the brain in older adults: the cardiovascular health study. Stroke. 2001 Sep;32(9):1939-46.

43. Mukamal KJ, Kuller LH, Fitzpatrick AL, Longstreth WT, Jr., Mittleman MA, Siscovick DS. Prospective study of alcohol consumption and risk of dementia in older adults. JAMA. 2003;289:1405–13.
44. Jagust W. Untangling vascular dementia. Lancet.2001;358:2097-2098.
45. Sabia S, Fayosse A, Dumurgier J, et al. Alcohol consumption and risk of dementia: 23 year follow-up of Whitehall II cohort study. BMJ. 2018;362:k2927. Published 2018 Aug 1. doi:10.1136/bmj.k2927.
46. Vliegenthart R, Geleijnse JM, Hofman A, Meijer WT, van Rooij FJ, Grobbee DE, et al. Alcohol consumption and risk of peripheral arterial disease: the Rotterdam study. Am J Epidemiol. 2002;155:332–338.
47. Mukamal KJ, Kennedy M, Cushman M, Kuller LH, Newman AB, Polak J, Criqui MH, Siscovick DS. Alcohol consumption and lower extremity arterial disease among older adults: the cardiovascular health study. Am J Epidemiol 2008;167:34–41.
48. Camargo CA Jr, Stampfer MJ, Glynn RJ, Gaziano JM, Manson JE, Goldhaber SZ, Hennekens CH. Prospective study of moderate alcohol consumption and risk of peripheral arterial disease in US male physicians. Circulation 1997;95:577–80.
49. Djoussé L, Levy D, Murabito JM, Cupples LA, Ellison RC. Alcohol consumption and risk of intermittent claudication in the Framingham Heart Study. Circulation 2000;102:3092–7.
50. Ogilvie RP, Lutsey PL, Heiss G, Folsom AR, Steffen LM. Dietary intake and peripheral arterial disease incidence in middle-aged adults: the Atherosclerosis Risk in Communities (ARIC) Study. Am J Clin Nutr. 2017;105(3):651-659.
51. Wakabayashi I, Sotoda Y. [Alcohol drinking and peripheral arterial disease of lower extremity]. Nihon Arukoru Yakubutsu Igakkai Zasshi. 2014 Feb;49(1):13-27.
52. Mendelson JH, Mello NK. Medical progress, Biologic concomitants of Alcoholism. N Engl J Med. 1979;301:912–21.
53. Van Thiel DH, Lester R. The effect of chronic alcohol abuse on sexual function. th Clin Endocrinol Metab. 1979; 8:499–510.
54. Fahrner EM. Sexual dysfunction in male alcohol addicts, prevalence and treatment. Arch Sex Behav. 1987;16:247–57.
55. Miller NS, Gold MS. The human sexual response and alcohol and drugs. J Subst Abuse Treat. 1988;5:171–7.
56. Vijayasenan ME. Alcohol and sex. N Z Med J. 1981;93:18–20.
57. Ahti TM, Mäkivaara LA, Luukkaala T, Hakama M, Laurikka JO. Lifestyle factors and varicose veins: does cross-sectional design result in underestimate of the risk? Phlebology. 2010 Aug;25(4):201-6. doi: 10.1258/phleb.2009.009031.
58. Pahor M., Guralnik J.M., Havlik R.J., Carbonin P., Salive M.E., Ferrucci L., Corti M.C., Hennekens C.H. Alcohol consumption and risk of deep venous thrombosis and pulmonary embolism in older persons. J. Am. Geriatr. Soc. 1996;44:1030–1037.
59. Pomp E.R., Rosendaal F.R., Doggen C.J. Alcohol consumption is associated with a decreased risk of venous thrombosis. Thromb. Haemost. 2008;99:59–63.
60. Hansen-Krone I.J., Braekkan S.K., Enga K.F., Wilsgaard T., Hansen J.B. Alcohol consumption, types of alcoholic beverages and risk of venous thromboembolism—the Tromso Study. Thromb. Haemost. 2011;106:272–278.
61. Ross A, Friedmann E, Bevans M, Thomas S. National survey of yoga practitioners: mental and physical health benefits. Complement Ther Med. 2013;21(4):313-23.

Alcoholism

1. https://www.samhsa.gov/data/sites/default/files/NSDUH-DetTabs-2015/NSDUH-DetTabs-2015/NSDUH-DetTabs-2015.htm.
2. Tannapfel A, Denk H, Dienes HP, Langner C, Schirmacher P, Trauner M, Flott-Rahmel B. Histopathological diagnosis of non-alcoholic and alcoholic fatty liver disease. Virchows Arch. 2011 May;458(5):511-23. doi: 10.1007/s00428-011-1066-1. Epub 2011 Mar 26.
3. Aday AW, Mitchell MC, Casey LC. Alcoholic hepatitis: current trends in management. Curr Opin Gastroenterol. 2017 May;33(3):142-148. doi: 10.1097/MOG.0000000000000359.

4. Burnett DA, Sorell MF. Alcoholic cirrhosis. Clin Gastroenterol 1981;10:443-55.
5. Lahnborg G, Friman L, Berghem L. Reticuloendothelial function in patients with alcoholic liver cirrhosis. Scand J Gastroenterol 1981;16:481-9.
6. Mendenhall CL. Alcoholic hepatitis. Clin Gastroenterol 1981;10:417-419–11.
7. Mezey E. Alcoholic liver disease: roles of alcohol and malnutrition. Am J Clin Nutr. 1980 Dec;33(12):2709-18.
8. Wienbeck M, Berges W. Oesophageal lesions in the alcoholic.Clin Gastroenterol 1981;10:375-88.
9. Valencia-Parparcen J. Alcoholic gastritis. Clin Gastroenterol.1981;10:389-99.
10. Kanagasundaram N, Leevy CM. Ethanol immune reactions and the digestive system. Clin Gastroenterol 1981;10:295- 306.
11. Sarles H, Laugier R. Alcoholic pancreatitis. Clin Gastroenterol. 1981;10:401.
12. Morgan TR, Mandayam S, Jamal MM. Alcohol and hepatocellular carcinoma. Gastroenterology. 2004;127(5 Suppl 1):S87–S96.
13. Seitz HK, Becker P. Alcohol metabolism and cancer risk. Alcohol Res Health. 2007;30:38–41. 4–7.
14. Chomet B, Gach HM. Lobar pneumonia and alcoholism: an analysis of thirty-seven cases. Am J Med Sci 1967;253:300- 4.
15. Green GM, Kass EH. Factors influencing the clearance of bacteria by the lung. J Clin Invest 1964;43:769-76.
16. Victor M, Adams RD. The effect of alcohol on the nervous system. Res Publ Assoc Res Nerv Ment Dis 1953;32:526-73.
17. Mellion M, Gilchrist JM, de la Monte S. Alcohol-related peripheral neuropathy: nutritional, toxic, or both?. Muscle Nerve. 2011;43(3):309-16.
18. Rogers DG, Des Prfz RM, Heller P, Brawald E, Greenberger NJ. Bondy PRK, et al. Year book of medicine 1976. Chicago:Year Book Medical Publishers; 1976.
19. Hingson, R.W.; Zha, W.; and Weitzman, E.R. Magnitude of and trends in alcohol-related mortality and morbidity among U.S. college students ages 18–24, 1998–2005. Journal of Studies on Alcohol and Drugs (Suppl. 16):12–20, 2009.
20. Rehm J, Baliunas D, Borges GL, Graham K, Irving H, Kehoe T, et al. The relation between different dimensions of alcohol consumption and burden of disease: an overview. Addiction. 2010;105(5):817-43.
21. Mäkelä P. Alcohol-related mortality as a function of socio-economic status. Addiction. 1999 Jun;94(6):867-86.
22. Mäkelä P. Ramstedt M (2002) Alcohol-related mortality in 15 European countries in the postwar period In: Norstrom T, editor. Alcohol in postwar Europe: consumption, drinking patterns, consequences and policy responses in 15 European countries. Stockholm: National Institute of Public Health.
23. Whitman IR, Agarwal V, Nah G, et al. Alcohol Abuse and Cardiac Disease. J Am Coll Cardiol. 2017;69(1):13-24.
24. Costanzo S, Di Castelnuovo A, Donati MB, Iacoviello L, de Gaetano G. Alcohol consumption and mortality in patients with cardiovascular disease: a meta-analysis. J Am Coll Cardiol. 2010;55:1339–47.
25. Larsson SC, Drca N, Wolk A. Alcohol consumption and risk of atrial fibrillation: a prospective study and dose-response meta-analysis. J Am Coll Cardiol. 2014;64:281–9.
26. Regan TJ. Alcohol and the cardiovascular system. JAMA. 1990;264:377–81.
27. Urbano-Marquez A, Estruch R, Navarro-Lopez F, Grau JM, Mont L, Rubin E. The effects of alcoholism on skeletal and cardiac muscle. N Engl J Med. 1989;320:409–15.
28. Rehm J, Hasan OSM, Imtiaz S, Neufeld M. Quantifying the contribution of alcohol to cardiomyopathy: A systematic review. Alcohol. 2017 Jun;61:9-15. doi: 10.1016/j alcohol.2017.01.011. Epub 2017 Apr 20.
29. Mostofsky E, Chahal HS, Mukamal KJ, et al. Alcohol and Immediate Risk of Cardiovascular Events: A Systematic Review and Dose-Response Meta-Analysis. Circulation. 2016;133:979–87.

30. Klatsky AL, Armstrong MA, Friedman GD. Alcohol and mortality. Annals of internal medicine. 1992;117:646–54.
31. Caicoya M, Rodriguez T, Corrales C, Cuello R, Lasheras C. Alcohol and stroke. A community case control study in Astrurias, Spain. J Clin Epidemiol. 1999;52:677–684. doi: 10.1016/S0895-4356(98)00074-2.
32. Donahue RP, Abbott RD, Reed DM, Yano K. Alcohol and hemorrhagic stroke: the Honolulu Heart Program. JAMA. 1986;255:2311–2314. doi: 10.1001/jama.255.17.2311.
33. Thrift A, Donnan G, McNeil J. Heavy drinking, but not moderate or intermediate drinking, increases the risk of intracerebral hemorrhage. Epidemiol. 1999;10:307–312. doi: 10.1097/00001648-199905000-00020.
34. Patra J, Taylor B, Irving H, Roerecke M, Baliunas D, Mohapatra S, et al. Alcohol consumption and the risk of morbidity and mortality for different stroke types--a systematic review and meta-analysis. BMC Public Health. 2010;10:258.
35. Hallgren M, Romberg K, Bakshi AS, Andréasson S. Yoga as an adjunct treatment for alcohol dependence: a pilot study. Complement Ther Med. 2014 Jun;22(3):441-5. doi: 10.1016/j.ctim.2014.03.003. Epub 2014 Mar 15.
36. Shafil M. Lavely R, Jaffe R. Meditation and the prevention of alcohol abuse. Am J Psychiatry. 1975 Sep;132(9):942-5.
37. Reddy S, Dick AM, Gerber MR, Mitchell K. The Effect of a Yoga Intervention on Alcohol and Drug Abuse Risk in Veteran and Civilian Women with Posttraumatic Stress Disorder. Journal of Alternative and Complementary Medicine. 2014;20(10):750-756. doi:10.1089/acm.2014.0014.

Anti-oxidants

1. Griendling KK, Touyz RM, Zweier JL, et al. Measurement of Reactive Oxygen Species, Reactive Nitrogen Species, and Redox-Dependent Signaling in the Cardiovascular System: A Scientific Statement From the American Heart Association. Circ Res. 2016;119(5):e39-75.
2. R Kohen, A Nyska. Oxidation of biological systems: oxidative stress phenomena, antioxidants, redox reactions, and methods for their quantification. Toxicol Pathol. 2002;30:620–50.
3. Gori T, Münzel T. Oxidative stress and endothelial dysfunction: therapeutic implications. Ann Med. 2011;43:259–72. ; Münzel T, Gori T, Bruno RM, Taddei S. Is oxidative stress a therapeutic target in cardiovascular disease? Eur Heart J. 2010;31:2741–8.
4. A Ceriello. Possible role of oxidative stress in the pathogenesis of hypertension. Diabetes Care. 2008;2:S181–84.
5. PJ Mateos-Caceres, JJ Zamorano-Leon, P Rodriquez-Sierra, C Macaya, AJ Lopez- Farre. New and old mechanism associated with hypertension in the elderly. Int J Hypertens. 2012;2012(150107).
6. AM Briones, RM Touyz. Oxidative stress and hypertension: current concepts. Curr Hypertens Rep. 2010;12:135–42. ;E Grossman. Does increased oxidative stress cause hypertension? Diabetes Care. 2008;31:S185–89.
7. Touyz RM, Briones AM. Reactive oxygen species and vascular biology: implications in human hypertension. Hypertens Res. 2011 Jan;34(1):5-14. doi: 10.1038/hr.2010.201. Epub 2010 Oct 28.
8. RC Jin, J Loscalzo. Vascular nitric oxide: Formation and function. J Blood Med. 2010;2010:147–62.].; E Schulz, T Gori, T Munzel. Oxidative stress and endothelial dysfunction in hypertension. Hypertens Res. 2011;34:665–73.
9. BR Silva, L Pernomian, LM Bendhack. Contribution of oxidative stress to endothelial dysfunction in hypertension. Front Physiol. 2012;3(441.].
10. Sinha N, Dabla PK. Oxidative stress and antioxidants in hypertension-a current review. Curr Hypertens Rev. 2015;11(2):132-42.
11. Camici GG, Schiavoni M, Francia P, et al. Genetic deletion of p66Shc adaptor protein prevents hyperglycemia-induced endothelial dysfunction and oxidative stress. Proc Natl Acad Sci U S A. 2007;104:5217–22.
12. Warolin J., Coenen K.R., Kantor J.L., Whitaker L.E., Wang L., Acra S.A., Roberts L.J.,

2nd, Buchowski M.S. The relationship of oxidative stress, adiposity and metabolic risk factors in healthy Black and White American youth. Pediatr. Obes. 2013 doi: 10.1111/j.2047-6310.2012.00135.
13. Savini I, Catani MV, Evangelista D, Gasperi V, Avigliano L. Obesity-associated oxidative stress: strategies finalized to improve redox state. Int J Mol Sci. 2013;14(5):10497-538. Published 2013 May 21. doi:10.3390/ijms140510497.
14. Csiszar A, Podlutsky A, Wolin MS, Losonczy G, Pacher P, Ungvari Z. Oxidative stress and accelerated vascular aging: implications for cigarette smoking. Front Biosci (Landmark Ed) 2009;14:3128–44.
15. Niemann B, Rohrbach S, Miller MR, Newby DE, Fuster V, Kovacic JC. Oxidative Stress and Cardiovascular Risk: Obesity, Diabetes, Smoking, and Pollution: Part 3 of a 3-Part Series. J Am Coll Cardiol. 2017;70(2):230-251.
16. Pritchard KA, Jr, Groszek L, Smalley DM, et al. Native low-density lipoprotein increases endothelial cell nitric oxide synthase generation of superoxide anion. Circ Res. 1995;77:510–8.
17. Camici GG, Savarese G, Akhmedov A, Lüscher TF. Molecular mechanism of endothelial and vascular aging: implications for cardiovascular disease. Eur Heart J. 2015;36:3392–403.
18. Evrard SM, Lecce L, Michelis KC, et al. Endothelial to mesenchymal transition is common in atherosclerotic lesions and is associated with plaque instability. Nat Commun. 2016;7:11853.
19. Mitra S, Goyal T, Mehta JL. Oxidized LDL, LOX-1 and atherosclerosis. Cardiovasc Drugs Ther. 2011 Oct;25(5):419-29. doi: 10.1007/s10557-011-6341-5.
20. Usman A, Ribatti D, Sadat U, Gillard JH. From Lipid Retention to Immune-Mediate Inflammation and Associated Angiogenesis in the Pathogenesis of Atherosclerosis. J Atheroscler Thromb. 2015 Aug 26;22(8):739-49. doi: 10.5551/jat.30460. Epub 2015 Jul 8.
21. Ross R. Atherosclerosis, an inflammatory disease. N Eng J. 1999; 340:115-26.
22. Guzik TJ, Sadowski J, Guzik B, et al. Coronary artery superoxide production and nox isoform expression in human coronary artery disease. Arterioscler Thromb Vasc Biol. 2006;26:333–9.
23. Münzel T, Camici GG, Maack C, Bonetti NR, Fuster V, Kovacic JC. Impact of Oxidative Stress on the Heart and Vasculature: Part 2 of a 3-Part Series. J Am Coll Cardiol. 2017;70(2):212-229.
24. Maack C, Kartes T, Kilter H, et al. Oxygen free radical release in human failing myocardium is associated with increased activity of rac1-GTPase and represents a target for statin treatment. Circulation. 2003;108:1567–74.
25. Mollnau H, Oelze M, August M, et al. Mechanisms of increased vascular superoxide production in an experimental model of idiopathic dilated cardiomyopathy. Arterioscler Thromb Vasc Biol. 2005;25:2554–9.
26. Belch JJ, Bridges AB, Scott N, Chopra M. Oxygen free radicals and congestive heart failure. Br Heart J. 1991;65:245–8.; Faria A, Persaud SJ. Cardiac oxidative stress in diabetes: Mechanisms and therapeutic potential. Pharmacol Ther. 2017 Apr; 172:50-62. doi: 10.1016/j.pharmthera.2016.11.013. Epub 2016 Dec 1.
27. Rodrigo R, Fernández-Gajardo R, Gutiérrez R, Matamala JM, Carrasco R, Miranda-Merchak A, Feuerhake W. Oxidative stress and pathophysiology of ischemic stroke: novel therapeutic opportunities. CNS Neurol Disord Drug Targets. 2013 Aug;12(5):698-714.
28. Ismaeel A, Brumberg RS, Kirk JS, et al. Oxidative Stress and Arterial Dysfunction in Peripheral Artery Disease. Antioxidants (Basel). 2018;7(10):145. Published 2018 Oct 19. doi:10.3390/antiox7100145.
29. Musicki B, Bella AJ, Bivalacqua TJ, et al. Basic Science Evidence for the Link Between Erectile Dysfunction and Cardiometabolic Dysfunction. J Sex Med. 2015;12(12):2233-55.
30. Pal R, Gupta N. Yogic practices on oxidative stress and of antioxidant level: a systematic review of randomized controlled trials. J Complement Integr Med. 2017 Oct 25. pii: /j/jcim.ahead-of-print/jcim-2017-0079/jcim-2017-0079.xml. doi: 10.1515/jcim-2017-0079.

Atherosclerosis

1. Falk E. Pathogenesis of Atherosclerosis. J. Am. Coll. Cardiol. 2006;47:C7–C12. doi: 10.1016/j.jacc.2005.09.068.
2. Mallika V, Goswami B, Rajappa M. Atherosclerosis pathophysiology and the role of novel risk factors: a clinicobiochemical perspective. Angiology 2007;58:513-22.
3. Marulanda-Londoño E, Chaturvedi S. Stroke due to large vessel atherosclerosis: Five new things. Neurol Clin Pract. 2016;6(3):252-258.
4. Newman B, Siscovick S, Manolio A, et al. Ankle-arm index as a marker of atherosclerosis in the Cardiovascular Health Study. Cardiovascular Heart Study (CHS) Collaborative Research Group. Circulation 1993;88:837–45.
5. Bonetti PO, Lerman LO, Lerman A. Endothelial dysfunction: A marker of atherosclerotic risk. Arterioscler Thromb Vasc Biol. 2003;23:168–175.
6. Ibrahim A, Ali M, Kiernan TJ, Stack AG. Erectile Dysfunction and Ischaemic Heart Disease. Eur Cardiol. 2018;13(2):98-103.
7. Viola J, Soehnlein O. Atherosclerosis - A matter of unresolved inflammation. Semin Immunol. 2015 May;27(3):184-93. doi: 10.1016/j.smim.2015.03.013. Epub 2015 Apr 10.
8. Tuttolomondo A., Di Raimondo D., Pecoraro R., et al. Atherosclerosis as an inflammatory disease. Curr. Pharm. Des. 2012;18:4266–4288.
9. Hansson GK. Inflammation, atherosclerosis, and coronary artery disease. N Engl J Med. 2005;352:1685–95.
10. Catapano AL, Pirillo A, Norata GD. Vascular inflammation and low-density lipoproteins: is cholesterol the link? A lesson from the clinical trials. Br J Pharmacol. 2017 Nov;174(22):3973-3985. doi: 10.1111/bph.13805. Epub 2017 May 5.
11. A.J. Lusis. Atherosclerosis. Nature, 407 (2000), pp. 233-241
12. Wiśniewska A., Olszanecki R., Totoń-Żurańska J., Kuś K., Stachowicz A., Suski M., Gębska A., Gajda M., Jawień J., Korbut R. Anti-Atherosclerotic Action of Agmatine in ApoE-Knockout Mice. Int. J. Mol. Sci. 2017;18:1706 doi: 10.3390/ijms18081706.
13. Bloomer R.J. Decreased Blood Antioxidant Capacity and Increased Lipid Peroxidation in Young Cigarette Smokers Compared to Nonsmokers: Impact of Dietary Intake. Nutr. J. 2007;6:39. doi: 10.1186/1475-2891-6-39.
14. Frostegård J., Ruihua W.U., Lemne C., Thulin T., Witztum J.L., de Faire U. Circulating Oxidized Low-Density Lipoprotein Is Increased in Hypertension. Clin. Sci. 2003;105:615–620. doi: 10.1042/CS20030152
15. Badrnya S., Assinger A., Volf I. Native High Density Lipoproteins (HDL) Interfere with Platelet Activation Induced by Oxidized Low Density Lipoproteins (OxLDL) Int. J. Mol. Sci. 2013;14:10107 doi: 10.3390/ijms140510107.
16. Moore KJ, Tabas I. Macrophages in the pathogenesis of atherosclerosis. Cell. 2011;145(3):341-55.
17. K. Sakakura, M. Nakano, F. Otsuka, E. Ladich, F.D. Kolodgie, R. Virmani. Pathophysiology of atherosclerosis plaque progression. Heart Lung Circ., 22 (2013), pp. 399-411.
18. Kunjathoor VV, Febbraio M, Podrez EA, Moore KJ, Andersson L, Koehn S, Rhee JS, Silverstein R, Hoff HF, Freeman MW. Scavenger receptors class A-I/II and CD36 are the principal receptors responsible for the uptake of modified low density lipoprotein leading to lipid loading in macrophages. J Biol Chem. 2002;277:49982–49988.
19. Usman A, Ribatti D, Sadat U, Gillard JH. From Lipid Retention to Immune-Mediate Inflammation and Associated Angiogenesis in the Pathogenesis of Atherosclerosis. J Atheroscler Thromb. 2015 Aug 26;22(8):739-49. doi: 10.5551/jat.30460. Epub 2015 Jul 8.
20. Rudijanto A. The role of vascular smooth muscle cells on the pathogenesis of atherosclerosis. Acta Med Indones. 2007 Apr-Jun;39(2):86-93.
21. Ross R. Atherosclerosis, an inflammatory disease. N Eng J. 1999; 340:115-26.
22. Kolodgie FD, Burke AP, Farb A, Gold HK, Yuan J, Narula J, Finn AV, Virmani R. The thin-cap fibroatheroma: a type of vulnerable plaque: the major precursor lesion to acute coronary syndromes. Curr Opin Cardiol. 2001;16:285–92.

23. Geng Y-J, Wu Q, Muszynski M, Hansson G, Libby P. Apoptosis of vascular smooth muscle cells induced by in vitro stimulation with interferon-gamma, tumor necrosis factor-alpha, and interleukin-1-beta. Arteriosclerosis, Thrombosis, and Vascular Biology. 1996;16:19–27.
24. Geng Y-J, Libby P. Evidence for apoptosis in advanced human atheroma. Co-localization with interleukin-1 β-converting enzyme. Am J Pathol. 1995;147:251–266.
25. Libby P. Inflammation in atherosclerosis. Arterioscler Thromb Vasc Biol. 2012;32(9):2045-51.
26. Scalone G, Niccoli G, Refaat H, Vergallo R, Porto I, Leone AM, Burzotta F, D'Amario D, Liuzzo G, Fracassi F, Trani C, Crea F. Not all plaque ruptures are born equal: an optical coherence tomography study. Eur Heart J Cardiovasc Imaging. 2017 Nov 1;18(11):1271-1277. doi: 10.1093/ehjci/jew208.
27. Sakakura K, Nakano M, Otsuka F, Ladich E, Kolodgie FD, Virmani R. Pathophysiology of atherosclerosis plaque progression. Heart Lung Circ. 2013 Jun;22(6):399-411. doi: 10.1016/j.hlc.2013.03.001. Epub 2013 Mar 29.
28. Otsuka F, Yasuda S, Noguchi T, Ishibashi-Ueda H. Pathology of coronary atherosclerosis and thrombosis. Cardiovasc Diagn Ther. 2016 Aug;6(4):396-408. doi: 10.21037/cdt.2016.06.01.
29. Mackman N. Triggers, targets and treatments for thrombosis. Nature. 2008;451(7181):914-8.
30. J.A. Berliner, M. Navab, A.M. Fogelman, J.S. Frank, L.L. Demer, P.A. Edwards, A.D. Watson, A.J. Lusis. Atherosclerosis: basic mechanisms: oxidation, inflammation, and genetics. Circulation, 91 (1995), pp. 2488-2496.
31. Tegos TJ, Kalodiki E, Sabetai MM, et al. The genesis of atherosclerosis and risk factors: A review. Angiology. 2001;52:89–98.
32. Manchanda SC, Narang R, Reddy KS, Sachdeva U, Prabhakaran D, Dharmanand S, Rajani M, Bijlani R. Retardation of coronary atherosclerosis with yoga lifestyle intervention. J Assoc Physicians India. 2000. Jul; 48(7): 687-94.
33. Yogendra J, Yogendra HJ, Ambardekar S, Lele RD, Shetty S, Dave M, Husein N. Beneficial effects of yoga lifestyle on reversibility of ischaemic heart disease: caring heart project of International Board of Yoga. J Assoc Physicians India. 2004 Apr;52:283-9.
34. Manchanda SC, Mehrotra UC, Makhija A, Mohanty A, Dhawan S, et al. (2013) Reversal of Early Atherosclerosis in Metabolic Syndrome by Yoga – A Randomized Controlled Trial. J Yoga Phys Ther 3:132. doi: 10.4172/2157-7595.1000132.

Autonomic Nervous System

1. Goyal RK, Hirano I. The enteric nervous system. N Engl J Med (1996) 334(17):1106–15.10.1056/ NEJM199604253341707.
2. https://opentextbc.ca/anatomyandphysiology/chapter/15-1-divisions-of-the-autonomic-nervous-system/.
3. Wehrwein EA, Orer HS, Barman SM. Overview of the Anatomy, Physiology, and Pharmacology of the Autonomic Nervous System. Compr Physiol. 2016 Jun 13;6(3):1239-78. doi: 10.1002/cphy.c150037.
4. McLeod JG. Autonomic dysfunction in peripheral nerve disorders. Curr Opin Neurol Neurosurg. 1992 Aug;5(4):476-81.
5. Hu Y, Converse C, Lyons MC, Hsu WH. Neural control of sweat secretion: a review. Br J Dermatol. 2018 Jun;178(6):1246-1256. doi: 10.1111/bjd.15808. Epub 2018 Apr 25.
6. Biaggioni I. The Pharmacology of Autonomic Failure: From Hypotension to Hypertension. Pharmacol Rev. 2017;69(1):53-62.
7. Jardine DL, Wieling W, Brignole M, Lenders JWM, Sutton R, Stewart J. The pathophysiology of the vasovagal response. Heart Rhythm. 2018 Jun;15(6):921-929. doi: 10.1016/j.hrthm.2017.12.013. Epub 2017 Dec 12.
8. Affoo RH, Foley N, Rosenbek J, Shoemaker JK, Martin RE. Swallowing dysfunction and autonomic nervous system dysfunction in Alzheimer's disease: a scoping review of the evidence. J Am Geriatr Soc. 2013 Dec;61(12):2203-13.
9. Goldstein DS. Dysautonomia in Parkinson disease. Compr Physiol. 2014;4(2):805-26.

10. Bujnakova I, Ondrejka I, Mestanik M, Visnovcova Z, Mestanikova A, Hrtanek I, Fleskova D, Calkovska A, Tonhajzerova I. Autism spectrum disorder is associated with autonomic underarousal. Physiol Res. 2016 Dec 22;65 (Supplementum 5):S673-S682.
11. Koopman FA, Tang MW, Vermeij J, et al. Autonomic Dysfunction Precedes Development of Rheumatoid Arthritis: A Prospective Cohort Study. EBioMedicine. 2016;6:231-237.
12. Aydemir M., Yazisiz V., Basarici I. Cardiac autonomic profile in rheumatoid arthritis and systemic lupus erythematosus. Lupus. 2010;19(3):255–261.
13. Sternberg Z. Promoting sympathovagal balance in multiple sclerosis; pharmacological, non-pharmacological, and surgical strategies. Autoimmun Rev. 2016 Feb;15(2):113-23. doi: 10.1016/j.autrev.2015.04.012. Epub 2015 May 3.
14. Sharma P., Makharia G.K., Ahuja V., Dwivedi S.N., Deepak K.K. Autonomic dysfunctions in patients with inflammatory bowel disease in clinical remission. Dig. Dis. Sci. 2009;54(4):853–861.
15. Schlaich M, Straznicky N, Lambert E, Lambert G. Metabolic syndrome: a sympathetic disease? Lancet Diabetes Endocrinol (2015) 3(2):148–58.10.1016/S2213-8587(14)70033-6.
16. Vinik A. I., Maser R. E., Mitchell B. D., Freeman R. (2003). Diabetic autonomic neuropathy. Diabetes Care 26 1553–1579. 10.2337/diacare.26.5.1553.
17. Lambert E, Straznicky N, Sari C, Eikelis N, Hering D, Head G, et al. Dyslipidemia is associated with sympathetic nervous activation and impaired endothelial function in young females. Am J Hypertens (2013) 26:250–6.10.1093/ajh/hps016.
18. Tentolouris N, Liatis S, Katsilambros N. Sympathetic system activity in obesity and metabolic syndrome. Ann N Y Acad Sci. 2006 Nov;1083:129-52.
19. Miu AC, Heilman RM, Miclea M. Reduced heart rate variability and vagal tone in anxiety: trait versus state, and the effects of autogenic training. Auton Neurosci. 2009 Jan 28;145(1-2):99-103. doi: 10.1016/j.autneu.2008.11.010. Epub 2008 Dec 6.
20. Won E, Kim YK. Stress, the Autonomic Nervous System, and the Immune-kynurenine Pathway in the Etiology of Depression. Curr Neuropharmacol. 2016;14(7):665-73.
21. Schulz S, Bolz M, Bär KJ, Voss A. Central- and autonomic nervous system coupling in schizophrenia. Philos Trans A Math Phys Eng Sci. 2016;374(2067):20150178.
22. Lakoski SG, Jones LW, Krone RJ, Stein PK, Scott JM. Autonomic dysfunction in early breast cancer: Incidence, clinical importance, and underlying mechanisms. Am Heart J. 2015;170(2):231-41.
23. Tsuji H, Venditti FJ, Jr, Manders ES, Evans JC, Larson MG, Feldman CL. Levy D. Reduced heart rate variability and mortality risk in an elderly cohort. The Framingham Heart Study. Circulation. 1994;90:878–883.
24. Dekker JM, Schouten EG, Klootwijk P, Pool J, Swenne CA. Kromhout D. Heart rate variability from short electrocardiographic recordings predicts mortality from all causes in middle-aged and elderly men. The Zutphen Study. Am J Epidemiol. 1997;145:899–908.
25. Lymperopoulos A. Physiology and pharmacology of the cardiovascular adrenergic system. Front Physiol. 2013;4:240. Published 2013 Sep 4. doi:10.3389/fphys.2013.00240.
26. McCorry LK. Physiology of the autonomic nervous system. Am J Pharm Educ. 2007;71(4):78.
27. Glick D. Autonomic nervous system. In: Miller RD, Pardo MC Jr, editors. Basics of anesthesia. 6. Philadelphia: Elsevier Saunders; 2011.
28. Maron BA, Leopold JA. Emerging concepts in the molecular basis of pulmonary arterial hypertension. Circulation. 2015;131:2079–2091. doi: 10.1161/CIRCULATIONAHA.114.006980.
29. Levy MN. Autonomic interactions in cardiac control. Ann N Y Acad Sci. 1990;601:209–221.
30. Caetano J, Delgado Alves J. Heart rate and cardiovascular protection. European journal of internal medicine. 2015;26:217–222.
31. Palatini P, Julius S. The role of cardiac autonomic function in hypertension and cardiovascular disease. Curr Hypertens Rep (2009) 11(3):199–205.10.1007/s11906-009-0035-4.
32. Grassi G, Ram VS. Evidence for a critical role of the sympathetic nervous system in hypertension. J Am Soc Hypertens. 2016;10:457–66.

33. Wellen KE, Hotamisligil GS. Inflammation, stress, and diabetes. J Clin Invest (2005) 115(5):1111–9.10.1172/JCI200525102.
34. Schlaich M, Straznicky N, Lambert E, Lambert G. Metabolic syndrome: a sympathetic disease? Lancet Diabetes Endocrinol (2015) 3(2):148–58.10.1016/S2213-8587(14)70033-6.
35. Carnethon MR, Golden SH, Folsom AR, Haskell W, Liao D. Prospective investigation of autonomic nervous system function and the development of type 2 diabetes: the atherosclerosis risk in communities study, 1987–1998. Circulation (2003) 107(17):2190–5.10.1161/01.CIR.0000066324.74807.95.
36. Lambert E, Straznicky N, Sari C, Eikelis N, Hering D, Head G, et al. Dyslipidemia is associated with sympathetic nervous activation and impaired endothelial function in young females. Am J Hypertens (2013) 26:250–6.10.1093/ajh/hps016.
37. Kimura T, Matsumoto T, Akiyoshi M, Owa Y, Miyasaka N, Aso T, et al. Body fat and blood lipids in postmenopausal women are related to resting autonomic nervous system activity. Eur J Appl Physiol (2006) 97(5):542–7.10.1007/s00421-006-0207-8.
38. Saini S, Saxena Y, Gupta R. Arterial compliance and autonomic functions in adult male smokers. J Clin Diagn Res (2016) 10(5):CC12–6.10.7860/JCDR/2016/19547.7831.
39. Harvey RE, Barnes JN, Hart ECJ, Nicholson WT, Joyner MJ, Casey DP. Influence of sympathetic nerve activity on aortic hemodynamics and pulse wave velocity in women. Am J Physiol Hear Circ Physiol (2017) 312(2):H340–6.10.1152/ajpheart.00447.2016.
40. Dishman RK, Nakamura Y, Garcia ME, Thompson RW, Dunn AL, Blair SN. Heart rate variability, trait anxiety, and percieved stress among physically fit men and women. Int J Psychophysiol (2000) 37:121–33.10.1016/S0167-8760(00)00085-4.
41. Miu AC, Heilman RM, Miclea M. Reduced heart rate variability and vagal tone in anxiety: trait versus state, and the effects of autogenic training. Auton Neurosci. 2009 Jan 28;145(1-2):99-103. doi: 10.1016/j.autneu.2008.11.010. Epub 2008 Dec 6.
42. Webster J. I., Tonelli L., Sternberg E. M. (2002). Neuroendocrine regulation of immunity. Annu. Rev. Immunol. 20, 125–163 10.1146/annurev.immunol.20.082401.104914.
43. Bernstein IM, Damron D, Schonberg AL, Shapiro R. The relationship of plasma volume, sympathetic tone, and proinflammatory cytokines in young healthy nonpregnant women. Reprod Sci. 2009;16:980–985. doi: 10.1177/1933719109338876.
44. Shebuski RJ, Kilgore KS. Role of inflammatory mediators in thrombogenesis. J Pharmacol Exp Ther (2002) 300:729–35.10.1124/jpet.300.3.729.
45. Ellestad MH. Chronotropic incompetence. The implications of heart rate response to exercise (compensatory parasympathetic hyperactivity?) Circulation. 1996;93(8):1485–7. https://doi.org/10.1161/01.CIR.93.8.1485.
46. Curtis BM, O'Keefe JH. Autonomic tone as a cardiovascular risk factor: the dangers of chronic fight or flight. Mayo Clin Proc (2002) 77(1):45–54.10.4065/77.1.45.
47. Huikuri HV, Stein PK. Heart rate variability in risk stratification of cardiac patients. Prog Cardiovasc Dis (2013) 56(2):153–9.10.1016/j.pcad.2013.07.003.
48. Ross R. Inflammation or atherogenesis. N Engl J Med (1999) 340(2):115–26.10.1056/NEJM199901143400207.
49. Tracey KJ. The inflammatory reflex. Nature (2002) 420(6917):853–9.10.1038/nature01321.
50. Chistiakov DA, Ashwell KW, Orekhov AN, Bobryshev YV. Innervation of the arterial wall and its modification in atherosclerosis. Auton Neurosci. 2015 Dec;193:7-11. doi: 10.1016/j.autneu.2015.06.005. Epub 2015 Jun 19.
51. Huikuri HV, Jokinen V, Syva M, Nieminen MS, Airaksinen KEJ, Koistinen JM, et al. Heart rate variability and progression of coronary atherosclerosis. Arterioscler Thromb Vasc Biol (1999) 19:1979–85.10.1161/01.ATV.19.8.1979.
52. Manfrini O, Pizzi C, Viecca M, Bugiardini R. Abnormalities of cardiac autonomic nervous activity correlate with expansive coronary artery remodeling. Atherosclerosis (2008) 197(1):183–9.10.1016/j.atherosclerosis.2007.03.013.
53. Wennerblom B, Lurje L, Tygesen H, Vahisalo R, Hjalmarson A. Patients with uncomplicated coronary artery disease have reduced heart rate variability mainly affecting vagal tone. Heart. 2000;83:290–294. doi: 10.1136/heart.83.3.290.

54. Hayano J, Sakakibara Y, Yamada A, Ohte N, Fujinami T, Yokohama K, Watanabe Y, Takata K. Decreased magnitude of heart rate spectral components in coronary artery disease. Its Relation to Angiographic Severity. Circulation. 1990;81:1217–1224. doi: 10.1161/01.CIR.81.4.1217.
55. van Boven AJ, Jukema JW, Haaksma J, Zwinderman AH, Crijns HJ. Lie KI. Depressed heart rate variability is associated with events in patients with stable coronary artery disease and preserved left ventricular function. REGRESS Study Group. Am Heart J. 1998;135:571–576.
56. Rich MW, Saini JS, Kleiger RE, Carney RM, teVelde A, Freeland KE. Correlation of heart rate variability with clinical and angiographic variables and late mortality after coronary angiography. Am J Cardiol. 1988;62:714–717. doi: 10.1016/0002-9149(88)91208-8.
57. Lymperopoulos A, Rengo G, Koch WJ. Adrenergic nervous system in heart failure: pathophysiology and therapy. Circ Res. 2013;113(6):739-53.
58. Bilchick KC, Fetics B, Djoukeng R, Fisher SG, Fletcher RD, Singh SN, Nevo E, Berger RD. Prognostic value of heart rate variability in chronic congestive heart failure (Veterans Affairs' Survival Trial of Antiarrhythmic Therapy in Congestive Heart Failure) Am J Cardiol. 2002;90:24–28.
59. Goldsmith R. L., Bigger J. T., Bloomfield D. M., Krum H., Steinman R. C., Sackner-Bernstein J., et al. (1997). Long-term carvedilol therapy increases parasympathetic nervous system activity in chronic heart failure. Am. J. Cardiol. 80, 1101–1104 10.1016/S0002-9149(97)00616-4.
60. Shen MJ, Choi E-K, Tan AY, Lin S-F, Fishbein MC, Chen LS, et al. Neural mechanisms of atrial arrhythmias. Nat Rev Cardiol (2012) 9(1):30–9.10.1038/nrcardio.2011.139.
61. Kleiger RE, Miller JP, Bigger JT, Moss AJ. Decreased heart rate variability and its association with increased mortality after acute myocardial infarction. Am J Cardiol. 1987;59:256–262.
62. Guan L, Collet JP, Mazowita G, Claydon VE. Autonomic Nervous System and Stress to Predict Secondary Ischemic Events after Transient Ischemic Attack or Minor Stroke: Possible Implications of Heart Rate Variability. Front Neurol. 2018;9:90. Published 2018 Mar 5. doi:10.3389/fneur.2018.00090.
63. Tokgozoglu SL, Batur MK, Top uoglu MA, Saribas O, Kes S, Oto A. Effects of stroke localization on cardiac autonomic balance and sudden death. Stroke. 1999;30(7):1307–11.
64. Sander D, Winbeck K, Klingelhofer J, Etgen T, Conrad B. Prognostic relevance of pathological sympathetic activation after acute thromboembolic stroke. Neurology. 2001;57(5):833–8.
65. Kleiger RE, Miller JP, Bigger JT, Jr, Moss AJ. Decreased heart rate variability and its association with increased mortality after acute myocardial infarction. Am J Cardiol. 1987;59:256–262.
66. La Rovere M.T., Bigger J.T., Jr., Marcus F.I., Mortara A., Schwartz P.J. Baroreflex sensitivity and heart-rate variability in prediction of total cardiac mortality after myocardial infarction. ATRAMI (Autonomic Tone and Reflexes After Myocardial Infarction) Investigators. Lancet. 1998;351:478–484. doi: 10.1016/S0140-6736(97)11144-8.
67. Curtis BM. Autonomic tone as a cardiovascular risk factor: the dangers of chronic fight or flight. Mayo Clin Proc. 2002;77:45–54.
68. Gehi A, Mangano D, Pipkin S, Browner WS, Whooley MA. Depression and heart rate variability in patients with stable coronary heart disease: findings from the Heart and Soul Study. Arch Gen Psychiatry. 2005;62:661–666.
69. Mathias CJ. Autonomic nervous system disorders and erectile dysfunction. Int J STD AIDS. 1996;7 Suppl 3:5-8.
70. Norman EC, Mary AC. Erectile Dysfunction and Diabetes Mellitus: Mechanistic Considerations from Studies in Experimental Models. Current Diabetes Reviews. 2007;3:149.
71. Fedele D, Coscelli C, Santeusanio F, et al. Erectile dysfunction in diabetic subjects in Italy. Gruppo Italiano Studio Deficit Erettile nei Diabetici. Diabetes Care. 1998;21:1973.

72. Muralikrishnan K, Balakrishnan B, Balasubramanian K, Visnegarawla F. Measurement of the effect of Isha Yoga on cardiac autonomic nervous system using short-term heart rate variability. J Ayurveda Integr Med. 2012;3:91–6.
73. Vinay AV, Venkatesh D, Ambarish V. Impact of short-term practice of yoga on heart rate variability. Int J Yoga. 2016;9(1):62-6.; Khattab K. Khattab AA. Ortak J, et al. Iyengar yoga increases cardiac parasympathetic nervous modulation among healthy yoga practitioners. Evid Based Complement Alternat Med. 2007;4:511–517.
74. Jerath R, Edry JW, Barnes VA, Jerath V. Physiology of long pranayamic breathing: neural respiratory elements may provide a mechanism that explains how slow deep breathing shifts the autonomic nervous system. Med Hypotheses. 2006;67(3):566-71. Epub 2006 Apr 18.
75. Nivethitha L, Mooventhan A, Manjunath NK. Effects of Various Prāṇāyāma on Cardiovascular and Autonomic Variables. Anc Sci Life. 2016;36(2):72-77.
76. Pal K, Vekumary S, Madan Mohan. Effect of short term practice of breathing exercises on autonomic functions in normal human. Indian J Med Res. 2001;120:115–21.
77. Pramanik T., Pudasaini B., Prajapati R. Immediate effect of a slow pace breathing exercise Bhramari Pranayama on blood pressure and heart rate. Nepal Med Coll J. 2010;12(3):154–157.
78. Sinha AN, Deepak D, Gusain VS. Assessment of the effects of pranayama/alternate nostril breathing on the parasympathetic nervous system in young adults. J Clin Diagn Res. 2013;7(5):821-3.
79. Bhaskar L, Kharya C, Deepak KK, Kochupillai V. Assessment of Cardiac Autonomic Tone Following Long Sudarshan Kriya Yoga in Art of Living Practitioners. J Altern Complement Med. 2017 Sep;23(9):705-712. doi: 10.1089/acm.2016.0391. Epub 2017 Jul 10.
80. Orme-Johnson DW. Autonomic stability and Transcendental Meditation. Psychosom Med. 1973;35:341–349.; Anand BK. Yoga and medical sciences. Indian Journal of Physiology and Pharmacology. 1991;35(2):84–87.
81. Telles S, Raghavendra BR, Naveen KV, Manjunath NK, Kumar S, Subramanya P. Changes in Autonomic Variables Following Two Meditative States Described in Yoga Texts. Journal of Alternative and Complementary Medicine. 2013;19(1):35-42. doi:10.1089/acm.2011.0282.
82. Markil N, Whitehurst M, Jacobs PL, Zoeller RF. Yoga Nidra relaxation increases heart rate variability and is unaffected by a prior bout of Hatha yoga. Altern Complement Med. 2012 Oct;18(10):953-8. doi: 10.1089/acm.2011.0331. Epub 2012 Aug 6.
83. Dhikav V, Karmarkar G, Verma M, Gupta R, Gupta S, Mittal D, and Anand K. Yoga in male sexual functioning: A noncompararive pilot study. J Sex Med 2010;7:3460–3466.

BNDF

1. Barde YA, Edgar D, Thoenen H. (1982) Purification of a new neurotrophic factor from mammalian brain. EMBO J 1:549–553.
2. Tyler WJ, Pozzo-Miller LD. BDNF enhances quantal neurotransmitter release and increases the number of docked vesicles at the active zones of hippocampal excitatory synapses. J Neurosci. 2001;21(12):4249-58.
3. Siuda J, Patalong-Ogiewa M, Żmuda W, Targosz-Gajniak M, Niewiadomska E, Matuszek I, Jędrzejowska-Szypułka H, Lewin-Kowalik J, Rudzińska-Bar M. Cognitive impairment and BDNF serum levels. Neurol Neurochir Pol. 2017 Jan - Feb;51(1):24-32. doi: 10.1016/j.pjnns.2016.10.001. Epub 2016 Oct 21.
4. Jiang L, Zhang H, Wang C, Ming F, Shi X Yang M. Serum level of brain-derived neurotrophic factor in Parkinson's disease: a meta-analysis. Prog Neuropsychopharmacol Biol Psychiatry. 2019 Jan 10;88:168-174. doi: 10.1016/j.pnpbp.2018.07.010. Epub 2018 Jul 11.
5. Green MJ, Matheson SL, Shepherd A, Weickert CS, Carr VJ. Brain-derived neurotrophic factor levels in schizophrenia: a systematic review with meta-analysis. Mol Psychiatry. 2011 Sep;16(9):960-72. doi: 10.1038/mp.2010.88. Epub 2010 Aug 24.
6. Duman RS, Monteggia LM. (2006) A neurotrophic model for stress-related mood disorders. Biol Psychiatry 59:1116–1127; Martinowich K, Manji H, Lu B. (2007) New insights into BDNF function in depression and anxiety. Nat Neurosci 10:1089–1093.

7. Castrén E, Kojima M. Brain-derived neurotrophic factor in mood disorders and antidepressant treatments. Neurobiol Dis. 2017 Jan;97(Pt B):119-126. doi: 10.1016/j.nbd.2016.07.010. Epub 2016 Jul 15.
8. Jonas BS, Lando JF. Negative affect as a prospective risk factor for hypertension. Psychosomatic Medicine. 2000;62:188–196.
9. Rugulies R. Depression as a Predictor for Coronary Heart Disease A Review and Meta-Analysis. American Journal of Preventative Medicine. 2002;23:51–61.
10. Jonas BS, Lando JF. Negative affect as a prospective risk factor for hypertension. Psychosomatic Medicine. 2000;62:188–196.
11. Gump BB, Matthews KA, Eberly LE, Chang YF MRFIT Research Group. Depressive symptoms and mortality in men: results from the Multiple Risk Factor Intervention Trial. Stroke. 2005;36:98–102.
12. Jiang H, Liu Y, Zhang Y, Chen ZY. Association of plasma brain-derived neurotrophic factor and cardiovascular risk factors and prognosis in angina pectoris. Biochem Biophys Res Commun. 2011; 415:99-103.
13. Kaess BM, Preis SR, Lieb W, et al. Circulating brain-derived neurotrophic factor concentrations and the risk of cardiovascular disease in the community. J Am Heart Assoc. 2015;4(3):e001544. Published 2015 Mar 11. doi:10.1161/JAHA.114.001544.
14. Ejiri J, Inoue N, Kobayashi S, Shiraki R, Otsui K, Honjo T, Takahashi M, Ohashi Y, Ichikawa S, Terashima M, Mori T, Awano K, Shinke T, Shite J, Hirata K, Yokozaki H, Kawashima S, Yokoyama M. Possible role of brain-derived neurotrophic factor in the pathogenesis of coronary artery disease. Circulation. 2005; 112:2114-2120.
15. Krabbe KS, Mortensen EL, Avlund K, Pedersen AN, Pedersen BK, Jorgensen T, Bruunsgaard H. Brain-derived neurotrophic factor predicts mortality risk in older women. J Am Geriatr Soc. 2009; 57:1447-1452.
16. Pal R, Singh SN, Chatterjee A, Saha M. Age-related changes in cardiovascular system, autonomic functions, and levels of BDNF of healthy active males: role of yogic practice. Age (Dordr). 2014;36(4):9683.
17. Naveen GH, Varambally S, Thirthalli J, Rao M, Christopher R, Gangadhar BN. Serum cortisol and BDNF in patients with major depression-effect of yoga. Int Rev Psychiatry. 2016 Jun;28(3):273-8. doi: 10.1080/09540261.2016.1175419. Epub 2016 May 13.
18. Naveen GH, Thirthalli J, Rao MG, Varambally S, Christopher R, Gangadhar BN. Positive therapeutic and neurotropic effects of yoga in depression: A comparative study. Indian J Psychiatry. 2013 Jul;55(Suppl 3):S400-4. doi: 10.4103/0019-5545.116313.
19. Lee M, Moon W, Kim J. Effect of yoga on pain, brain-derived neurotrophic factor, and serotonin in premenopausal women with chronic low back pain. Evid Based Complement Alternat Med. 2014;2014:203173. doi: 10.1155/2014/203173. Epub 2014 Jul 10.
20. Halappa NG, Thirthalli J, Varambally S, Rao M, Christopher R, Nanjundaiah GB. Improvement in neurocognitive functions and serum brain-derived neurotrophic factor levels in patients with depression treated with antidepressants and yoga. Indian J Psychiatry. 2018 Jan-Mar;60(1):32-37. doi: 10.4103/psychiatry.IndianJPsychiatry_154_17.
21. Pedersen BK, Pedersen M, Krabbe KS, Bruunsgaard H, Matthews VB, Febbraio MA. Role of exercise-induced brain-derived neurotrophic factor production in the regulation of energy homeostasis in mammals. Exp Physiol. 2009;94:1153–1160. doi: 10.1113/expphysiol.2009.048561.
22. Rasmussen P, Brassard P, Adser H, Pedersen MV, Leick L, Hart E, et al. Evidence for a release of brain-derived neurotrophic factor from the brain during exercise. Exp Physiol. 2009;94:1062–1069. doi: 10.1113/expphysiol.2009.048512.
23. Larson-Meyer DE. A Systematic Review of the Energy Cost and Metabolic Intensity of Yoga. Med Sci Sports Exerc. 2016 Aug;48(8):1558-69. doi: 10.1249/MSS.0000000000000922.
24. Hagins M, Moore W, Rundle A. Does practicing hatha yoga satisfy recommendations for intensity of physical activity which improves and maintains health and cardiovascular fitness? BMC Complementary and Alternative Medicine. 2007;7, article 40.
25. Ray US, Pathak A, Tomer OS. Hatha yoga practices: energy expenditure. Evidence-Based Complementary and Alternative Medicine. 2011;2011:12 pages.24129452–56.

Cortisol

1. Chan S, Debono M. Replication of cortisol circadian rhythm: new advances in hydrocortisone replacement therapy. Ther Adv Endocrinol Metab. 2010;1(3):129-38.
2. Debono M., Ghobadi C., Rostami-Hodjegan A., Huatan H., Campbell M.J., Newell-Price J., et al. (2009) Modified-release hydrocortisone to provide circadian cortisol profiles. J Clin Endocrinol Metab 94: 1548–1554.
3. Adam EK, Kumari M. Assessing salivary cortisol in large-scale, epidemiological research. Psychoneuroendocrinology. 2009;34:1423–1436.
4. Anagnostis P, Athyros VG, Tziomalos K, Karagiannis A, Mikhailidis DP. Clinical review: The pathogenetic role of cortisol in the metabolic syndrome: A hypothesis. J Clin Endocrinol Metab. 2009;94(8):2692–2701.
5. Filipovsky J, Ducimetiere P, Eschwege E, Richard JL, Rosselin G, Claude JR. The relationship of blood pressure with glucose, insulin, heart rate, free fatty acids and plasma cortisol levels according to degree of obesity in middle-aged men. J Hypertens. 1996;14:229–235.
6. Whitworth JA, Williamson PM, Mangos G, Kelly JJ. Cardiovascular consequences of cortisol excess. Vasc Health Risk Manag. 2005;1(4):291-9.
7. Olnes MJ, Kotliarov Y, Biancotto A, et al. Effects of Systemically Administered Hydrocortisone on the Human Immunome. Sci Rep. 2016;6:23002. Published 2016 Mar 14. doi:10.1038/srep23002.
8. Hakamata Y, Komi S, Moriguchi Y, Izawa S, Motomura Y, Sato E, Mizukami S, Kim Y, Hanakawa T, Inoue Y, Tagaya H. Amygdala-centred functional connectivity affects daily cortisol concentrations: a putative link with anxiety. Sci Rep. 2017 Aug 16;7(1):8313.
9. Chrousos GP, Gold PW. The concepts of stress and stress system disorders. Overview of physical and behavioral homeostasis. Journal of American Medical Association. 1992; 267: 1244–1252.
10. Doane LD, Mineka S, Zinbarg RE, Craske M, Griffith JW, Adam EK. Are flatter diurnal cortisol rhythms associated with major depression and anxiety disorders in late adolescence? The role of life stress and daily negative emotion. Development and psychopathology. 2013;25:629–642.
11. Bower JE, Ganz PA, Dickerson SS, Petersen L, Aziz N, Fahey JL. Diurnal cortisol rhythm and fatigue in breast cancer survivors. Psychoneuroendocrinology. 2005b;30:92–100.
12. Matthews K, Schwartz J, Cohen S, Seeman T. Diurnal cortisol decline is related to coronary calcification: CARDIA study. Psychosomatic Medicine. 2006;68:657–661.
13. Phillips DI, Barker DJ, Fall CH, Seckl JR, Whorwood CB, Wood PJ, Walker BR. Elevated plasma cortisol concentrations: a link between low birth weight and the insulin resistance syndrome? J Clin Endocrinol Metab. 1998;83:757–760.
14. Reynolds RM, Walker BR. Human insulin resistance: the role of glucocorticoids. Diabetes Obes Metab. 2003;5:5–12.
15. Stetler C, Miller GE. Depression and Hypothalamic-Pituitary-Adrenal Activation: A Quantitative Summary of Four Decades of Research. Psychosom Med. 2011;73:114–126. doi: 10.1097/PSY.0b013e31820ad12b.
16. Björntorp P, Rosmond R. Obesity and cortisol. Nutrition. 2000;16:924–936.
17. Whitworth JA, Brown MA, Kelly JJ, Williamson PM. Mechanisms of cortisol-induced hypertension in humans. Steroids. 1995;60:76–80.
18. Whitworth JA, Williamson PM, Mangos G, Kelly JJ 2005 Cardiovascular consequences of cortisol excess. Vasc Health Risk Manag 1:291–299.
19. Petrovsky N, McNair P, Harrison LC. Diurnal rhythms of pro-inflammatory cytokines: regulation by plasma cortisol and therapeutic implications. Cytokine. 1998;10:307–312.
20. Korte SM. Corticosteroids in relation to fear, anxiety and psychopathology. Neurosci Biobehav Rev. 2001;25(2):117–142.
21. Sapolsky RM. Glucocorticoids and hippocampal atrophy in neuropsychiatric disorders. Arch Gen Psychiatry. 2000;57(10):925–935.

22. Kumari M, Badrick E, Chandola T, Adam EK, Stafford M, Marmot MG, Kirschbaum C, Kivimaki M. Cortisol secretion and fatigue: associations in a community based cohort. Psychoneuroendocrinology. 2009;34:1476–1485.
23. Coates JM, Herbert J. Endogenous steroids and financial risk taking on a London trading floor. Proc Natl Acad Sci USA. 2008;105(16):6167–6172.
24. Doane LD, Adam EK. Loneliness and cortisol: Momentary, day-to-day, and trait associations. Psychoneuroendocrinology. 2010;35:430–441.
25. Herman JP, McKlveen JM, Ghosal S, et al. Regulation of the Hypothalamic-Pituitary-Adrenocortical Stress Response. Compr Physiol. 2016;6(2):603-21. Published 2016 Mar 15. doi:10.1002/cphy.c150015.
26. Richardson S, Shaffer JA, Falzon L, Krupka D, Davidson KW, Edmondson D. Meta-analysis of perceived stress and its association with incident coronary heart disease. Am J Cardiol. 2012; 110:1711–6.
27. Fantidis P. The role of the stress-related anti-inflammatory hormones ACTH and cortisol in atherosclerosis. Curr Vasc Pharmacol. 2010;8:517–525.
28. Broadley AJ, Korszun A, Abdelaal E, Moskvina V, Jones CJ, Nash GB, Ray C, Deanfield J, Frenneaux MP. Inhibition of cortisol production with metyrapone prevents mental stress-induced endothelial dysfunction and baroreflex impairment. J Am Coll Cardiol. 2005;46:344–350.
29. Broadley AJM, Korszun A, Abdelaal E, Moskvina V, Deanfield J, Jones CJH, Frenneaux MP. Metyrapone improves endothelial dysfunction in patients with treated depression. J Am Coll Cardiol. 2006;48:170–175.
30. Fantidis P. The role of the stress-related anti-inflammatory hormones ACTH and cortisol in atherosclerosis. Curr Vasc Pharmacol. 2010;8:517–525.
31. Violanti JM, Burchfiel CM, Fekedulegn D, Andrew ME, Dorn J, Hartley TA, Charles LE, Miller DB. Cortisol patterns and brachial artery reactivity in a high stress environment. Psychiatry Res. 2009;169:75–81.
32. Dekker MJ, Koper JW, van Aken MO, Pols HA, Hofman A, de Jong FH, Kirschbaum C, Witteman JC, Lamberts SW, Tiemeier H. Salivary cortisol is related to atherosclerosis of carotid arteries. J Clin Endocrinol Metab. 2008;93:3741–3747.
33. Matthews K, Schwartz J, Cohen S, Seeman T. Diurnal cortisol decline is related to coronary calcification: CARDIA study. Psychosom Med. 2006;68:657–661.
34. Hajat A, Diez-Roux AV, Sánchez BN, et al. Examining the association between salivary cortisol levels and subclinical measures of atherosclerosis: the Multi-Ethnic Study of Atherosclerosis. Psychoneuroendocrinology. 2012;38(7):1036-46.
35. Dekker MJ, Koper JW, van Aken MO, Pols HA, Hofman A, de Jong FH, Kirschbaum C, Witteman JC, Lamberts SW, Tiemeier H 2008 Salivary cortisol is related to atherosclerosis of carotid arteries. J Clin Endocrinol Metab 93:3741–3747.
36. Hamer M, Endrighi R, Venuraju SM, Lahiri A, Steptoe A. Cortisol Responses to Mental Stress and the Progression of Coronary Artery Calcification in Healthy Men and Women. PloS One. 2012;7:e31356.
37. Dekker MJ, Koper JW, van Aken MO, Pols HA, Hofman A, de Jong FH, Kirschbaum C, Witteman JC, Lamberts SW, Tiemeier H. Salivary cortisol is related to atherosclerosis of carotid arteries. J Clin Endocrinol Metab. 2008;93:3741–3747.
38. Matthews K, Schwartz J, Cohen S, Seeman T. Diurnal cortisol decline is related to coronary calcification: CARDIA study. Psychosom Med. 2006;68:657–661.
39. Eller N, Netterstrøm B, Marie Hansen Å. Cortisol in urine and saliva: relations to the intima media thickness, IMT. Atherosclerosis. 2001;159:175–185.
40. Hamer M, Endrighi R, Venuraju SM, Lahiri A, Steptoe A. Cortisol Responses to Mental Stress and the Progression of Coronary Artery Calcification in Healthy Men and Women. PloS One. 2012;7:e31356.
41. Hamer M, O'Donnell K, Lahiri A, Steptoe A. Salivary cortisol responses to mental stress are associated with coronary artery calcification in healthy men and women. European Heart Journal. 2010;31:424–429.

42. Matthews K, Schwartz J, Cohen S, Seeman T. Diurnal cortisol decline is related to coronary calcification: CARDIA study. Psychosom Med. 2006;68:657–661.
43. Zipursky RT, Press MC, Srikanthan P, Gornbein J, McClelland R, Watson K, Horwich TB. Relation of Stress Hormones (Urinary Catecholamines/Cortisol) to Coronary Artery Calcium in Men Versus Women (from the Multi-Ethnic Study of Atherosclerosis [MESA]). Am J Cardiol. 2017 Jun 15;119(12):1963-1971. doi: 10.1016/j.amjcard.2017.03.025. Epub 2017 Mar 29.
44. Alevizaki M, Cimponeriu A, Lekakis J, Papamichael C, Chrousos GP. High anticipatory stress plasma cortisol levels and sensitivity to glucocorticoids predict severity of coronary artery disease in subjects undergoing coronary angiography. Metabolism. 2007;56:222–226.
45. Dekker MJ, Koper JW, van Aken MO, Pols HA, Hofman A, de Jong FH, Kirschbaum C, Witteman JC, Lamberts SW, Tiemeier H. Salivary cortisol is related to atherosclerosis of carotid arteries. J Clin Endocrinol Metab. 2008;93:3741–3747.
46. Koertge J, Al-Khalili F, Ahnve S, Janszky I, Svane B, Schenck-Gustafsson K. Cortisol and vital exhaustion in relation to significant coronary artery stenosis in middle-aged women with acute coronary syndrome. Psychoneuroendocrinology. 2002;27:893–906.
47. Izawa S, Miki K, Tsuchiya M, Yamada H, Nagayama M. Hair and fingernail cortisol and the onset of acute coronary syndrome in the middle-aged and elderly men. Psychoneuroendocrinology. 2019 Mar;101:240-245. doi: 10.1016/j.psyneuen.2018.11.021. Epub 2018 Nov 15.
48. Wilkowska A, Rynkiewicz A, Wdowczyk J, Landowski J. Morning and afternoon serum cortisol level in patients with post-myocardial infarction depression. Cardiol J. 2017 Oct 24. doi: 10.5603/CJ.a2017.0123.
49. Sundbøll J, Schmidt M, Adelborg K, Pedersen L, Bøtker HE, Videbech P, Sørensen HT. Impact of pre-admission depression on mortality following myocardial infarction. Br J Psychiatry. 2017 May;210(5):356-361. doi: 10.1192/bjp.bp.116.194605. Epub 2017 Mar 2.
50. Whitworth JA, Williamson PM, Mangos G, Kelly JJ. Cardiovascular consequences of cortisol excess. Vasc Health Risk Manag. 2005;1(4):291-9.
51. Walker BR. Glucocorticoids and cardiovascular disease. Eur J Endocrinol. 2007;157:545–559.
52. Manenschijn L, Schaap L, van Schoor NM, van der Pas S, Peeters GM, Lips P, Koper JW, van Rossum EF. High long-term cortisol levels, measured in scalp hair, are associated with a history of cardiovascular disease. J Clin Endocrinol Metab. 2013 May;98(5):2078-83. doi: 10.1210/jc.2012-3663. Epub 2013 Apr 17.
53. Kumari M, Shipley M, Stafford M, Kivimaki M. Association of diurnal patterns in salivary cortisol with all-cause and cardiovascular mortality: findings from the Whitehall II study. J Clin Endocrinol Metab. 2011;96:1478–1485.
54. Vogelzangs N, Beekman AT, Milaneschi Y, Bandinelli S, Ferrucci L, Penninx BW. Urinary cortisol and six-year risk of all-cause and cardiovascular mortality. J Clin Endocrinol Metab. 2010;95:4959–4964.
55. Guder G, Bauersachs J, Frantz S, Weismann D, Allolio B, Ertl G, Angermann CE, Stork S. Complementary and incremental mortality risk prediction by cortisol and aldosterone in chronic heart failure. Circulation. 2007;115:1754–1761.
56. Yamaji M, Tsutamoto T, Kawahara C, Nishiyama K, Yamamoto T, Fujii M, Horie M. Serum cortisol as a useful predictor of cardiac events in patients with chronic heart failure: the impact of oxidative stress. Circ Heart Fail. 2009;2:608–615.
57. Barugh AJ, Gray P, Shenkin SD, MacLullich AM, Mead GE. Cortisol levels and the severity and outcomes of acute stroke: a systematic review. J Neurol. 2014;261(3):533-45.
58. Granath J, Ingvarsson S, von Thiele U, Lundberg U. Stress management: a randomized study of cognitive behavioural therapy and yoga. Cognitive Behaviour Therapy. 2006;35:3–10. doi: 10.1080/16506070500401292.
59. West J, Otte C, Geher K, Johnson J, Mohr DC. Effects of Hatha yoga and African dance on perceived stress, affect, and salivary cortisol. Annals of Behavioral Medicine: A Publication of the Society of Behavioral Medicine. 2004;28:114–118. doi: 10.1207/s15324796abm2802_6.

60. Pal R, Singh SN, Chatterjee A, Saha M. Age-related changes in cardiovascular system, autonomic functions, and levels of BDNF of healthy active males: role of yogic practice. Age (Dordr). 2014;36(4):9683.
61. Pascoe MC, Thompson DR, Ski CF. Yoga, mindfulness-based stress reduction and stress-related physiological measures: A meta-analysis. Psychoneuroendocrinology. 2017 Dec;86:152-168. doi: 10.1016/j.psyneuen.2017.08.008. Epub 2017 Aug 30.
62. Oka T, Tanahashi T, Sudo N, Lkhagvasuren B, Yamada Y. Changes in fatigue, autonomic functions, and blood biomarkers due to sitting isometric yoga in patients with chronic fatigue syndrome. Biopsychosoc Med. 2018;12:3. Published 2018 Apr 10. doi:10.1186/s13030-018-0123-2.
63. Fujisawa A, Ota A, Matsunaga M, Li Y, Kakizaki M, Naito H, Yatsuya H. Effect of laughter yoga on salivary cortisol and dehydroepiandrosterone among healthy university students: A randomized controlled trial. Complement Ther Clin Pract. 2018 Aug;32:6-11. doi: 10.1016/j.ctcp.2018.04.005. Epub 2018 Apr 12.
64. Vedamurthachar A, Janakiramaiah N, Hegde JM, Shetty TK, Subbakrishna DK, Sureshbabu SV, et al. Antidepressant efficacy and hormonal effects of Sudarshana Kriya Yoga (SKY) in alcohol dependent individuals. J Affect Disord. 2006;94:249–53.
65. Michaels RR, Parra J, McCann DS, Vander AJ. Renin, cortisol, and aldosterone during transcendental meditation. Psychosom Med. 1979 Feb;41(1):50–54.
66. Walton KG, Fields JZ, Levitsky DK, Harris DA, Pugh ND, Schneider RH. Lowering cortisol and CVD risk in postmenopausal women: a pilot study using the Transcendental Meditation program. Ann N Y Acad Sci. 2004 Dec;1032:211-5.

DHEA

1. Yen SS, Laughlin GA. Aging and the adrenal cortex. Experimental Gerontology. 1998;33(7-8):281–287.
2. Webb SJ, Geoghegan TE, Prough RA, Michael Miller KK. The biological actions of dehydroepiandrosterone involves multiple receptors. Drug Metab Rev. 2006;38(1-2):89-116.
3. Parker CR, Jr., Mixon RL, Brissie RM, Grizzle WE. Aging alters zonation in the adrenal cortex of men. The Journal of Clinical Endocrinology and Metabolism. 1997;82(11):3898–3901.
4. Genazzani AD. Lanzoni C. Genazzani AR. Might DHEA be considered a beneficial replacement therapy in the elderly? Drugs Aging. 2007;24:173–185.
5. Kostka T. Aging and so called "youth hormones". Potential influence of exercise training. Przeglad Lekarski. 2001;58(1):25–27.
6. Perrini S, Laviola L, Natalicchio A, Giorgino F. Associated hormonal declines in aging: DHEAS. Journal of Endocrinological Investigation. 2005;28(3, supplement):85–93.
7. Dennis TV, John OH. DHEA enhances effects of weight training on muscle mass and strength in elderly women and men. American Journal of Physiology—Endocrinology and Metabolism. 2006;291(5):E1003–E1008.
8. Roberts E, Bologa L, Flood JF, Smith GE. Effects of dehydroepiandrosterone and its sulfate on brain tissue in culture and on memory in mice. Brain Res. 1987;406(1–2):357–362. doi: 10.1016/0006-8993(87)90807-9.
9. Morgan CA, 3rd, Southwick S, Hazlett G, Rasmusson A, Hoyt G, Zimolo Z, Charney D. Relationships among plasma dehydroepiandrosterone sulfate and cortisol levels, symptoms of dissociation, and objective performance in humans exposed to acute stress. Arch Gen Psychiatry. 2004;61(8):819–825. doi: 10.1001/archpsyc.61.8.819.
10. Scott LV, Salahuddin F, Cooney J, Svec F, Dinan TG. Differences in adrenal steroid profile in chronic fatigue syndrome, in depression and in health. J Affect Disord. 1999;54(1–2):129–137. doi: 10.1016/S0165-0327(98)00169-4.
11. Wolkowitz OM et al. Dehydroepiandrosterone (DHEA) treatment of depression. Biol Psychiatry 1997 Feb 1;41(3):311-8.

12. Wang L. Hao Q. Wang YD. Wang WJ. Li DJ. Protective effects of dehydroepiandrosterone on atherosclerosis in ovariectomized rabbits via alleviating inflammatory injury in endothelial cells. Atherosclerosis. 2011;214:47–57.
13. Yoshida S. Aihara K. Azuma H. Uemoto R. Sumitomo-Ueda Y. Yagi S. Ikeda Y. Iwase T. Nishio S. Kawano H. Miki J. Yamada H. Hirata Y. Akaike M. Sata M. Matsumoto T. Dehydroepiandrosterone sulfate is inversely associated with sex-dependent diverse carotid atherosclerosis regardless of endothelial function. Atherosclerosis. 2010;212:310–315.
14. Barrett-Cnnor E, Khaw KT, Yen SS. A prospective study of dehydroepiandrosterone sulfate, mortality, and cardiovascular disease. N Engl J Med. 1986;315(24):1519–24. doi: 10.1056/NEJM198612113152405.6).
15. Hak AE, Witteman JC, de Jong FH, Geerlings MI, Hofman A, Pols HA. Low levels of endogenous androgens increase the risk of atherosclerosis in elderly men: the Rotterdam study. J Clin Endocrinol Metab. 2002;87(8):3632–9. doi: 10.1210/jcem.87.8.8762.
16. Herrington DM. Dehydroepiandrosterone and coronary atherosclerosis. Ann N Y Acad Sci. 1995;774:271–80.
17. Feldman HA, Johannes CB, Araujo AB, Mohr BA, Longcope C, McKinlay JB. Low dehydroepiandrosterone and ischemic heart disease in middle-aged men: prospective results from the Massachusetts Male Aging Study. Am J Epidemiol. 2001;153(1):79–89.
18. Feldman HA. Johannes CB. Araujo AB. Mohr BA. Longcope C. McKinlay JB. Low dehydroepiandrosterone and ischemic heart disease in middle-aged men: Prospective results from the Massachusetts Male Aging Study. Am J Epidemiol. 2001;153:79–89.
19. Herrington DM. Dehydroepiandrosterone and coronary atherosclerosis. Ann NY Acad Sci. 1995;774:271–280.
20. Barrett-Cnnor E, Khaw KT, Yen SS. A prospective study of dehydroepiandrosterone sulfate, mortality, and cardiovascular disease. N Engl J Med. 1986;315(24):1519–24. doi: 10.1056/NEJM198612113152405.6.
21. Shufelt C, Bretsky P, Almeida CM, Johnson BD, Shaw LJ, Azziz R, et al. Dhea-s levels and cardiovascular disease mortality in postmenopausal women: Results from the national institutes of health--national heart, lung, and blood institute (nhlbi)-sponsored women's ischemia syndrome evaluation (wise) J Clin Endocrinol Metab. 2010;95:4985–4992.
22. Nakamura S. Yoshimura M. Nakayama M. Ito T. Mizuno Y. Harada E. Sakamoto T. Saito Y. Nakao K. Yasue H. Ogawa H. Possible association of heart failure status with synthetic balance between aldosterone and dehydroepiandrosterone in human heart. Circulation. 2004;110:1787–1793.
23. Jankowska EA. Biel B. Majda J. Szklarska A. Lopuszanska M. Medras M. Anker SD. Banasiak W. Poole-Wilson PA. Ponikowski P. Anabolic deficiency in men with chronic heart failure: prevalence and detrimental impact on survival. Circulation. 2006;114:1829–1837.
24. Herrington DM. Nanjee N. Achuff SC. Cameron DE. Dobbs B. Baughman KL. Dehydroepiandrosterone and cardiac allograft vasculopathy. J Heart Lung Transplant. 1996;15:88–93.
25. Mannic T, Viguie J, Rossier MF. In vivo and in vitro evidences of dehydroepiandrosterone protective role on the cardiovascular system. Int J Endocrinol Metab. 2015;13(2):e24660. Published 2015 Apr 30. doi:10.5812/ijem.24660.
26. Wu TT, Chen Y, Zhou Y, et al. Prognostic Value of Dehydroepiandrosterone Sulfate for Patients With Cardiovascular Disease: A Systematic Review and Meta-Analysis. J Am Heart Assoc. 2017;6(5):e004896. Published 2017 May 5. doi:10.1161/JAHA.116.004896.
27. Jiménez MC, Sun Q, Schürks M, et al. Low dehydroepiandrosterone sulfate is associated with increased risk of ischemic stroke among women. Stroke. 2013;44(7):1784-9.
28. Blum CA, Mueller C, Schuetz P, et al. Prognostic value of dehydroepiandrosterone-sulfate and other parameters of adrenal function in acute ischemic stroke. PLoS One. 2013;8(5):e63224. Published 2013 May 1. doi:10.1371/journal.pone.0063224.
29. Basar MM. Aydin G. Mert HC. Keles I. Caglayan O. Orkun S. Batislam E. Relationship between serum sex steroids and Aging Male Symptoms score and International Index of Erectile Function. Urology. 2005;66:597–601. ;108.

30. Alexopoulou O. Jamart J. Maiter D. Hermans MP. De Hertogh R. De Nayer P. Buysschaert M. Erectile dysfunction and lower androgenicity in type 1 diabetic patients. Diabetes Metab. 2001;27:329–336.
31. Feldman HA. Goldstein I. Hatzichristou DG. Krane RJ. McKinlay JB. Impotence and its medical and psychosocial correlates: Results of the Massachusetts Male Aging Study. J Urol. 1994;151:54–61.
32. El-Sakka AI. Dehydroepiandrosterone and Erectile Function: A Review. World J Mens Health. 2018;36(3):183-191.
33. Reiter WJ. Pycha A. Schatzl G. Klingler HC. Märk I. Auterith A. Marberger M. Serum dehydroepiandrosterone sulfate concentrations in men with erectile dysfunction. Urology. 2000;55:755–758.
34. Reiter WJ. Pycha A. Schatzl G. Pokorny A. Gruber DM. Huber JC. Marberger M. Dehydroepiandrosterone in the treatment of erectile dysfunction: A prospective, double-blind, randomized, placebo-controlled study. Urology. 1999;53:590–594.
35. Reiter WJ. Schatzl G. Mark I. Zeiner A. Pycha A. Marberger M. Dehydroepiandrosterone in the treatment of erectile dysfunction in patients with different organic etiologies. Urol Res. 2001;29:278–281.
36. Vera FM, Manzaneque JM, Maldonado EF, et al. Subjective Sleep Quality and hormonal modulation in long-term yoga practitioners. Biological Psychology. 2009;81(3):164–168.
37. Chatterjee S, Mondal S. Effect of regular yogic training on growth hormone and dehydroepiandrosterone sulfate as an endocrine marker of aging. Evid Based Complement Alternat Med. 2014;2014:240581.
38. Glaser JL, Brind JL, Vogelman JH, et al. Elevated serum dehydroepiandrosterone sulfate levels in practitioners of the Transcendental Meditation (TM) and TM-Sidhi programs. Journal of Behavioral Medicine. 1992;15(4):327–341.

Dopamine

1. Hornykiewicz O. Dopamine miracle: from brain homogenate to dopamine replacement. Mov Disord. 2002;17:501–8. doi: 10.1002/mds.10115.
2. Treadway MT, Zald DH. (2011) Reconsidering anhedonia in depression: lessons from translational neuroscience. Neurosci Biobehav Rev 35:537–555.
3. Sherdell L, Waugh CE, Gotlib IH. (2012) Anticipatory pleasure predicts motivation for reward in major depression. J Abnorm Psychol 121:51–60.
4. Vrieze E, Pizzagalli DA, Demyttenaere K, Hompes T, Sienaert P, de Boer P, Schmidt M, Claes S. (2013) Reduced reward learning predicts outcome in major depressive disorder. Biol Psychiatry 73:639–645.
5. Meyer JH, Kruger S, Wilson AA, Christensen BK, Goulding VS, Schaffer A, Minifie C, Houle S, Hussey D, Kennedy SH. (2001) Lower dopamine transporter binding potential in striatum during depression. Neuroreport 12:4121–4125.
6. Sarchiapone M, Carli V, Camardese G, Cuomo C, Di Giuda D, Calcagni ML, Focacci C, De Risio S. (2006) Dopamine transporter binding in depressed patients with anhedonia. Psychiatry Res 147:243–248.
7. Kilbourn MR, Sherman PS, Pisani T. (1992) Repeated reserpine administration reduces in vivo [18F]GBR 13119 binding to the dopamine uptake site. Eur J Pharmacol 216:109–112.
8. Ikawa K, Watanabe A, Motohashi N, Kaneno S. (1994) The effect of repeated administration of methamphetamine on dopamine uptake sites in rat striatum. Neurosci Lett 167:37–40.
9. Gordon I, Weizman R, Rehavi M. (1996) Modulatory effect of agents active in the presynaptic dopaminergic system on the striatal dopamine transporter. Eur J Pharmacol 298:27–30.
10. Rugulies R. Depression as a predictor for coronary heart disease. a review and meta-analysis. Am J Prev Med. 2002;23: 51–61.
11. Dong J-Y, Zhang Y-H, Tong J, Qin L-Q. Depression and risk of stroke: a meta-analysis of prospective studies. Stroke. 2012;43: 32–7. 10.1161/STROKEAHA.111.630871.

12. Daskalopoulou M, George J, Walters K, et al. Depression as a Risk Factor for the Initial Presentation of Twelve Cardiac, Cerebrovascular, and Peripheral Arterial Diseases: Data Linkage Study of 1.9 Million Women and Men. PLoS One. 2016;11(4):e0153838. Published 2016 Apr 22. doi:10.1371/journal.pone.0153838.
13. Ma BO, Shim SG, Yang HJ. Association of erectile dysfunction with depression in patients with chronic viral hepatitis. World J Gastroenterol. 2015;21(18):5641-6.
14. Christopher L, Duff-Canning S, Koshimori Y, et al. Salience network and parahippocampal dopamine dysfunction in memory-impaired Parkinson disease. Ann Neurol. 2014;77(2):269-80.
15. Howes O, McCutcheon R, Stone J. Glutamate and dopamine in schizophrenia: an update for the 21st century. J Psychopharmacol. 2015;29(2):97-115.
16. Calipari ES, Ferris MJ, Jones SR. Extended access of cocaine self-administration results in tolerance to the dopamine-elevating and locomotor-stimulating effects of cocaine. J Neurochem. 2013;128(2):224-32.
17. Drozak J, Bryła J. Dopamine: not just a neurotransmitter. [Article in Polish] Postepy Hig Med Dosw (Online). 2005;59:405-20.
18. Pal R, Singh SN, Chatterjee A, Saha M. Age-related changes in cardiovascular system, autonomic functions, and levels of BDNF of healthy active males: role of yogic practice. Age (Dordr). 2014;36(4):9683.
19. Troels W. Kjaer, Camilla Bertelsen, et al. Increased dopamine tone during meditation-induced change of consciousness. Cognitive Brain Research 13 (2002) 255–259.

GABA

1. Enna SJ, Maggi A. Minireview: Biochemical pharmacology of GABA-ergic agonists. Life Sci. 1979;24:1727.
2. Tappaz M, Brownstein MJ, Kopin IJ. Glutamate decarboxylase (GAD) and gamma-aminobutyric acid (GABA) in discrete nuclei of hypothalamus and substantia nigra. Brain Res. 1977;125:109.
3. Brambilla P. Perez J. Barale F, et al. GABAergic dysfunction in mood disorders. Mol Psychiatry. 2003;8:721–737.
4. Houser CR. GABA neurons in seizure disorders: A review of immunocytochemical studies. Neurochem Res. 1991;16:295–308.
5. Breier A. Paul S. The GABAa/benzodiazepine receptor: Implications for the molecular basis of anxiety. J Psychiatr Res. 1990;24:91–104.
6. Streeter CC, Whitfield TH, Owen L, et al. Effects of yoga versus walking on mood, anxiety, and brain GABA levels: a randomized controlled MRS study. J Altern Complement Med. 2010;16(11):1145-52.
7. Lim DY, Suh J, Yoo HJ, et al. Influence of gamma-aminobutyric acid on the changes of blood pressure in rats. Korean J Intern Med. 1990;5(1):23-33.
8. Allen AM. Inhibition of the hypothalamic paraventricular nucleus in spontaneously hypertensive rats dramatically reduces sympathetic vasomotor tone. Hypertension 39: 275–280, 2002.
9. Haywood JR, Mifflin SW, Craig T, Calderon A, Hensler JG, Hinojosa-Laborde C. gamma-Aminobutyric acid (GABA)-A function and binding in the paraventricular nucleus of the hypothalamus in chronic renal-wrap hypertension. Hypertension 37: 614–618, 2001.
10. Reynolds AY, Zhang K, Patel KP. Renal sympathetic nerve discharge mediated by the paraventricular nucleus is altered in STZ induced diabetic rats. Nebraska Med J 81: 419–423, 1996.
11. Zhang K, Li YF, Patel KP. Reduced endogenous GABA-mediated inhibition in the PVN on renal nerve discharge in rats with heart failure.11 Am J Physiol Regul Integr Comp Physiol 282: R1006–R1015, 2002.
12. Pandit S, Jo JY, Lee SU, et al. Enhanced astroglial GABA uptake attenuates tonic GABAA inhibition of the presympathetic hypothalamic paraventricular nucleus neurons in heart failure. J Neurophysiol. 2015;114(2):914-26.

13. Streeter CC. Jensen JE. Perlmutter RM, et al. Yoga Asana sessions increase brain GABA levels: A pilot study. J Altern Complement Med. 2007;13:419–426.
14. Streeter CC, Whitfield TH, Owen L, et al. Effects of yoga versus walking on mood, anxiety, and brain GABA levels: a randomized controlled MRS study. J Altern Complement Med. 2010;16(11):1145-52.

Growth Hormone

1. Lanfranco F, Gianotti L, Giordano R, Pellegrino M, Maccario M, Arvat E. Ageing, growth hormone and physical performance. Journal of Endocrinological Investigation. 2003;26(9):861–872.
2. Stokes K. Growth hormone responses to sub-maximal and sprint exercise. Growth Hormone and IGF Research. 2003;13(5):225–238.
3. Stokes KA, Nevill ME, Cherry PW, Lakomy HKA, Hall GM. Effect of 6 weeks of sprint training on growth hormone responses to sprinting. European Journal of Applied Physiology. 2004;92(1-2):26–32.1–3.
4. Brook CGD, Hindmarsh PC. The somatotropic axis in puberty. Endocrinology and Metabolism Clinics of North America. 1992;21(4):767–782.
5. Bidlingmaier M, Strasburger CJ. Growth hormone. Handb Exp Pharmacol. 2010;(195):187-200. doi: 10.1007/978-3-540-79088-4_8.
6. Sacca L, Cittadini A, Fazio S. Growth hormone and the heart. Endocr. Rev. 1994;15:555–573. ; Ren J, Samson WK, Sowers JR. Insulin-like growth factor I as a cardiac hormone: physiological and pathophysiological implications in heart disease. J. Mol. Cell. Cardiol. 1999;31:2049–2061.
7. Johansson J-O, Fowelin J, Landin K, Lager I, Bengtsson B-Å. Growth hormone-deficient adults are insulin-resistant. Metabolism. 1995;44:1126–1129.
8. Hew F, Koschmann M, Christopher M, Rantzau C, Vaag A, Ward G, Beck-Nielsen H, Alford F. Insulin resistance in growth hormone-deficient adults: defects in glucose utilization and glycogen synthase activity. J. Clin. Endocrinol. Metab. 1996;81:555–564.
9. Lanes R, Soros A, Gunczler P, Paoli M, Carrillo E, Villaroel O, Palacios A. Growth hormone deficiency, low levels of adiponectin, and unfavorable plasma lipid and lipoproteins. J Pediatr. 2006 Sep;149(3):324-9.
10. Johansson J-O, Landin K, Tengborn L, Rosén T, Bengtsson B-Å. High fibrinogen and plasminogen activator inhibitor activity in growth hormone-deficient adults. Arterioscler. Thromb. 1994;14:434–437.
11. Sverrisdóttir Y, Elam M, Bengtsson B-Å, Johannsson G. Intense sympathetic nerve activity in adults with hypopituitarism and untreated growth hormone deficiency. J. Clin. Endocrinol. Metab. 1998;83:1881–1885.
12. Gola M, Bonadonna S, Doga M, Giustina A. Clinical review. Growth hormone and cardiovascular risk factors. J. Clin. Endocrinol. Metab. 2005;90(3):1864–1870.
13. Tivesten Å., Barlind A., Caidahl K., Klintland N., Cittadini A., Ohlsson C., Isgaard J. Growth hormone-induced blood pressure decrease is associated with increased mRNA levels of the vascular smooth muscle KATP channel. J. Endocrinol. 2004;183:195–202. doi: 10.1677/joe.1.05726.
14. Devesa J., Almengló C., Devesa P. Multiple Effects of Growth Hormone in the Body: Is it Really the Hormone for Growth? Clin. Med. Insights. Endocrinol. Diabetes. 2016;9:47–71. doi: 10.4137/CMED.S38201.
15. Colao A. The GH-IGF-I axis and the cardiovascular system: Clinical implications. Clin. Endocrinol. (Oxf). 2008;69:347–358. doi: 10.1111/j.1365-2265.2008.03292.x.
16. Isgaard J., Arcopinto M., Karason K., Cittadini A. GH and the cardiovascular system: An update on a topic at heart. Endocrine. 2014;48:25–35. doi: 10.1007/s12020-014-0327-6.
17. Le Corvoisier P., Hittinger L., Chanson P., Montagne O., Macquin-Mavier I., Maison P. Cardiac effects of growth hormone treatment in chronic heart failure: A meta-analysis. J. Clin. Endocrinol. Metab. 2007;92:180–185. doi: 10.1210/jc.2006-1313.

18. Rosén T, Edén S, Larsson G, Wilhelmsen L, Bengtsson B-Å. Cardiovascular risk factors in adult patients with growth hormone deficiency. Acta Endocrinol. 1993;129:195–200.
19. Leinninger G.M., Vincent A.M., Feldman E.L. The role of growth factors in diabetic peripheral neuropathy. J. Peripher. Nerv. Syst. 2004;9:26–53. doi: 10.1111/j.1085-9489.2004.09105.x.
20. Chatterjee S, Mondal S. Effect of regular yogic training on growth hormone and dehydroepiandrosterone sulfate as an endocrine marker of aging. Evid Based Complement Alternat Med. 2014;2014:240581.
21. Yu AP, Ugwu FN, Tam BT, et al. One Year of Yoga Training Alters Ghrelin Axis in Centrally Obese Adults With Metabolic Syndrome. Front Physiol. 2018;9:1321. Published 2018 Sep 20. doi:10.3389/fphys.2018.01321.
22. Hurel SJ, Koppiker N, Newkirk J, et al. Relationship of physical exercise and ageing to growth hormone production. Clinical Endocrinology. 1999;51(6):687–691.
23. Ari Z, Kutlu N, Uyanik BS, Taneli F, Buyukyazi G, Tavli T. Serum testosterone, growth hormone, and insulin-like growth factor-1 levels, mental reaction time, and maximal aerobic exercise in sedentary and long-term physically trained elderly males. International Journal of Neuroscience. 2004;114(5):623–637.
24. Hagins M, Moore W, Rundle A. Does practicing hatha yoga satisfy recommendations for intensity of physical activity which improves and maintains health and cardiovascular fitness? BMC Complementary and Alternative Medicine. 2007;7, article 40.
25. Sinha B, Ray US, Pathak A, Selvamurthy W. Energy cost and cardiorespiratory changes during the practice of Surya Namaskar. Indian Journal of Physiology and Pharmacology. 2004;48(2):184–190.
26. Ray US, Pathak A, Tomer OS. Hatha yoga practices: energy expenditure. Evidence-Based Complementary and Alternative Medicine. 2011;2011:12 pages.24129452–56.
27. Larson-Meyer DE. A Systematic Review of the Energy Cost and Metabolic Intensity of Yoga. Med Sci Sports Exerc. 2016 Aug;48(8):1558-69. doi: 10.1249/MSS.0000000000000922.

Melatonin

1. Sapède D, Cau E. The pineal gland from development to function. Curr Top Dev Biol. 2013;106:171-215. doi: 10.1016/B978-0-12-416021-7.00005-5.
2. Tricoire H., Locatelli A., Chemineau P., & Malpaux B. (2002). Melatonin Enters the Cerebrospinal Fluid through the Pineal Recess. Endocrinology, Volume 143, Issue 1, 1 January 2002, Pages 84–90,
3. Tan D. X., Manchester L. C., Terron M. P., Flores L. J., & Reiter R. J. (2007). One molecule, many derivatives: a never-ending interaction of melatonin with reactive oxygen and nitrogen species? Journal of Pineal Research, 42(1), 28–42. https://doi.org/10.1111/j.1600-079X.2006.00407.x.
4. Li R., Luo X., Li L., Peng Q., Yang Y., Zhao L., Ma M., Hou Z. The protective effects of melatonin against oxidative stress and inflammation induced by acute cadmium exposure in mice testis. Biol. Trace Elem. Res. 2016;170:152–164. doi: 10.1007/s12011-015-0449-6.
5. De Pedro N., Martinez-Alvarez R. M., & Delgado M. J. (2008). Melatonin reduces body weight in goldfish (Carassius auratus): effects on metabolic resources and some feeding regulators. Journal of Pineal Research, 45(1), 32–39. https://doi.org/10.1111/j.1600-079X.2007.00553.x.
6. Chen S.J., Huang S.H., Chen J.W., Wang K.C., Yang Y.R., Liu P.F., Lin G.J., Sytwu H.K. Melatonin enhances interleukin-10 expression and suppresses chemotaxis to inhibit inflammation in situ and reduce the severity of experimental autoimmune encephalomyelitis. Int. Immunopharmacol. 2016;31:169–177. doi: 10.1016/j.intimp.2015.12.020.)
7. Li F., Li S., Li H.B., Deng G.F., Ling W.H., Wu S., Xu X.R., Chen F. Antiproliferative activity of peels, pulps and seeds of 61 fruits. J. Funct. Foods. 2013;5:1298–1309. doi: 10.1016/j.jff.2013.04.016.

8. Carrillo-Vico A, Lardone PJ, Alvarez-Sánchez N, Rodríguez-Rodríguez A, Guerrero JM. Melatonin: buffering the immune system. Int J Mol Sci. 2013;14(4):8638-83. Published 2013 Apr 22. doi:10.3390/ijms14048638.
9. Karasek M, Reiter RJ. Melatonin and aging. Neuro Endocrinol Lett. 2002;23(Suppl 1):14–6.
10. Zhdanova IV. Melatonin as a hypnotic: Pro. Sleep Med Rev. 2005 Feb;9(1):51–65.
11. Brzezinksi A. Melatonin in Humans. N Engl J Med. 1997 Jan;336(3):186.
12. Sack RL, Brandes RW, Kendall AR, Lewy AJ. Entrainment of free-running circadian rhythms by melatonin in blind people. N Engl J Med. 2000;343(15):1070–1077.
13. Brown G.M., Pandi-Perumal S.R., Trakht I., Cardinali D.P. Melatonin and its relevance to jet lag. Travel Med. Infect. Dis. 2009;7:69–81. doi: 10.1016/j.tmaid.2008.09.004.
14. Pandi-Perumal S.R., Srinivasan V., Poeggeler B., Hardeland R., Cardinali D.P. Drug Insight: The use of melatonergic agonists for the treatment of insomnia-focus on ramelteon. Nat. Clin. Pract. Neurol. 2007;3:221–228. doi: 10.1038/ncpneuro0467.
15. Agil A., Elmahallawy E.K., Rodriguez-Ferrer J.M., Adem A., Bastaki S.M., Al-Abbadi I., Fino Solano Y.A., Navarro-Alarcon M. Melatonin increases intracellular calcium in the liver, muscle, white adipose tissues and pancreas of diabetic obese rats. Food Funct. 2015;6:2671–2678. doi: 10.1039/C5FO00590F.
16. Agil A., El-Hammadi M., Jimenez-Aranda A., Tassi M., Abdo W., Fernandez-Vazquez G., Reiter R.J. Melatonin reduces hepatic mitochondrial dysfunction in diabetic obese rats. J. Pineal Res. 2015;59:70–79. doi: 10.1111/jpi.12241.
17. Anisimov V.N., Popovich I.G., Zabezhinski M.A., Anisimov S.V., Vesnushkin G.M., Vinogradova I.A. Melatonin as antioxidant, geroprotector and anticarcinogen. Biochim. Biophys. Acta. 2006;1757:573–589. doi: 10.1016/j.bbabio.2006.03.012.
18. Chenevard R., Suter Y., Erne P. Effects of the heart-lung machine on melatonin metabolism and mood disturbances. Eur. J. Cardiothorac. Surg. 2008;34:338–343. doi: 10.1016/j.ejcts.2008.03.035.
19. Yousaf F, Seet E, Venkatraghavan L, Abrishami A, Chung F. Efficacy and safety of melatonin as an anxiolytic and analgesic in the perioperative period. Anesthesiology. 2010;113:968–976.
20. Hansen MV, Halladin NL, Rosenberg J, Gögenur I, Møller AM. Melatonin for pre- and postoperative anxiety in adults. Cochrane Database Syst Rev. 2015 Apr 9;(4):CD009861. doi: 10.1002/14651858.CD009861.pub2.
21. Hu Z. P., Fang X. L., Fang N., et al. Melatonin ameliorates vascular endothelial dysfunction, inflammation, and atherosclerosis by suppressing the tlr4/nf-κb system in high-fat-fed rabbits. Journal of Pineal Research. 2013;55:388–398. doi: 10.1111/jpi.12085.
22. Tan DX, Manchester LC, Esteban-Zubero E, Zhou Z, Reiter RJ. Melatonin as a Potent and Inducible Endogenous Antioxidant: Synthesis and Metabolism. Molecules. 2015;20(10):18886-906. Published 2015 Oct 16. doi:10.3390/molecules201018886.
23. Yang Y., Sun Y., Yi W., et al. A review of melatonin as a suitable antioxidant against myocardial ischemia-reperfusion injury and clinical heart diseases. Journal of Pineal Research. 2014;57(4):357–366. doi: 10.1111/jpi.12175.
24. Zhang H. M., Zhang Y. Melatonin: a well-documented antioxidant with conditional pro-oxidant actions. Journal of Pineal Research. 2014;57(2):131–146. doi: 10.1111/jpi.12162.
25. Favero G., Rodella L. F., Reiter R. J., Rezzani R. Melatonin and its atheroprotective effects: a review. Molecular and Cellular Endocrinology. 2014;382(2):926–937. doi: 10.1016/j.mce.2013.11.016.
26. Ma S, Chen J, Feng J, et al. Melatonin Ameliorates the Progression of Atherosclerosis via Mitophagy Activation and NLRP3 Inflammasome Inhibition. Oxid Med Cell Longev. 2018;2018:9286458. Published 2018 Sep 4. doi:10.1155/2018/9286458.
27. Reiter RJ, Tan DX, Paredes SD, Fuentes-Broto L. Beneficial effects of melatonin in cardiovascular disease. Ann Med. 2010 May 6;42(4):276-85. doi: 10.3109/07853890903485748.
28. Pandi-Perumal S.R., Zisapel N., Srinivasan V., Cardinali D.P. Melatonin and sleep in aging population. Exp. Gerontol. 2005;40:911–925. doi: 10.1016/j.exger.2005.08.009.

29. Tengattini S., Reiter R. J., Tan D. X., Terron M. P., Rodella L. F., Rezzani R. Cardiovascular diseases: protective effects of melatonin. Journal of Pineal Research. 2008;44(1):16–25. doi: 10.1111/j.1600-079x.2007.00518.x.
30. Reiter R. J., Tan D. X., Paredes S. D., Fuentes-Broto L. Beneficial effects of melatonin in cardiovascular disease. Annals of Medicine. 2010;42(4):276–285. doi: 10.3109/07853890903485748.
31. Brugger P, Marktl W, Herold M. Impaired nocturnal secretion of melatonin in coronary heart disease. Lancet. 1995 Jun;345(8962):1408.
32. Reiter R. J., Tan D. X. Melatonin: a novel protective agent against oxidative injury of the ischemic/reperfused heart. Cardiovascular Research. 2003;58(1):10–19. doi: 10.1016/S0008-6363(02)00827-1.
33. Yu L., Gong B., Duan W., et al. Melatonin ameliorates myocardial ischemia/reperfusion injury in type 1 diabetic rats by preserving mitochondrial function: role of ampk-pgc-1α-sirt3 signaling. Scientific Reports. 2017;7(1, article 41337) doi: 10.1038/srep41337.
34. Simko F, Bednarova KR, Krajcirovicova K, Hrenak J, Celec P, Kamodyova N, Gajdosechova L, Zorad S, Adamcova M. Melatonin reduces cardiac remodeling and improves survival in rats with isoproterenol-induced heart failure. J Pineal Res. 2014 Sep;57(2):177-84. doi: 10.1111/jpi.12154. Epub 2014 Jul 10.
35. Nduhirabandi F, Maarman GJ. Melatonin in Heart Failure: A Promising Therapeutic Strategy?. Molecules. 2018;23(7):1819. Published 2018 Jul 22. doi:10.3390/molecules23071819.
36. Fiorina P, Lattuada G, Silvestrini C, Ponari O, Dall'Aglio P. Disruption of nocturnal melatonin rhythm and immunological involvement in ischaemic stroke patients. Scand J Immunol. 1999 Aug;50(2):228–231.
37. Harinath K, Malhotra AS, Pal K, Prasad R, Kumar R, Kain TC, Rai L, Sawhney RC. Effects of Hatha yoga and Omkar meditation on cardiorespiratory performance, psychologic profile, and melatonin secretion. J Altern Complement Med. 2004 Apr;10(2):261-8.
38. Tooley GA, Armstrong SM, Norman TR, Sali A. Acute increases in night-time plasma melatonin levels following a period of meditation. Biol Psychol. 2000 May;53(1):69-78.

Catecholamines

1. Tank AW, Lee Wong D. Peripheral and central effects of circulating catecholamines. Compr Physiol. 2015 Jan;5(1):1-15. doi: 10.1002/cphy.c140007.
2. Goldstein DS. Plasma catecholamines and essential hypertension. An analytical review. Hypertension. 1983 Jan-Feb;5(1):86-99.
3. Nezu M, Miura Y, Adachi M, Adachi M, Kimura S, Toriyabe S, Ishizuka Y, Ohashi H, Sugawara T, Takahashi M, et al. The effects of epinephrine on norepinephrine release in essential hypertension. Hypertension. 1985 Mar-Apr;7(2):187-95.
4. Missouris, Constantinos G.; Markandu, Nirmala D.; He, Feng J.; Papavasileiou, Maria V.; Sever, Peter; MacGregor, Graham A. Urinary catecholamines and the relationship with blood pressure and pharmacological therapy. Journal of Hypertension. 34(4):704–709, APR 2016.
5. Parmley WW. Pathophysiology and current therapy of congestive heart failure. J Am Coll Cardiol. 1989 Mar 15;13(4):771-85.
6. Y-Hassan S. Plasma epinephrine levels and its causal link to takotsubo syndrome revisited: Critical review with a diverse conclusion. Cardiovasc Revasc Med. 2018 Nov 7. pii: S1553-8389(18)30466-4. doi: 10.1016/j.carrev.2018.10.026.
7. Pelliccia F, Kaski JC, Crea F, Camici PG. Pathophysiology of Takotsubo Syndrome. Circulation. 2017 Jun 13;135(24):2426-2441. doi: 10.1161/circulationaha.116.027121.
8. Pal R, Singh SN, Chatterjee A, Saha M. Age-related changes in cardiovascular system, autonomic functions, and levels of BDNF of healthy active males: role of yogic practice. Age (Dordr). 2014;36(4):9683.
9. Lim SA, Cheong KJ. Regular Yoga Practice Improves Antioxidant Status, Immune Function, and Stress Hormone Releases in Young Healthy People: A Randomized, Double-Blind,

Controlled Pilot Study. J Altern Complement Med. 2015 Sep;21(9):530-8. doi: 10.1089/acm.2014.0044. Epub 2015 Jul 16.
10. Curiati JA, Bocchi E, Freire JO, Arantes AC, Braga M, Garcia Y, Guimarães G, Fo WJ. Meditation reduces sympathetic activation and improves the quality of life in elderly patients with optimally treated heart failure: a prospective randomized study. Journal of Alternative & Complementary Medicine. 2005;11:465–472.
11. Infante JR, Torres-Avisbal M, Pinel P, Vallejo JA, Peran F, Gonzalez F, Contreras P, Pacheco C, Latre JMa, Roldan A. Catecholamine levels in practitioners of the transcendental meditation technique. Physiology & behavior. 2001;72:141–146.

Oxytocin

1. Swaab DF, Pool CW, Nijveldt F. Immunofluorescence of vasopressin and oxytocin in the rat hypothalamo-neurohypophypopseal system. J Neural Transm. 1975;36(3–4):195–215.
2. Pittman QJ, Blume HW, Renaud LP. Connections of the hypothalamic paraventricular nucleus with the neurohypophysis, median eminence, amygdala, lateral septum and midbrain periaqueductal gray: An electrophysiological study in the rat. Brain Res. 1981;215(1–2):15–28.
3. Du Vigneaud V (1956). Hormones of the posterior pituitary gland. Oxytocin and vasopressin. Harvey Lectures, 51: 1-26.
4. Insel TR, Young LJ. The neurobiology of attachment. Nat Rev Neurosci. 2001;2(2):129–136.
5. Macdonald K, Macdonald TM. The peptide that binds: A systematic review of oxytocin and its prosocial effects in humans. Harv Rev Psychiatry. 2010;18(1):1–21.
6. Jones C, Barrera I, Brothers S, Ring R, Wahlestedt C. Oxytocin and social functioning. Dialogues Clin Neurosci. 2017;19(2):193-201.
7. Heinrichs M, Baumgartner T, Kirschbaum C, Ehlert U. Social support and oxytocin interact to suppress cortisol and subjective responses to psychosocial stress. Biol Psychiatry. 2003;54(12):1389–1398.
8. Kirsch P, Esslinger C, Chen Q, et al. Oxytocin modulates neural circuitry for social cognition and fear in humans. J Neurosci. 2005;25(49):11489–11493.
9. Lawson EA. The effects of oxytocin on eating behaviour and metabolism in humans. Nat Rev Endocrinol. 2017;13(12):700-709.
10. Ott V, et al. Oxytocin reduces reward-driven food intake in humans. Diabetes. 2013;62:3418–3425. doi: 10.2337/db13-0663.
11. Lawson EA, et al. Oxytocin reduces caloric intake in men. Obesity. 2015;23:950–956. doi: 10.1002/oby.21069.
12. Gutkowska, J., Jankowski, M., Mukaddam-Daher, S., & McCann, S.M.. (2000). Oxytocin is a cardiovascular hormone. Brazilian Journal of Medical and Biological Research, 33(6), 625-633.
13. Alizadeh AM, Mirzabeglo P. Is oxytocin a therapeutic factor for ischemic heart disease? Peptides. 2013;45:66–72. doi: 10.1016/j.peptides.2013.04.016.
14. Gonzalez-Reyes A, Menaouar A, Yip D, Danalache B, Plante E, Noiseux N, et al. Molecular mechanisms underlying oxytocin-induced cardiomyocyte protection from simulated ischemia-reperfusion. Mol Cell Endocrinol. 2015;412:170–81. doi: 10.1016/j.mce.2015.04.028.
15. Jankowski M, Broderick TL, Gutkowska J. Oxytocin and cardioprotection in diabetes and obesity. BMC Endocr Disord. 2016;16(1):34. Published 2016 Jun 7. doi:10.1186/s12902-016-0110-1.
16. Gutkowska J, Jankowski M. Oxytocin revisited: its role in cardiovascular regulation. J Neuroendocrinol. 2012;24(4):599–608. doi: 10.1111/j.1365-2826.2011.02235.x.
17. Kirsch P, Esslinger C, Chen Q, Mier D, Lis S, Siddhanti S, Gruppe H, Mattay VS, Gallhofer B, Meyer-Lindenberg A. Oxytocin modulates neural circuitry for social cognition and fear in humans. Journal of Neuroscience. 2005;25(49):11489–11493.
18. Kosfeld M, Heinrichs M, Zak PJ, Fischbacher U, Fehr E. Oxytocin increases trust in humans. Nature. 2005;435(7042):673–676.

19. Heinrichs M, Baumgartner T, Kirschbaum C, Ehlert U. Social support and oxytocin interact to suppress cortisol and subjective responses to psychosocial stress. Biological Psychiatry. 2003;54(12):1389–1398.
20. Kubzansky LD, Mendes WB, Appleton AA, Block J, Adler GK. A heartfelt response: Oxytocin effects in response to social stress in men and women. Biol Psychol. 2012;90(1):1-9.
21. Jayaram N, Varambally S, Behere RV, et al. Effect of yoga therapy on plasma oxytocin and facial emotion recognition deficits in patients of schizophrenia. Indian J Psychiatry. 2013;55(Suppl 3):S409-13.

Prolactin

1. Ben-Jonathan N, Hugo ER, Brandebourg TD, LaPensee CR. Focus on prolactin as a metabolic hormone. Trends Endocrinol Metab. 2006;17:110–116.
2. Therkelsen KE, Abraham TM, Pedley A, et al. Association Between Prolactin and Incidence of Cardiovascular Risk Factors in the Framingham Heart Study. J Am Heart Assoc. 2016;5(2):e002640. Published 2016 Feb 23. doi:10.1161/JAHA.115.002640.
3. Haring R, Friedrich N, Völzke H, Vasan RS, Felix SB, Dörr M, Meyer zu Schwabedissen HE, Nauck M, Wallaschofski H. Positive association of serum prolactin concentrations with all-cause and cardiovascular mortality. Eur Heart J. 2014 May;35(18):1215-21. doi: 10.1093/eurheartj/ehs233. Epub 2012 Jul 26.
4. Oka T, Tanahashi T, Sudo N, Lkhagvasuren B, Yamada Y. Changes in fatigue, autonomic functions, and blood biomarkers due to sitting isometric yoga in patients with chronic fatigue syndrome. Biopsychosoc Med. 2018 Apr 10;12:3. doi: 10.1186/s13030-018-0123-2. eCollection 2018.
5. Rani M, Singh U, Agrawal GG, Natu SM, Kala S, Ghildiyal A, Srivastava N. Impact of Yoga Nidra on menstrual abnormalities in females of reproductive age. J Altern Complement Med. 2013 Dec;19(12):925-9. doi: 10.1089/acm.2010.0676. Epub 2013 May 6.

Serotonin

1. Haduch, A. , Bromek, E. , Kot, M. , Kamińska, K. , Gołembiowska, K. and Daniel, W. A. (2015), The cytochrome P450 2D-mediated formation of serotonin from 5-methoxytryptamine in the brain in vivo: a microdialysis study. J. Neurochem., 133: 83-92. doi:10.1111/jnc.13031.
2. Merens W., Willem Van der Does A.J., Spinhoven P. The effects of serotonin manipulations on emotional information processing and mood. J. Affect. Disord. 2007;103:43–62.
3. Young S.N., Leyton M. The role of serotonin in human mood and social interaction: Insight from altered tryptophan levels. Pharmacol. Biochem. Behav. 2002;71:857–86.
4. Monti J.M. Serotonin control of sleep-wake behavior. Sleep Med. Rev. 2011;15:269–281.
5. Lam D.D., Garfield A.S., Marston O.J., Shaw J., Heisler L.K. Brain serotonin system in the coordination of food intake and body weight. Pharmacol. Biochem. Behav. 2010;97:84–91.
6. Keszthelyi D., Troost F.J., Masclee A.A.M. Understanding the role of tryptophan and serotonin metabolism in gastrointestinal function. Neurogastroenterol. Motil. 2009;21:1239–1249.
7. Gershon M.D., Ross L.L. Location of sites of 5-hydroxytryptamine storage and metabolism by radioautography. J. Physiol. 1966;186:477–492.
8. Matsuda M., Imaoka T., Vomachka A.J., Gudelsky G.A., Hou Z., Mistry M., Bailey J.P., Nieport K.M., Walther D.J., Bader M., et al. Serotonin regulates mammary gland development via an autocrine-paracrine loop. Dev. Cell. 2004;6:193–203.
9. Lesurtel M., Graf R., Aleil B., Walther D.J., Tian Y., Jochum W., Gachet C., Bader M., Clavien P.A. Platelet-derived serotonin mediates liver regeneration. Science. 2006;312:104–107.
10. Yadav V.K., Ryu J.H., Suda N., Tanaka K.F., Gingrich J.A., Schutz G., Glorieux F.H., Chiang C.Y., Zajac J.D., Insogna K.L., et al. Lrp5 controls bone formation by inhibiting serotonin synthesis in the duodenum. Cell. 2008;135:825–837.

11. Kim H., Toyofuku Y., Lynn F.C., Chak E., Uchida T., Mizukami H., Fujitani Y., Kawamori R., Miyatsuka T., Kosaka Y., et al. Serotonin regulates pancreatic beta cell mass during pregnancy. Nat. Med. 2010;16:804–808.
12. Ohara-Imaizumi M., Kim H., Yoshida M., Fujiwara T., Aoyagi K., Toyofuku Y., Nakamichi Y., Nishiwaki C., Okamura T., Uchida T. Serotonin regulates glucose-stimulated insulin secretion from pancreatic β cells during pregnancy. Proc. Natl. Acad. Sci. USA. 2013;110:19420–19425.
13. Brown GL, Goodwin FK, Ballenger JC, Goyer PF, Major LF. Aggression in humans correlates with cerebrospinal fluid amine metabolites. Psychiatry Res. 1979;1:131–139.
14. Roy A, De Jong J, Linnoila M. Cerebrospinal fluid monoamine metabolites and suicidal behavior in depressed patients. A 5-year follow-up study. Arch Gen Psychiatry. 1989;46:609–612.
15. Kim J, Gorman J. The psychobiology of anxiety. Clinical Neuroscience Research. 2005;4:335–347.
16. Traskman L, Asberg M, Bertilsson L, Sjostrand L. Monoamine metabolites in CSF and suicidal behavior. Arch Gen Psychiatry. 1981;38:631–636.
17. Kubzansky LD, Kawachi I. Going to the heart of the matter: do negative emotions cause coronary heart disease? J Psychosom Res. 2000 Apr-May;48(4-5):323-37.
18. Sirois BC, Burg MM. Negative emotion and coronary heart disease. A review. Behav Modif. 2003 Jan;27(1):83-102.
19. Rosengren A, Hawken S, Ounpuu S, et al. Association of psychosocial risk factors with risk of acute myocardial infarction in 11119 cases and 13648 controls from 52 countries (INTERHEART study): case-control study. Lancet. 2004;364:953–962.
20. May M. Does psychological distress predict the risk of ischemic stroke and transient ischemic attack? The Caerphilly Study. Stroke. 2002;33:7–12.
21. Van Dooren FEP, Nefs G, Schram MT, Verhey FRJ, Denollet J, Pouwer F. Depression and Risk of Mortality in People with Diabetes Mellitus: A Systematic Review and Meta-Analysis. Berthold HK, ed. PLoS ONE. 2013;8(3): e57058.
22. Chida Y, Steptoe A. The association of anger and hostility with future coronary heart disease: a meta-analytic review of prospective evidence. J Am Coll Cardiol. 2009;53:936–946.
23. Saran RK, Puri A, Agarwal M. Depression and the heart. Indian Heart Journal. 2012;64(4):397-401.
24. Pal R, Singh SN, Chatterjee A, Saha M. Age-related changes in cardiovascular system, autonomic functions, and levels of BDNF of healthy active males: role of yogic practice. Age (Dordr). 2014;36(4):9683.
25. Lim SA, Cheong KJ, Regular Yoga Practice Improves Antioxidant Status, Immune Function, and Stress Hormone Releases in Young Healthy People: A Randomized, Double-Blind, Controlled Pilot Study. J Altern Complement Med 2015 Sep;21(9):530-8.
26. Bujatti M, Biederer P. Serotonin, noradrenaline, dopamine metabolites in transcendental meditation-technique. Journal of Neural Transmission. 1976;39:257–267.

Blood pressure/Hypertension

1. https://www.heart.org/en/health-topics/high-blood-pressure/understanding-blood-pressure-readings/monitoring-your-blood-pressure-at-home.
2. Whelton PL, Carey RM, Aronow WS, et al. ACC/AHA/AAPA/ABC/ACPM/AGS/APhA/ASH/ASPC/NMA/PCNA. Guideline for the Prevention, Detection, Evaluation, and Management of High Blood Pressure in Adults 2017. Executive Summary: A Report of the American College of Cardiology/American Heart Association Task Force on Clinical Practice Guidelines. Hypertension. 2018 Jun;71(6):1269-1324. doi: 10.1161/HYP.0000000000000066. Epub 2017 Nov 13.
3. Benjamin EJ, Virani SS, Callaway CW, Chamberlain AM, et al. Heart Disease and Stroke Statistics-2018 Update: A Report From the American Heart Association. Circulation. 2018 Mar 20;137(12):e67-e492. doi: 10.1161/CIR.0000000000000558. Epub 2018 Jan 31.
4. Chobanian AV, Bakris GL, Black HR, et al. The Seventh Report of the Joint National Committee on Prevention, Detection, Evaluation, and Treatment of High Blood Pressure: the

JNC 7 report. JAMA. 2003;289:2560–2572.
5. Rapsomaniki E, Timmis A, George J, et al. Blood pressure and incidence of twelve cardiovascular diseases: lifetime risks, healthy life-years lost, and age-specific associations in 1·25 million people. Lancet. 2014 May 31;383(9932):1899-911. doi: 10.1016/S0140-6736(14)60685-1.
6. Aidietis A, Laucevicius A, Marinskis G. Hypertension and cardiac arrhythmias. Curr Pharm Des. 2007;13(25):2545-55.
7. Connor A. Emdin, Peter M. Rothwell, Gholamreza Salimi-Khorshidi, Amit Kiran, Nathalie Conrad, Thomas Callender, Ziyah Mehta, Sarah T. Pendlebury, Simon G. Anderson, Hamid Mohseni, Mark Woodward, Kazem Rahimi. Blood Pressure and Risk of Vascular Dementia. Stroke, 2016; STROKEAHA.116.012658 doi: 10.1161/STROKEAHA.116.012658.
8. Bhargava M, Ikram MK, Wong TY. How does hypertension affect your eyes? J Hum Hypertens. 2012 Feb;26(2):71-83. doi: 10.1038/jhh.2011.37. Epub 2011 Apr 21.
9. Nunes KP, Labazi H, Webb RC. New insights into hypertension-associated erectile dysfunction. Curr Opin Nephrol Hypertens. 2012 Mar;21(2):163-70. doi: 10.1097/MNH.0b013e32835021bd.
10. https://www.heart.org/-/media/data-import/downloadables/heart-disease-and-stroke-statistics-2018---at-a-glance-ucm_498848.pdf.
11. Lewington S, Clarke R, Qizilbash N, Peto R, Collins R; Prospective Studies Collaboration . Age-specific relevance of usual blood pressure to vascular mortality: a meta-analysis of individual data for one million adults in 61 prospective studies. Lancet. 2002;360:1903–1913014;383:1899-911.
12. Vasan RS, Larson MG, Leip EP, et al. Impact of high-normal blood pressure on the risk of cardiovascular disease. N Engl J Med. 2001;345(18):1291-1297.
13. The SPRINT Research Group. A Randomized Trial of Intensive versus Standard Blood-Pressure Control. N Engl J Med 2015; 373:2103-2116. DOI: 10.1056/NEJMoa1511939.
14. Gueyffier, F. et al. Effect of antihypertensive drug treatment on cardiovascular outcomes in women and men. A meta-analysis of individual patient data from randomized, controlled trials. The INDANA Investigators. Ann Intern Med 126, 761–767 (1997).
15. Hardy ST, Loehr LR, Butler KR, et al. Reducing the Blood Pressure-Related Burden of Cardiovascular Disease: Impact of Achievable Improvements in Blood Pressure Prevention and Control. J Am Heart Assoc. 2015;4(10):e002276. Published 2015 Oct 27. doi:10.1161/JAHA.115.002276.
16. Cook NR, Cohen J, Hebert PR, et al. Implications of small reductions in diastolic blood pressure for primary prevention. Arch Intern Med. 1995;155(7):701–709.
17. Lewington S, Clarke R, Qizilbash N, Peto R, Collins R. Age-specific relevance of usual blood pressure to vascular mortality: a meta-analysis of individual data for one million adults in 61 prospective studies. The Lancet. 2002;360(9349):1903–1913.
18. Hackam DG, Khan NA, Hemmelgarn BR, et al. The 2010 Canadian Hypertension Education Program recommendations for the management of hypertension: part 2 - therapy. Can J Cardiol. 2010 May;26(5):249-58.; NIHCG, 2013.
19. Erdine S, Ari O, Zanchetti A, Cifkova R et al. ESH-ESC guidelines for the management of hypertension. Herz. 2006 Jun;31(4):331-8.
20. Nicoll R, Henein MY. Hypertension and lifestyle modification: how useful are the guidelines? The British Journal of General Practice. 2010;60(581):879-880. doi:10.3399/bjgp10X544014.
21. Wanpen Vongpatanasin. Resistant Hypertension.A Review of Diagnosis and Management. JAMA. 2014;311(21):2216-2224.
22. Persell SD. Prevalence of resistant hypertension in the United States, 2003-2008. Hypertension. 2011;57:1076–1080.
23. Egan BM, Zhao Y, Axon RN, Brzezinski WA, Ferdinand KC. Uncontrolled and apparent treatment resistant hypertension in the United States, 1988-2008. Circulation. 2011;124:1046–1058.
24. de la Sierra A, Segura J, Banegas JR, Gorostidi M, de la Cruz JJ, Armario P, Oliveras A, Ruilope LM. Clinical features of 8295 patients with resistant hypertension classified on the basis of ambulatory blood pressure monitoring. Hypertension. 2011;57:898–902.
25. Roberie DR, Elliott WJ. What is the prevalence of resistant hypertension in the United States. Curr Opin Cardiol. 2012;27:386–391.
26. Calhoun DA, Jones D, Textor S, Goff DC, Murphy TP, Toto RD, White A, Cushman WC,

White WB, Sica D, Ferdinand K, Giles TD, Falkner B, Carey RM. American Heart Association Scientific statement on resistant hypertension: diagnosis, evaluation, and treatment. Hypertension. 2008;51:1403–1419.
27. Pierdomenico SD, Lapenna D, Bucci A, Di Tommaso R, Di Mascio R, Manente BM, Caldarella MP, Neri M, Cuccurullo F, Mezzettti A. Cardiovascular outcome in treated hypertensive patients with responder, masked, false resistant and true resistant hypertension. Am J Hypertens. 2005;18:1422–1428.
28. Isaksson H, Ostergren J. Prognosis in therapy-resistant hypertension. J Intern Med. 1994;236:643–649.
29. NIH 2015: http://www.nhlbi.nih.gov/news/press-releases/2015/landmark-nih-study-shows-intensive-blood-pressure-management-may-save-lives. Accessed 1/19/18.
30. Selvin E, Erlinger TP. Prevalence of and risk factors for peripheral arterial disease in the United States: results from the National Health and Nutrition Examination Survey, 1999-2000. Circulation 2004;110:738-43.
31. Rahimi K, Emdin C, MacMahon S. The epidemiology of blood pressure and its worldwide management. Circ Res 2015;116:925-36.
32. Emdin CA, Anderson SG, Callender T, et al. Usual blood pressure, peripheral arterial disease, and vascular risk: cohort study of 4.2 million adults. BMJ. 2015;351:h4865. Published 2015 Sep 29. doi:10.1136/bmj.h4865.
33. Ning L, Yang L. Hypertension might be a risk factor for erectile dysfunction: a meta-analysis. Andrologia. 2017 May;49(4). doi: 10.1111/and.12644. Epub 2016 Aug 5.
34. Sarma AV, Hotaling JM, de Boer IH, et al. Blood pressure, antihypertensive medication use, and risk of erectile dysfunction in men with type I diabetes. J Hypertens. 2019 May;37(5):1070-1076. doi: 10.1097/HJH.0000000000001988.
35. Papatsoris AG, Korantzopoulos PG. Hypertension, antihypertensive therapy, and erectile dysfunction. Angiology. 2006 Jan-Feb;57(1):47–52.
36. Osamor PE, Owumi BE. Complementary and alternative medicine in the management of hypertension in an urban Nigerian community. BMC Complementary and Alternative Medicine. 2010;10:36. doi:10.1186/1472-6882-10-36.
37. Wang J, Xiong X. Evidence-Based Chinese Medicine for Hypertension. Evidence-based Complementary and Alternative Medicine : eCAM. 2013;2013:978398. doi:10.1155/2013/978398.
38. Cohen D, Townsend RR. Yoga and hypertension. The Journal of Clinical Hypertension. 2007;9:800–801.
39. Wolff M, Sundquist K, Larsson Lönn S, Midlöv P. Impact of yoga on blood pressure and quality of life in patients with hypertension – a controlled trial in primary care, matched for systolic blood pressure. BMC Cardiovascular Disorders. 2013;13:111. doi:10.1186/1471-2261-13-111.nces
40. Chauhan A, Semwal DK, Mishra SP, Semwal RB. Yoga Practice Improves the Body Mass Index and Blood Pressure: A Randomized Controlled Trial. Int J Yoga. 2017;10(2):103-106.
41. Hagins M, States R, Selfe T, et al. Effectiveness of Yoga for Hypertension: Systematic Review and Meta-Analysis Evidence-Based Complementary and Alternative Medicine. Volume 2013 (2013), Article ID 649836.
42. Yang H, Wu X, Wang M. The Effect of Three Different Meditation Exercises on Hypertension: A Network Meta-Analysis. Evidence-based Complementary and Alternative Medicine: eCAM. 2017;2017:9784271.
43. Shirley Telles, Sadhana Verma, Sachin Kumar Sharma, Ram Kumar Gupta, and Acharya Balkrishna. Alternate-Nostril Yoga Breathing Reduced Blood Pressure While Increasing Performance in a Vigilance Test. Med Sci Monit Basic Res. 2017; 23: 392–398.
44. Tyagi A, Cohen M. Yoga and hypertension: a systematic review. Altern Ther Health Med. 2014 Mar-Apr;20(2):32-59.
45. Devasena I., Narhare P. Effect of yoga on heart rate and blood pressure and its clinical significance. International Journal of Biological & Medical Research. 2011;2:750–753.
46. Wolff M, Sundquist K, Larsson Lönn S, et al. Impact of yoga on blood pressure and quality of life in patients with hypertension - a controlled trial in primary care, matched for systolic blood pressure. BMC Cardiovasc Disord. 2013 Dec 7;13: 111.
47. Wolff M, Ashfaque A. Memon, John P, et al. Yoga's effect on inflammatory biomarkers and metabolic risk factors in a high-risk population - a controlled trial in primary care. BMC Cardiovasc Disord. 2015 Aug 19; 15:91.

Blood sugar/Diabetes

1. http://www.diabetes.org/diabetes-basics/statistics/?referrer=https://www.google.com/- accessed 1/1/18).
2. Danaei G, Finucane MM, Lu Y, et al. National, regional, and global trends in fasting plasma glucose and diabetes prevalence since 1980: systematic analysis of health examination surveys and epidemiological studies with 370 country-years and 2.7 million participants. Lancet. 2011;378:31–40.
3. Go AS, Mozaffarian D, Roger VL, et al. Heart Disease and Stroke Statistics—2014 Update: A Report From the American Heart Association. Circulation. 2014;129:e28–e292.
4. Lam D. W., LeRoith D. The worldwide diabetes epidemic. Current Opinion in Endocrinology, Diabetes and Obesity. 2012;19(2):93–96.
5. Boyle JP, Thompson TJ, Gregg EW, Barker LE, Williamson DF. Projection of the year 2050 burden of diabetes in the US adult population: dynamic modeling of incidence, mortality, and prediabetes prevalence. Popul Health Metr 2010;8:29.
6. Bhutani J, Bhutani S. Worldwide burden of diabetes. Indian Journal of Endocrinology and Metabolism. 2014;18(6):868-870.
7. Maahs DM, West NA, Lawrence JM, Mayer-Davis EJ. Epidemiology of type 1 diabetes. Endocrinol Metab Clin North Am. 2010;39:481–497.
8. Daneman D. Type 1 diabetes. Lancet. 2006;367:847–858.;Devendra D, Liu E, Eisenbarth GS. Type 1 diabetes: recent developments. BMJ. 2004;328:750–754.
9. Dabelea D, Mayer-Davis EJ, Saydah S, Imperatore G, Linder B, Divers J, Bell R, Badaru A, Talton JW, Crume T, et al. Prevalence of type 1 and type 2 diabetes among children and adolescents from 2001 to 2009. JAMA. 2014;311:1778–1786.
10. https://www.niddk.nih.gov/health-information/diabetes/overview/symptoms-causes.
11. American Diabetes Association. Diagnosis and classification of diabetes mellitus. Diabetes Care. 2013;36 Suppl 1:S67–S74.
12. American Diabetes Association. Diagnosis and classification of diabetes mellitus. Diabetes Care. 2012;36 Suppl 1(Suppl 1):S67-74.
13. Buysschaert M, Bergman M. Definition of prediabetes. Med Clin North Am. 2011;95:289–297.
14. https://www.cdc.gov/media/releases/2017/p0718-diabetes-report.html.
15. Giovannucci E, Harlan DM, Archer MC, Bergenstal RM, Gapstur SM, Habel LA, et al. Diabetes and cancer: a consensus report. Diabetes Care. 2010 Jul. 33(7):1674-85.
16. Murphy HR, Steel SA, Roland JM, Morris D, Ball V, Campbell PJ, et al. Obstetric and perinatal outcomes in pregnancies complicated by Type 1 and Type 2 diabetes: influences of glycaemic control, obesity and social disadvantage. Diabet Med. 2011 Sep. 28(9):1060-7.
17. Skyler JS, Bakris GL, Bonifacio E, et al. Differentiation of Diabetes by Pathophysiology, Natural History, and Prognosis. Diabetes. 2016;66(2):241-255.
18. Shah CP, Chen C. Review of therapeutic advances in diabetic retinopathy. Ther Adv Endocrinol Metab. 2011;2(1):39-53.
19. United States Renal Data System. 2016 USRDS Annual Data Report: Epidemiology of Kidney Disease in the United States.
20. Junmei Miao Jonasson, Weimin Ye, Pär Sparén, Jan Apelqvist, Olof Nyrén, Kerstin Brismar. Risks of Nontraumatic Lower-Extremity Amputations in Patients with Type 1 Diabetes. Diabetes Care Aug 2008, 31 (8) 1536-1540; DOI: 10.2337/dc08-0344.
21. DeFronzo RA, Abdul-Ghani M. Assessment and treatment of cardiovascular risk in prediabetes: impaired glucose tolerance and impaired fasting glucose. Am J Cardiol. 2011;108:3B–24B.
22. Preis SR, Pencina MJ, Hwang SJ, et al. Trends in cardiovascular disease risk factors in individuals with and without diabetes mellitus in the Framingham Heart Study. Circulation. 2009;120:212–220.
23. Martin-Timon I, Sevillano-Collantes C, Segura-Galindo A, Del Canizo-Gomez FJ. Type 2 diabetes and cardiovascular disease: have all risk factors the same strength? World J Diabetes. 2014;5(4):444–470. doi: 10.4239/wjd.v5.i4.444.

24. Lloyd-Jones, D.M., Leip, E.P., Larson, M.G. et al. Prediction of lifetime risk for cardiovascular disease by risk factor burden at 50 years of age. Circulation. 2006; 113: 791–798.
25. Berry C, Tardif JC, Bourassa MG. Coronary heart disease in patients with diabetes: part II: recent advances in coronary revascularization. J Am Coll Cardiol. 2007;49:643–656.
26. Smith JW, Marcus F, Serokman R. Prognosis of patients with diabetes mellitus after acute myocardial infarction. Am J Cardiol.1984;54:718–721.
27. Aronson D, Rayfield EJ, Chesebro JH. Mechanisms determining course and outcome of diabetic patients who have had acute myocardial infarction. Ann Intern Med. 1997;126:296–306. Donahoe SM, Stewart GC, McCabe CH, et al. Diabetes and mortality following acute coronary syndromes. JAMA. 2007;298:765–775.
28. Berry C, Tardif JC, Bourassa MG. Coronary heart disease in patients with diabetes: part II: recent advances in coronary revascularization. J Am Coll Cardiol. 2007;49:643–656. D Lau, G Shen. Cardiovascular Complications of Diabetes. Canadian Journal of Diabetes. October 2013 Volume 37, Issue 5, Pages 279–281.
29. Barr EL, Zimmet PZ, Welborn TA, et al. Risk of cardiovascular and all-cause mortality in individuals with diabetes mellitus, impaired fasting glucose, and impaired glucose tolerance: the Australian Diabetes, Obesity, and Lifestyle Study (AusDiab) Circulation. 2007;116:151–157.
30. https://www.heart.org/en/health-topics/diabetes/why-diabetes-matters/cardiovascular-disease--diabetes.
31. Stamler J, Vaccaro O, Neaton JD, Wentworth D. Diabetes, other risk factors, and 12-year cardiovascular mortality for men screened in the Multiple Risk Factor Intervention Trial (MRFIT). Diabetes Care. 1993;16:434–444.
32. Huxley, R., Barzi, F., and Woodward, M. Excess risk of fatal coronary heart disease associated with diabetes in men and women: meta-analysis of 37 prospective cohort studies. BMJ. 2006; 332: 73–78.
33. Huxley, R., Barzi, F., and Woodward, M. Excess risk of fatal coronary heart disease associated with diabetes in men and women: meta-analysis of 37 prospective cohort studies. BMJ. 2006; 332: 73–78.
34. Haffner SM, Lehto S, Rönnemaa T, Pyörälä K, Laakso M. Mortality from coronary heart disease in subjects with type 2 diabetes and in nondiabetic subjects with and without prior myocardial infarction. N Engl J Med. 1998;339:229–34.
35. Schramm TK, Gislason GH, Kober L, et al. Diabetes patients requiring glucose-lowering therapy and nondiabetics with a prior myocardial infarction carry the same cardiovascular risk: a population study of 3.3 million people. Circulation. 2008;117:1945–1954.
36. Hajar R. Diabetes as "Coronary Artery Disease Risk Equivalent": A Historical Perspective. Heart Views. 2017;18(1):34-37.
37. Petar M. Seferović, Mark C. Petrie, Gerasimos S. Filippatos, et al. Type 2 diabetes mellitus and heart failure: a position statement from the Heart Failure Association of the European Society of Cardiology. European J of Heart Failure. Volume 20, Issue 5. May 2018. Pages 853-872.
38. Díaz-Redondo A, Giráldez-García C, Carrillo L, et al. Modifiable risk factors associated with prediabetes in men and women: a cross-sectional analysis of the cohort study in primary health care on the evolution of patients with prediabetes (PREDAPS-Study). BMC Family Practice. 2015;16:5.
39. The Emerging Risk Factors Collaboration. Diabetes mellitus, fasting blood glucose concentration, and risk of vascular disease: a collaborative meta-analysis of 102 prospective studies. Lancet. 2010;375: 2215–2222.
40. Yamini S. Levitzky, Michael J. Pencina, et al. Impact of Impaired Fasting Glucose on Cardiovascular Disease. JACC, 2008. Volume 51, Issue 3, Pages 264-270.
41. Huang Y, Cai X, Mai W, Li M, Hu Y. Association between prediabetes and risk of cardiovascular disease and all cause mortality: systematic review and meta-analysis. The BMJ. 2016;355: i5953.

42. Fonville S, Zandbergen AA, Koudstaal PJ, den Hertog HM. Prediabetes in patients with stroke or transient ischemic attack: prevalence, risk and clinical management. Cerebrovasc Dis. 2014;37(6):393–400.
43. Criqui MH. Peripheral arterial disease--epidemiological aspects. Vasc Med. 2001;6:3–7.; Shah B, Rockman CB, Guo Y, Chesner J, Schwartzbard AZ, Weintraub HS, et al. Diabetes and vascular disease in different arterial territories. Diabetes Care. American Diabetes Association. 2014 Jun;37(6):1636–1642.
44. Golomb BA, Dang TT, Criqui MH. Peripheral arterial disease: morbidity and mortality implications. Circulation 2006;114:688–699. ;Berger JS, Hochman J, Lobach I, Adelman MA, Riles TS, Rockman CB.Modifiable risk factor burden and the prevalence of peripheral artery disease in different vascular territories. J Vasc Surg 2013;58:673–681.
45. Ness J, Aronow WS. Prevalence of coexistence of coronary artery disease, ischemic stroke, and peripheral arterial disease in older persons, mean age 80 years, in an academic hospital-based geriatrics practice. J Am Geriatr Soc. 1999 Oct;47(10):1255-6.
46. Ankle Brachial Index Collaboration. Ankle brachial index combined with Framingham Risk Score to predict cardiovascular events and mortality: a meta-analysis. JAMA. 2008; 300:197-208.
47. Jeffrey I. Weitz , John Byrne , G. Patrick Clagett , et al. Diagnosis and Treatment of Chronic Arterial Insufficiency of the Lower Extremities: A Critical Review. Circulation. 1996;94:3026–3049.
48. Kannel WB, McGee DL. Update on some epidemiologic features of intermittent claudication: the Framingham Study. J Am Geriatr Soc..1985; 33:13-18.; Ankle Brachial Index Collaboration. Ankle brachial index combined with Framingham Risk Score to predict cardiovascular events and mortality: a meta-analysis. JAMA. 2008; 300:197-208.
49. Criqui MH, Langer RD, Fronek A, et al. Mortality over a period of 10 years in patients with peripheral arterial disease. N Engl J Med 1992;326:381–386.
50. Bosevski M, Peovska I. Clinical usefulness of assessment of ankle-brachial index and carotid stenosis in type 2 diabetic population—three-year cohort follow-up of mortality. Angiology 2013;64:64–68.
51. Giuliano FA, Leriche A, Jaudinot EO, de Gendre AS. Prevalence of erectile dysfunction among 7689 patients with diabetes or hypertension, or both. Urology. 2004;64:1196–1201.
52. Kalter-Leibovici O, Wainstein J, Ziv A, Harman-Bohem I, Murad H, Raz I. Clinical, socioeconomic, and lifestyle parameters associated with erectile dysfunction among diabetic men. Diabetes Care. 2005;28:1739–1744.
53. Yamada T, Hara K, Umematsu H, Suzuki R, Kadowaki T. Erectile dysfunction and cardiovascular events in diabetic men: a meta-analysis of observational studies. PLoS One. 2012;7:e43673.
54. UK Prospective Diabetes Study (UKPDS) Group Intensive blood-glucose control with sulphonylureas or insulin compared with conventional treatment and risk of complications in patients with type 2 diabetes (UKPDS 33) Lancet. 1998;352:837–53. UK Prospective Diabetes Study (UKPDS) Group.
55. Center for Disease Control and Prevention. (2012). Diabetes Public Health Resources: Staying Healthy with Diabetes. Retrieved from Atlanta, GA: http://www.cdc.gov/diabetes/consumer/healthy.htm.
56. The Diabetes Control and Complications Trial Research Group The effect of intensive treatment of diabetes on the development and progression of long-term complications in insulin-dependent diabetes mellitus. N Engl J Med 1993;329:977–986.
57. Nathan DM, Cleary PA, Backlund JY, et al. Diabetes Control and Complications Trial/Epidemiology of Diabetes Interventions and Complications (DCCT/EDIC) Study Research Group Intensive diabetes treatment and cardiovascular disease in patients with type 1 diabetes. N Engl J Med 2005;353:2643–2653.
58. UK Prospective Diabetes Study (UKPDS) Group Intensive blood-glucose control with sulphonylureas or insulin compared with conventional treatment and risk of complications in patients with type 2 diabetes (UKPDS 33). Lancet 1998;352:837–853.

59. Skyler JS, Bergenstal R, Bonow RO, et al. Intensive glycemic control and the prevention of cardiovascular events: implications of the ACCORD, ADVANCE, and VA diabetes trials: a position statement of the American Diabetes Association and a scientific statement of the American College of Cardiology Foundation and the American Heart Association. Circulation. 2009;119:351–357.
60. Ray KK, Seshasai SRK, Wijesuriya S, et al. Effect of intensive control of glucose on cardiovascular outcomes and death in patients with diabetes mellitus: a meta-analysis of randomised controlled trials. Lancet. 2009;373:1765–1772.
61. Kelly TN, Bazzano LA, Fonseca VA, et al. Systematic review: glucose control and cardiovascular disease in type 2 diabetes. Ann Intern Med. 2009;151:394–403.
62. Boussageon R, Bejan-Angoulvant T, Saadatian-Elahi M, et al. Effect of intensive glucose lowering treatment on all cause mortality, cardiovascular death, and microvascular events in type 2 diabetes: meta-analysis of randomised controlled trials. BMJ. 2011;343:d4169–d14169.
63. Alvarez CA, Lingvay I, Vuylsteke V, Koffarnus RL, McGuire DK. Cardiovascular Risk in Diabetes Mellitus: Complication of the Disease or of Antihyperglycemic Medications. Clin Pharmacol Ther. 2015;98(2):145-61.
64. Gore MO, McGuire DK. Drugs for type 2 diabetes mellitus: the imperative for cardiovascular outcome assessment. Diabetes & vascular disease research : official journal of the International Society of Diabetes and Vascular Disease. 2012;9:85–8.
65. Valeska Ormazabal, Soumyalekshmi Nair, Omar Elfeky, Claudio Aguayo, Carlos Salomon, Felipe A. Zuñiga. Association between insulin resistance and the development of cardiovascular disease. Cardiovascular Diabetology, 2018, Volume 17, Number 1, Page 1.
66. Chilton R, Wyatt J, Nandish S, Oliveros R, Lujan M. Cardiovascular comorbidities of type 2 diabetes mellitus: defining the potential of glucagonlike peptide-1-based therapies. Am J Med. 2011 Jan;124(1 Suppl):S35-53. doi: 10.1016/j.amjmed.2010.11.004.
67. Gillies CL, Abrams KR, Lambert PC, et al. Pharmacological and lifestyle interventions to prevent or delay type 2 diabetes in people with impaired glucose tolerance: systematic review and meta-analysis. BMJ. 2007;334:299.
68. Bantle JP, Wylie-Rosett J, Albright AL, et al. ; American Diabetes Association Nutrition recommendations and interventions for diabetes: a position statement of the American Diabetes Association. Diabetes Care 2008;31(Suppl. 1):S61–S78.
69. Boulé NG, Haddad E, Kenny GP, Wells GA, Sigal RJ. Effects of exercise on glycemic control and body mass in type 2 diabetes mellitus: a meta-analysis of controlled clinical trials. JAMA 2001;286:1218–1227.
70. Cohen RV, Pinheiro JC, Schiavon CA, et al. Effects of gastric bypass surgery in patients with type 2 diabetes and only mild obesity. Diabetes Care. 2012;35:1420–1428.
71. Hostalek U, Gwilt M, Hildemann S. Therapeutic Use of Metformin in Prediabetes and Diabetes Prevention. Drugs. 2015;75(10):1071-94.
72. Diabetes Prevention Program Research Group. Long-term effects of lifestyle intervention or metformin on diabetes development and microvascular complications over 15-year follow-up: the Diabetes Prevention Program Outcomes Study. The Lancet: Diabetes & Endocrinology. 2015;3(11):866–875.
73. Monro R, Power J, Coumar A, Dandona P. Yoga therapy for NIDDM: a controlled trial. Complementary Med Res 1992; 6: 66–8.
74. Jain S, Uppal A, Bhatnagar S, Talukdar B. A study of response pattern of non-insulin dependent diabetics to yoga therapy. Diabetes Res Clin Pract 1993; 19: 69–74.
75. Singh S, Malhotra V, Singh K, Sharma S. A preliminary report on the role of yoga asanas on oxidative stress in non-insulin dependent diabetes. Indian J Clin Biochem 2001; 16: 216–20.
76. Fields JZ, Walton KG, Schneider RH, et al. Effect of a multimodality natural medicine program on carotid atherosclerosis in older subjects: a pilot trial of Maharishi Vedic Medicine. Am J Cardiol 2002; 89: 952–8.
77. Jain S, Uppal A, Bhatnagar S, Talukdar B. A studyof response pattern of non-insulin dependent diabetics to yoga therapy. Diabetes Res Clin Pract1993;19:69 –74.; Divekar M,

Bhat M, Mulla A. Effect of yoga therapy in diabetes and obesity. J Diab Assoc Ind 1978;17:75– 8.
78. Innes KE, Bourguignon C, Taylor AG. Risk indices associated with the insulin resistance syndrome, cardiovascular disease and possible protection with yoga: a systematic review. J Am Board Fam Pract. 2005;18:491–519. doi: 10.3122/jabfm.18.6.491.
79. Innes KE, Selfe TK. Yoga for Adults with Type 2 Diabetes: A Systematic Review of Controlled Trials. Journal of Diabetes Research. 2016;2016:6979370. doi:10.1155/2016/6979370.
80. Cui J, Yan J, Yan L, Pan L, Le J, Guo Y. Effects of yoga in adults with type 2 diabetes mellitus: A meta-analysis. Journal of Diabetes Investigation. 2017;8(2):201-209. doi:10.1111/jdi.12548.
81. Manchanda S, Narang R, Reddy K, Sachdeva U, Prabhakaran D, Dharmanand S, et al. Retardation of coronary atherosclerosis with yoga lifestyle intervention. [Randomized Controlled Trial] J Assoc Physicians India. 2000;48:687–94.
82. Dash S., Thakur A. K. Effect of yoga in patient's with type-II diabetes mellitus. Journal of Evolution of Medical and Dental Sciences. 2014;3(7):1642–1655. doi: 10.14260/jemds/2014/2038.
83. Shantakumari N., Sequeira S., Eldeeb R. Effect of a yoga intervention on hypertensive diabetic patients. Journal of Advances in Internal Medicine. 2012;1(2):60–63. doi: 10.3126/jaim.v1i2.6526.
84. Balaji P. A., Varne S. R., Ali S. S. Effects of yoga—pranayama practices on metabolic parameters and anthropometry in type 2 diabetes. International Multidisciplinary Research Journal. 2011;1(10):1–4).
85. Shantakumari N, Sequeira S, El deeb R. Effects of a yoga intervention on lipid profiles of diabetes patients with dyslipidemia. Indian Heart J. 2013 Mar-Apr; 65(2):127-31.
86. Chohan IS, Nayar HS, Thomas P, Geetha NS. Influence of yoga on blood coagulation. Thromb Haemost. 1984;51:196–7.
87. Chohan IS, Nayar HS, Thomas P, Geetha NS. Influence of yoga on blood coagulation. Thromb Haemost. 1984;51:196–197.
88. Pullen PR, Nagamia SH, Mehta PK, Thompson WR, Benardot D, Hammoud R, et al. Effects of yoga on inflammation and exercise capacity in patients with chronic heart failure. J Card Fail. 2008;14:407–13.
89. Hunter, Stacy D. et al. The effect of Bikram yoga on endothelial function in young and middle-aged and older adults. Journal of Bodywork and Movement Therapies , Volume 21 , Issue 1 , 30 – 34.
90. Hegde S. V., Adhikari P., Kotian S., Pinto V. J., D'Souza S., D'Souza V. Effect of 3-month yoga on oxidative stress in type 2 diabetes with or without complications: a controlled clinical trial. Diabetes Care. 2011;34(10):2208–2210. doi: 10.2337/dc10-2430.
91. Yadav RK, Magan D, Mehta N, Sharma R, Mahapatra SC.Efficacy of a short term yoga based lifestyle intervention in reducing stress and inflammation: Preliminary results. J Altern Complement Med. 2012;18:662–7.
92. Innes KE, Bourguignon C, Taylor AG. Risk indices associated with the insulin resistance syndrome, cardiovascular disease, and possible protection with yoga: a systematic review. J Am Board Fam Pract. 2005;18:491–519.
93. Keerthi GS, Pal P, Pal GK, Sahoo JP, Sridhar MG, Balachander J. Effect of 12 Weeks of Yoga Therapy on Quality of Life and Indian Diabetes Risk Score in Normotensive Indian Young Adult Prediabetics and Diabetics: Randomized Control Trial. Journal of Clinical and Diagnostic Research : JCDR. 2017;11(9):CC10-CC14. doi:10.7860/JCDR/2017/29307.10633.

Cardiac Arrhythmias

1. Roberts-Thomson K. C., Lau D. H., Sanders P. (2011). The diagnosis and management of ventricular arrhythmias. Nat. Rev. Cardiol. 8, 311–321. 10.1038/nrcardio.2011.15.
2. Huang CL. Murine Electrophysiological Models of Cardiac Arrhythmogenesis. Physiol Rev. 2016;97(1):283-409. doi:10.1152/physrev.00007.2016.
3. Brugada P, Gursoy S, Brugada J, et al. Investigation of palpitations. Lancet 1993;341:1254–

8.
4. Jonsbu E, Dammen T, Morken G, Martinsen EW. Patients with noncardiac chest pain and benign palpitations referred for cardiac outpatient investigation: a 6-month follow-up. Gen Hosp Psychiatry. 2010;32:406–412. doi: 10.1016/j.genhosppsych.2010.03.003.
5. Nattel S., Guasch E., Savelieva I., Cosio F. G., Valverde I., Halperin J. L., et al. . (2014). Early management of atrial fibrillation to prevent cardiovascular complications. Eur. Heart J. 35, 1448–1456. 10.1093/eurheartj/ehu028.
6. Wolf PA, Abbott RD, Kannel WB. Atrial fibrillation as an independent risk factor for stroke: the Framingham Study. Stroke. 1991;22:983–988.
7. Kong MH, Fonarow GC, Peterson ED, et al. Systematic review of the incidence of sudden cardiac death in the United States. J Am Coll Cardiol. 2011;57:794–801.
8. Magnani JW, Rienstra M, Lin H, et al. Atrial fibrillation: current knowledge and future directions in epidemiology and genomics. Circulation. 2011;124:1982–93.
9. National Clinical Guideline Centre Atrial fibrillation: the management of atrial fibrillation. Clinical guideline: Methods, evidence and recommendations. London. National Institute for Health and Care Excellence, 2014.
10. Wolf PA, Abbott RD, Kannel WB. Atrial fibrillation as an independent risk factor for stroke: the Framingham Study. Stroke 1991;22:983-8. 10.1161/01.STR.22.8.983.
11. Kannel WB, Benjamin EJ. Status of the epidemiology of atrial fibrillation. Med Clin North Am. 2008;92:17–40. Ix.
12. Heron M. Deaths: leading causes for 2007. Natl Vital Stat Rep. 2011;59:1–95.
13. Adderley NJ, Nirantharakumar K, Marshall T. Risk of stroke and transient ischaemic attack in patients with a diagnosis of resolved atrial fibrillation: retrospective cohort studies. BMJ. 2018;361:k1717. Published 2018 May 9. Doi:10.1136/bmj.k1717.
14. G. Thrall, D. Lane, D. Carroll, G.Y. Lip.Quality of life in patients with atrial fibrillation: a systematic review.Am J Med, 119 (2006)448 e1-e19.
15. Pellman J, Sheikh F. Atrial fibrillation: mechanisms, therapeutics, and future directions. Compr Physiol. 2015;5(2):649–665. doi:10.1002/cphy.c140047.
16. Kirchhof P, Calkins H. Catheter ablation in patients with persistent atrial fibrillation. Eur Heart J. 2016;38(1):20–26. doi:10.1093/eurheartj/ehw260.
17. H. Calkins. Catheter ablation to maintain sinus rhythm. Circulation, 125 (2012), pp. 1439-1445.
18. Jalife J. Ventricular fibrillation: mechanisms of initiation and maintenance. Annu Rev Physiol. 2000;62:25–50.
19. Israel CW. Mechanisms of sudden cardiac death. Indian Heart J. 2014;66 Suppl 1:S10–S17.
20. Priori S.G., Aliot E., Blomstrom-Lundqvist C. Task force on sudden cardiac death of the European Society of Cardiology. Eur Heart J. 2001;22:1374–1450.
21. Whang W, Kubzansky LD, Kawachi I, Rexrode KM, Kroenke CH, Glynn RJ, et al. Depression and Risk of Sudden Cardiac Death and Coronary Heart Disease in Women. Results From the Nurses' Health Study. Journal of the American College of Cardiology. 2009;53(11):950–958.
22. van den Broek KC, Nyklicek I, van der Voort PH, Alings M, Meijer A, Denollet J. Risk of Ventricular Arrhythmia After Implantable Defibrillator Treatment in Anxious Type D Patients. Journal of the American College of Cardiology. 2009;54(6):531–537.
23. Burg MM, Lampert R, Joska T, Batsford W, Jain D. Psychological traits and emotion-triggering of ICD shock terminated arrhythmias. Psychosomatic Medicine. 2004;66(6):898–902.
24. CAST I. Effect of encainide and flecainide on mortality in a random trial of arrhythmia suppression after myocardial infarction. N Engl J Med. 1989;321:406–12.
25. Waldo AL, Camm AJ, deRuyter H, Friedman PL, Macneil DJ, et al. Effect of d-sotalol on mortality in patients with left ventricular dysfunction after recent and remote myocardial infarction. Lancet. 1996;348:7–12.
26. Tung R, Zimetbaum P, Josephson ME. A critical appraisal of implantable cardioverter-defibrillator therapy for the prevention of sudden cardiac death. J Am Coll Cardiol. 2008;52:1111–21.
27. Hughes S. Yoga found to reduce AF episodes. http://www.theheart.org/article/1204423.do (Accessed November 2012) 0;0:0–0.
28. Manchanda SC, Madan K. Yoga and meditation in cardiovascular disease. Clin Res Cardiol. 2014 Sep;103(9):675-80. doi: 10.1007/s00392-014-0663-9. Epub 2014 Jan 25.
29. Deutsch SB, Krivitsky EL. The impact of yoga on atrial fibrillation: A review of The Yoga My

Heart Study. J Arrhythm. 2015;31(6):337–338. doi:10.1016/j.joa.2015.05.001.
30. Dhanunjaya Lakkireddy, DonitaAtkins, JayasreePillarisett, et al. Effect of Yoga on Arrhythmia Burden, Anxiety, Depression, and Quality of Life in Paroxysmal Atrial Fibrillation: The YOGA My Heart Study. Journal of the American College of Cardiology. Volume 61, Issue 11, 19 March 2013, Pages 1177-1182.
31. L. Huang, Z.C. Wen, W.L. Lee, M.S. Chang, S.A. Chen. Changes of autonomic tone before the onset of paroxysmal atrial fibrillation. Int J Cardiol, 66 (1998), pp. 275-283.
32. K. Khattab, A.A. Khattab, J. Ortak, G. Richardt, H. Bonnemeier.Iyengar yoga increases cardiac parasympathetic nervous modulation among healthy yoga practitioners. Evid Based Complement Alternat Med, 4 (2007), pp. 511-517.
33. Sabzwari SRA, Garg L, Lakkireddy D, Day J. Ten Lifestyle Modification Approaches to Treat Atrial Fibrillation. Cureus. 2018;10(5):e2682. Published 2018 May 24. doi:10.7759/cureus.2682.
34. Menezes AR, Lavie CJ, De Schutter A, Milani RV, O'Keefe J, DiNicolantonio JJ, Morin DP, Abi-Samra FM. Lifestyle modification in the prevention and treatment of atrial fibrillation. Prog Cardiovasc Dis. 2015 Sep-Oct;58(2):117-25. doi: 10.1016/j.pcad.2015.07.001. Epub 2015 Jul 13.
35. Hong KL, Glover BM. The impact of lifestyle intervention on atrial fibrillation. Curr Opin Cardiol. 2018 Jan;33(1):14-19. doi: 10.1097/HCO.0000000000000470.
36. Abdul-Aziz AA, Altawil M, Lyon A, MacEachern M, Richardson CR, Rubenfire M, Pelosi F Jr, Jackson EA. Lifestyle Therapy for the Management of Atrial Fibrillation. Am J Cardiol. 2018 May 1;121(9):1112-1117. doi: 10.1016/j.amjcard.2018.01.023. Epub 2018 Feb 7.
37. Yoga and atrial fibrillation. Eur Heart J. 2016 Oct 7;37(38):2855.; Wahlstrom M, Rydell Karlsson M, Medin J, Frykman V. Effects of yoga in patients with paroxysmal atrial fibrillation - a randomized controlled study. Eur J Cardiovasc Nurs. 2017 Jan;16(1):57-63. doi: 10.1177/1474515116637734. Epub 2016 Jul 7.
38. Alcohol consumption and risk of atrial fibrillation: a prospective study and dose-response meta-analysis. Larsson SC, Drca N, Wolk A. J Am Coll Cardiol. 2014;64:281–289.
39. Diabetes mellitus glycemic control, and risk of atrial fibrillation. Dublin S, Glazer NL, Smith NL, et al. J Gen Intern Med. 2010;25:853–858.
40. Martínez-González MÁ, Toledo E, Arós F, et al. Extra virgin olive oil consumption reduces risk of atrial fibrillation: the PREDIMED (Prevención con Dieta Mediterránea) trial. Circulation. 2014;130:18–26.
41. Mattioli AV, Miloro C, Pennella S, Pedrazzi P, Farinetti A. Adherence to Mediterranean diet and intake of antioxidants influence spontaneous conversion of atrial fibrillation. Nutr Metab Cardiovasc Dis. 2013;23:115–121.
42. Huxley RR, Misialek JR, Agarwal SK, Loehr LR, Soliman EZ, Chen LY, Alonso A. Physical activity, obesity, weight change, and risk of atrial fibrillation: the atherosclerosis risk in communities study. Circ Arrhythm Electrophysiol. 2014;7:620–625.
43. Staerk L, Wang B, Preis SR, et al. Lifetime risk of atrial fibrillation according to optimal, borderline, or elevated levels of risk factors: cohort study based on longitudinal data from the Framingham Heart Study. BMJ. 2018;361:0.
44. Lampert R, Jamner L, Burg M, et al. Triggering of symptomatic atrial fibrillation by negative emotion. J Am Coll Cardiol. 2014;64:1533–1534.
45. Pathak RK, Middeldorp ME, Meredith M, et al. Long-term effect of goal-directed weight management in an atrial fibrillation cohort: a long-term follow-up study (LEGACY) J Am Coll Cardiol. 2015;65:2159–2169.
46. Guilleminault C, Connolly SJ, Winkle RA. Cardiac arrhythmia and conduction disturbances during sleep in 400 patients with sleep apnea syndrome. Am J Cardiol. 1983;52:490–494.
47. Heeringa J, Kors JA, Hofman A, van Rooij FJA, Witteman JCM. Cigarette smoking and risk of atrial fibrillation: the Rotterdam study.. Am Heart J. 2008;156:1163–1169.
48. Atrial fibrillation in healthy adolescents after highly caffeinated beverage consumption: two case reports. Di Rocco JR, During A, Morelli PJ, Heyden M, Biancaniello TA. J Med Case Rep. 2011;5:18.
49. No authors listed.Yoga may help reduce episodes of atrial fibrillation. The calming and balancing effects of yoga may cut down on common triggers for AF episodes and may have other health benefits, too. Heart Advis. 2011 Jun;14(6):7.
50. Wahlström M, Rydell Karlsson M, Medin J. Perceptions and experiences of MediYoga among patients with paroxysmal atrial fibrillation-An interview study. Complement Ther

Med. 2018 Dec;41:29-34. doi: 10.1016/j.ctim.2018.09.002. Epub 2018 Sep 5.
51. Dhanunjaya Lakkireddy, DonitaAtkins, JayasreePillarisett, et al. Effect of Yoga on Arrhythmia Burden, Anxiety, Depression, and Quality of Life in Paroxysmal Atrial Fibrillation: The YOGA My Heart Study. Journal of the American College of Cardiology. Volume 61, Issue 11, 19 March 2013, Pages 1177-1182.
52. Gard T, Noggle JJ, Park CL, Vago DR, Wilson A. Potential self-regulatory mechanisms of yoga for psychological health. Front Hum Neurosci. 2014;8:770. Published 2014 Sep 30. doi:10.3389/fnhum.2014.00770.
53. K. Khattab, A.A. Khattab, J. Ortak, G. Richardt, H. Bonnemeier.Iyengar yoga increases cardiac parasympathetic nervous modulation among healthy yoga practitioners. Evid Based Complement Alternat Med, 4 (2007), pp. 511-517.
54. Ravindra PN, Madanmohan, Pavithran P. Effect of pranayam (yoga breathing) and shavasan (relaxation training) on the frequency of benign ventricular ectopics in two patients with palpitations. Int J Cardiol. 2006 Mar 22;108(1):124-5.
55. Yetkin E, Aksoy Y, Yetkin O, Turhan H. Beneficial effect of deep breathing on premature ventricular complexes: can it be related to the decrease in QT dispersion? Int J Cardiol. 2006 Nov 18;113(3):417-8. Epub 2005 Dec 2.
56. Yogendra J, Yogendra H, Ambardekar S, et al. Beneficial effects of yoga lifestyle on reversibility of ischaemic heart disease: Caring Heart Project of International Board of Yoga. JAPI. 2004; 52:283.
57. Lau HL, Kwong JS, Yeung F, et al. Yoga for secondary prevention of coronary heart disease. Cochrane Database Syst Rev. 2012 Dec 12;12:CD009506.
58. Dwivedi U, Kumari S, Akhilesh KB, Nagendra HR. Well-being at workplace through mindfulness: Influence of Yoga practice on positive affect and aggression. Ayu. 2015;36(4):375-379. doi:10.4103/0974-8520.190693.
59. de Bruin EI, Formsma AR, Frijstein G, Bögels SM. Mindful2Work: Effects of Combined Physical Exercise, Yoga, and Mindfulness Meditations for Stress Relieve in Employees. A Proof of Concept Study. Mindfulness (N Y). 2016;8(1):204-217.
60. Pilkington K, Kirkwood G, Rampes H, Richardson J. Yoga for depression: The research evidence. J Affect Disord. 2005;89: 13–24. 10.1016/j.jad.2005.08.013.
61. Chong CS, Tsunaka M, Tsang HW, Chan EP, Cheung WM. Effects of yoga on stress management in healthy adults: a systematic review. Alternative Therapies in Health and Medicine. 2011;17(1):32–38.

Cardiac Output

1. Stringer W, Hansen J, Wasserman K (1997) Cardiac Output estimated non-invsively from oxygen uptake (VO2) during exercise. J Appl Physiol 1997 82: 908–912)
2. Ponikowski P, et al and ESC Scientific Document Group. ESC guidelines for the diagnosis and treatment of acute and chronic heart failure: The Task Force for the diagnosis and treatment of acute and chronic heart failure of the European Society of Cardiology (ESC). Developed with the special contribution of the Heart Failure Association (HFA) of the ESC. Eur J Heart Fail 2016; 18: 891–975.
3. Dunlay SM, Redfield MM, Weston SA, Therneau TM, Hall Long K, Shah ND, et al. Hospitalizations after heart failure diagnosis a com-munity perspective. J Am Coll Cardiol. 2009;54:1695–702.; Mosterd A, Hoes AW. Clinical epidemiology of heart failure. Heart. 2007;93:1137–46.
4. Miles SC, Chun-Chung C, Hsin-Fu L, Hunter SD, Dhindsa M, Nualnim N, Tanaka H. Arterial blood pressure and cardiovascular responses to yoga practice. Altern Ther Health Med. 2013 Jan-Feb;19(1):38-45.
5. Madhu D R; Ambarish Vijayaraghava; Venkatesh Doreswamy; Omkar Subbaramajois Narasipur. Comparison of cardiac output between practitioners and nonpractitioners of yoga before and after physical stress intervention. Natl J Physiol Pharm Pharmacol. 2017; 7(3): 317-322doi: 10.5455/njppp.2017.7.1234112122016.
6. Gomes-Neto M, Rodrigues ES, Silva WM, Carvalho VO. Effects of Yoga in Patients with Chronic Heart Failure: A Meta-Analysis. Arq Bras Cardiol. 2014;103(5):433-439.
7. Pullen PR, et al. Benefits of yoga for African American heart failure patients. Med Sci Sports Exerc. 2010 Apr;42(4):651-7.
8. Howie-Esquivel J, et al. Yoga in heart failure patients: a pilot study. J Card Fail. 2010

Sep;16(9):742-9. doi: 10.1016/j.cardfail.2010.04.011. Epub 2010 Jun 8.
9. Pullen PR, Seffens WS, Thompson WR. Yoga for Heart Failure: A Review and Future Research. Int J Yoga. 2018;11(2):91-98.
10. P. R. Pullen, S. H. Nagamia, P. K. Mehta et al., "Effects of yoga on inflammation and exercise capacity in patients with chronic heart failure," Journal of Cardiac Failure, vol. 14, no. 5, pp. 407–413, 2008.

Cardiac Rehabilitation

1. Hotta SS. Cardiac rehabilitation programs. Health Technol Assess Rep. 1991;(3):1-10.
2. Dalal HM, Doherty P, Taylor RS. Cardiac rehabilitation. BMJ. 2015 Sep 29;351:h5000.
3. Balraj S Heran, Jenny MH Chen, Shah Ebrahim, et al. Exercise-based cardiac rehabilitation for coronary heart disease. Cochrane Database Syst Rev. 2011; (7): CD001800.
4. Pashkow FJ. Issues in contemporary cardiac rehabilitation: a historical perspective. J Am Coll Cardiol. 1993 Mar 1;21(3):822-34.
5. Pasquali S.K., Karen P. Alexander, Laura P. Coombs et al. Effect of Cardiac Rehabilitation on Functional Outcomes After Coronary Revascularization. Am Heart J. 2003;145(3).
6. Ades PA, Keteyian SJ, Balady GJ et al. Cardiac rehabilitation exercise and self-care for chronic heart failure. JACC Heart Fail. 2013 Dec;1(6):540-7.
7. Jon A. Kobashigawa, M.D., David A. Leaf, M.D., Nancy Lee, P.T., Michael P. Gleeson, B.S., HongHu Liu, Ph.D., Michele A. Hamilton, M.D., Jaime D. Moriguchi, M.D., Nobuyuki Kawata, M.D., Kim Einhorn, B.S., Elise Herlihy, R.N., and Hillel Laks, M.D. A Controlled Trial of Exercise Rehabilitation after Heart Transplantation. N Engl J Med 1999; 340:272-277January 28, 1999DOI: 10.1056/NEJM199901283400404.
8. Balady GJ, et al. Referral, enrollment, and delivery of cardiac rehabilitation/secondary prevention programs at clinical centers and beyond: A presidential advisory from the American Heart Association. Circulation. 2011;124:2951–2960.
9. José M Maroto Monteroa, Rosario Artigao Ramíreza, María D Morales Durána, Carmen de Pablo Zarzosaa, Víctor Abrairab. Cardiac Rehabilitation in Patients With Myocardial Infarction: a 10-Year Follow-Up Study. Rev Esp Cardiol. 2005;58:1181-7. - Vol. 58 Num.10.
10. Pashkow FJ. Issues in contemporary cardiac rehabilitation: a historical perspective. J Am Coll Cardiol. 1993 Mar 1;21(3):822-34.
11. Shen BJ, Wachowiak PS, Brooks LG. Psychosocial factors and assessment in cardiac rehabilitation. Eura Medicophys. 2005 Mar;41(1):75-91.
12. Mayou RA1, Gill D, Thompson DR et al. Depression and anxiety as predictors of outcome after myocardial infarction. Psychosom Med. 2000 Mar-Apr;62(2):212-9.
13. Shen BJ, Wachowiak PS, Brooks LG. Psychosocial factors and assessment in cardiac rehabilitation. Eura Medicophys. 2005 Mar;41(1):75-91.
14. McGee HM, Hevey D, Horgan JH. Psychosocial outcome assessments for use in cardiac rehabilitation service evaluation: a 10-year systematic review. Soc Sci Med. 1999 May;48(10):1373-93.
15. Taylor-Piliae RE, Silva E, Sheremeta SP. Tai Chi as an adjunct physical activity for adults aged 45 years and older enrolled in phase III cardiac rehabilitation. European journal of cardiovascular nursing : journal of the Working Group on Cardiovascular Nursing of the European Society of Cardiology. 2012;11(1):34-43. doi:10.1016/j.ejcnurse.2010.11.001.
16. Nieva R, Safavynia SA, Bishop KL, Sperling L. Herbal, Vitamin, and Mineral Supplement Use in Patients Enrolled in a Cardiac Rehabilitation Program. Journal of cardiopulmonary rehabilitation and prevention. 2012;32(5):270-277.
17. Salmoirago-Blotcher E, Wayne P, Bock BC, et al. Design and methods of the Gentle Cardiac Rehabilitation Study – A behavioral study of tai chi exercise for patients not attending cardiac rehabilitation. Contemporary clinical trials. 2015;43:243-251.

18. Telles S, Naveen KV. Yoga for rehabilitation: an overview. Indian J Med Sci. 1997 Apr;51(4):123-7.
19. Raghuram N, Parachuri VR, Swarnagowri MV, et al. Yoga based cardiac rehabilitation after coronary artery bypass surgery: One-year results on LVEF, lipid profile and psychological states – A randomized controlled study. Indian Heart Journal. 2014;66(5):490-502. doi:10.1016/j.ihj.2014.08.007.
20. Delui MH, Yari M, khouyinezhad G, Amini M, Bayazi MH. Comparison of Cardiac Rehabilitation Programs Combined with Relaxation and Meditation Techniques on Reduction of Depression and Anxiety of Cardiovascular Patients. The Open Cardiovascular Medicine Journal. 2013;7:99-103. doi:10.2174/1874192401307010099.
21. Raghuram N, Parachuri VR, Swarnagowri MV, et al. Yoga based cardiac rehabilitation after coronary artery bypass surgery: One-year results on LVEF, lipid profile and psychological states – A randomized controlled study. Indian Heart Journal. 2014;66(5):490-502. doi:10.1016/j.ihj.2014.08.007.
22. Gomes-Neto M, Rodrigues-Jr ES, Silva-Jr WM, Carvalho VO. Effects of Yoga in Patients with Chronic Heart Failure: A Meta-Analysis. Arquivos Brasileiros de Cardiologia. 2014;103(5):433-439. doi:10.5935/abc.20140149.

Congestive Heart Failure

1. Bui AL, Horwich TB, Fonarow GC. Epidemiology and risk profile of heart failure. Nature reviews Cardiology. 2011;8(1):30-41. doi:10.1038/nrcardio.2010.165.
2. Lloyd-Jones D, et al. Heart disease and stroke statistics—2010 update: a report from the American Heart Association. Circulation. 2010;121:e46–e215.
3. McMurray JJ, Petrie MC, Murdoch DR, Davie AP. Clinical epidemiology of heart failure: public and private health burden. Eur Heart J. 1998;19 (Suppl P):P9–P16.
4. Lloyd-Jones D, et al. Heart disease and stroke statistics—2010 update: a report from the American Heart Association. Circulation. 2010;121:e46–e215.
5. Levy D, et al. Long-term trends in the incidence of and survival with heart failure. N Engl J Med. 2002;347:1397–1402.
6. Stewart S, MacIntyre K, Hole DJ, Capewell S, McMurray JJ. More 'malignant' than cancer? Five-year survival following a first admission for heart failure. Eur J Heart Fail. 2001;3:315–322.
7. Dunlay SM, Pereira NL, Kushwaha SS. Contemporary Strategies in the Diagnosis and Management of Heart Failure. Mayo Clinic proceedings. 2014;89(5):662-676. doi:10.1016/j.mayocp.2014.01.004.
8. Bernardo BC, Blaxall BC. From Bench to Bedside: New approaches to therapeutic discovery for heart failure. Heart, lung & circulation. 2016;25(5):425-434. doi:10.1016/j.hlc.2016.01.002.
9. Gheorghiade M, Vaduganathan M, Fonarow GC, Bonow RO. Rehospitalization for heart failure: problems and perspectives. J Am Coll Cardiol. 2013 Jan 29;61(4):391-403. doi: 10.1016/j.jacc.2012.09.038. Epub 2012 Dec 5.
10. Norton C, Georgiopoulou VV, Kalogeropoulos AP, Butler J. Epidemiology and cost of advanced heart failure. Prog Cardiovasc Dis. 2011 Sep-Oct;54(2):78-85. doi: 10.1016/j.pcad.2011.04.002.
11. Albert N, Rathman L, Ross D, Walker D, Bena J, McIntyre S, Philip D, Siedlecki S, Lovelace R, Fogarty A. et al. Predictors of Over-the-Counter Drug and Herbal Therapies Use in Elderly Patients with Heart Failure. J Card Fail. 2009;15(7):600–606. doi: 10.1016/j.cardfail.2009.02.001.
12. Pan L, Yan J, Guo Y, Yan J. Effects of Tai Chi training on exercise capacity and quality of life in patients with chronic heart failure: a meta-analysis. Eur J Heart Fail. 2013 Mar;15(3):316-23. doi: 10.1093/eurjhf/hfs170. Epub 2012 Oct 25.

13. Kubo A, Hung YY, Ritterman J. Yoga for heart failure patients: a feasibility pilot study with a multiethnic population. Int J Yoga Therap. 2011;(21):77-83.
14. Pullen PR, Nagamia SH, Mehta PK, Thompson WR, Benardot D, Hammoud R, Parrott JM, Sola S, Khan BV. Effects of yoga on inflammation and exercise capacity in patients with chronic heart failure. J Card Fail. 2008 Jun;14(5):407-13.
15. Howie-Esquivel J, et al. Yoga in heart failure patients: a pilot study. J Card Fail. 2010.
16. Pullen PR, Thompson WR, Benardot D, Brandon LJ, Mehta PK, Rifai L, Vadnais DS, Parrott JM, Khan BV. Benefits of yoga for African American heart failure patients. Med Sci Sports Exerc. 2010 Apr;42(4):651-7. doi: 10.1249/MSS.0b013e3181bf24c4.
17. Gomes-Neto M, Rodrigues-Jr ES, Silva-Jr WM, Carvalho VO. Effects of Yoga in Patients with Chronic Heart Failure: A Meta-Analysis. Arquivos Brasileiros de Cardiologia. 2014;103(5):433-439. doi:10.5935/abc.20140149.
18. Krishna BH, et al. Effect of yoga therapy on heart rate, blood pressure and cardiac autonomic function in heart failure. J Clin Diagn Res. 2014 Jan;8(1):14-6. doi: 10.7860/JCDR/2014/7844.3983. Epub 2014 Jan 12.

Coronary Artery Disease

1. http://www.who.int/mediacentre/factsheets/fs317/en/- accessed 1/12/18
2. Dalen JE, Alpert JS, Goldberg RJ, Weinstein RS. The epidemic of the 20(th) century: coronary heart disease. Am J Med. 2014;127:807–812.
3. Wong ND. Epidemiological studies of CHD and the evolution of preventive cardiology. Nat Rev Cardiol. 2014;11:276–289.
4. https://www.cdc.gov/heartdisease/facts.htm - accesed 1/16/18.
5. CDC, NCHS. Underlying Cause of Death 1999-2013 on CDC WONDER Online Database, released 2015. Data are from the Multiple Cause of Death Files, 1999-2013, as compiled from data provided by the 57 vital statistics jurisdictions through the Vital Statistics Cooperative Program. Accessed Feb. 3, 2015.
6. Go AS, Mozaffarian D, Roger VL, Benjamin EJ, Berry JD, Blaha MJ, Dai S, Ford ES, Fox CS, Franco S, et al. Heart disease and stroke statistics--2014 update: a report from the American Heart Association. Circulation. 2014;129: e28–e292.
7. CDC, NCHS. Underlying Cause of Death 1999-2013 on CDC WONDER Online Database, released 2015. Data are from the Multiple Cause of Death Files, 1999-2013, as compiled from data provided by the 57 vital statistics jurisdictions through the Vital Statistics Cooperative Program. Accessed October 21, 2015.CDC, 2015.
8. Mallika V, Goswami B, Rajappa M. Atherosclerosis pathophysiology and the role of novel risk factors: a clinicobiochemical perspective. Angiology 2007;58:513-22.
9. Ross R. Atherosclerosis--an inflammatory disease. N Engl J Med. 1999;340(2):115–126.
10. Mallika V, Goswami B, Rajappa M. Atherosclerosis pathophysiology and the role of novel risk factors: a clinicobiochemical perspective. Angiology 2007;58:513-22.
11. Wilson PW, et al. Prediction of coronary heart disease using risk factor categories. Circulation. 1998;97:1837–1847.
12. Berenson GS, Srinivasan SR, Bao W, Newman WP, 3rd, Tracy RE, Wattigney WA. Association between multiple cardiovascular risk factors and atherosclerosis in children and young adults. The Bogalusa Heart Study. N Engl J Med. 1998;338:1650–1656.
13. Winkelmann BR, Hager J. Genetic variation in coronary heart disease and myocardial infarction: methodological overview and clinical evidence. Pharmacogenomics. 2000 Feb;1(1):73-94.
14. https://www.nhlbi.nih.gov/health-topics/coronary-heart-disease - accessed 1/7/18.
15. Douglas P. Zipes, Hein J. J. Wellens. Sudden Cardiac Death. Circulation. 1998;98:2334-2351.
16. Infante T, Forte E, Schiano C, et al. An integrated approach to coronary heart disease diagnosis and clinical management. American Journal of Translational Research. 2017;9(7):3148-3166.

17. Gogas BD, Farooq V, Serruys PW, Garcìa-Garcìa HM. Assessment of coronary atherosclerosis by IVUS and IVUS-based imaging modalities: progression and regression studies, tissue composition and beyond. The International Journal of Cardiovascular Imaging. 2011;27(2):225-237. Doi:10.1007/s10554-010-9791-0.
18. Pathan F, Negishi K. Prediction of cardiovascular outcomes by imaging coronary atherosclerosis. Cardiovascular Diagnosis and Therapy. 2016;6(4):322-339. Doi:10.21037/cdt.2015.12.08.
19. Ornish D, Scherwitz LW, Billings JH, et al. Intensive lifestyle changes for reversal of coronary heart disease: five-year follow-up of the Lifestyle Heart Trial. JAMA. 1998;280(23):2001–2007.
20. Qaseem A, Fihn SD, Dallas P, Williams S, Owens DK, Shekelle P. Management of stable ischemic heart disease: summary of a clinical practice guideline from the American College of Physicians/American College of Cardiology Foundation/American Heart Association/American Association for Thoracic Surgery/Preventive Cardiovascular Nurses Association/Society of Thoracic Surgeons. Ann Intern Med. 2012;157(10):735–743.
21. Degrauwe S, Pilgrim T, Aminian A, Noble S, Meier P, Iglesias JF. Dual antiplatelet therapy for secondary prevention of coronary artery disease. Open Heart. 2017;4(2): e000651. doi:10.1136/openhrt-2017-000651.
22. Delui MH, Yari M, khouyinezhad G, Amini M, Bayazi MH. Comparison of Cardiac Rehabilitation Programs Combined with Relaxation and Meditation Techniques on Reduction of Depression and Anxiety of Cardiovascular Patients. The Open Cardiovascular Medicine Journal. 2013;7:99-103. doi:10.2174/1874192401307010099.
23. Raghuram N, Parachuri VR, Swarnagowri MV, et al. Yoga based cardiac rehabilitation after coronary artery bypass surgery: One-year results on LVEF, lipid profile and psychological states – A randomized controlled study. Indian Heart Journal. 2014;66(5):490-502. doi:10.1016/j.ihj.2014.08.007.
24. Gomes-Neto M, Rodrigues-Jr ES, Silva-Jr WM, Carvalho VO. Effects of Yoga in Patients with Chronic Heart Failure: A Meta-Analysis. Arquivos Brasileiros de Cardiologia. 2014;103(5):433-439. doi:10.5935/abc.20140149.
25. Lan C, Chen S-Y, Wong M-K, Lai JS. Tai Chi Chuan Exercise for Patients with Cardiovascular Disease. Evidence-based Complementary and Alternative Medicine : eCAM. 2013;2013:983208. doi:10.1155/2013/983208.
26. Bruning RS, Sturek M. Benefits of exercise training on coronary blood flow in coronary artery disease patients. Progress in cardiovascular diseases. 2015;57(5):443-453. doi:10.1016/j.pcad.2014.10.006.
27. Yu C, Ji K, Cao H, et al. Effectiveness of acupuncture for angina pectoris: a systematic review of randomized controlled trials. BMC Complementary and Alternative Medicine. 2015;15:90. doi:10.1186/s12906-015-0586-7.
28. Tupule TH, Shah HM, Shah SJ, et al. Yogic exercises in the management of ischaemic heart disease. Indian Heart Journal. 1971;23(4):259–264.
29. Tupule TH, Shah HM, Shah SJ, et al. Yogic exercises in the management of ischaemic heart disease. Indian Heart Journal. 1971;23(4):259–264.
30. Hagins M, States R, Selfe T, et al. Effectiveness of Yoga for Hypertension: Systematic Review and Meta-Analysis Evidence-Based Complementary and Alternative Medicine. Volume 2013 (2013), Article ID 649836.
31. Wang J, Xiong X, Liu W (2013) Yoga for Essential Hypertension: A Systematic Review. PLoS ONE 8(10): e76357. https://doi.org/10.1371/journal.pone.0076357.
32. Okonta Nkechi. Does yoga therapy reduce blood pressure in patients with hypertension? An integrative review. Holist Nurs Pract 2012; 26: 137-141.
33. Tyagi A, Cohen M. Yoga and hypertension: a systematic review. Altern Ther Health Med. 2014 Mar-Apr;20(2):32-59.
34. Manchanda SC, Narang R, Reddy KS, Sachdeva U, Prabhakaran D, Dharmanand S, et al. Retardation of coronary atherosclerosis with yoga lifestyle intervention. J Assoc Physicians India. 2000;48:687–94.

35. Siu PM, Yu AP, Benzie IF, Woo J. Effects of 1-year yoga on cardiovascular risk factors in middle-aged and older adults with metabolic syndrome: a randomized trial. Diabetology & Metabolic Syndrome. 2015;7:40. doi:10.1186/s13098-015-0034-3.
36. Ross A., Friedmann E., Bevans M., Thomas S. National survey of yoga practitioners: mental and physical health benefits. Complementary Therapies in Medicine. 2013;21(4):313–323. doi: 10.1016/j.ctim.2013.04.001.
37. Ross A., Friedmann E., Bevans M., Thomas S. Frequency of yoga practice predicts health: results of a national survey of yoga practitioners. Evidence-based Complementary and Alternative Medicine. 2012;2012:10. doi: 10.1155/2012/983258.983258).
38. Olson K. L., Emery C. F. Mindfulness and weight loss: a systematic review. Psychosomatic Medicine. 2015;77(1):59–67.; Rioux JG, Ritenbaugh C. Narrative review of yoga intervention clinical trials including weight-related outcomes. Altern Ther Health Med. 2013 May-Jun;19(3):32-46.
39. Acharya BK, AK Upadhyay, Ruchita T Upadhyay,et al. Effect of Pranayama (voluntary regulated breathing) and Yogasana (yoga postures) on lipid profile in normal healthy junior footballers. Int J Yoga. 2010 Jul-Dec; 3(2): 70.
40. Yadav RK, Magan D, Yadav R, et al. High-density lipoprotein cholesterol increases following a short-term yoga-based lifestyle intervention: a non-pharmacological modulation. Acta Cardiol. 2014 Oct;69(5):543-9.
41. Gokal R, Shillito L, Maharaj SR. Positive impact of yoga and pranayam on obesity, hypertension, blood sugar, and cholesterol: a pilot assessment. J Altern Complement Med. 2007 Dec;13(10):1056-7.
42. Mahajan A., Reddy K., Sachdeva U. Lipid profile of coronary risk subjects following yogic lifestyle intervention. Indian Heart J. 1999;51:37–40.
43. Shantakumari N, Sequeira S, El deeb R. Effects of a yoga intervention on lipid profiles of diabetes patients with dyslipidemia. Indian Heart Journal. 2013;65(2):127-131. doi:10.1016/j.ihj.2013.02.010.
44. Innes KE, Selfe TK. Yoga for Adults with Type 2 Diabetes: A Systematic Review of Controlled Trials. Journal of Diabetes Research. 2016;2016:6979370. doi:10.1155/2016/6979370.
45. Kelly A McDermott, Mohan Raghavendra Rao, Raghuram Nagarathna, Elizabeth J Murphy, Adam Burke, Ramarao Hongasandra Nagendra and Frederick M Hecht. A yoga intervention for type 2 diabetes risk reduction: a pilot randomized controlled trial. BMC Complementary and Alternative Medicine. 201414:212.
46. Innes KE, Selfe TK. Yoga for Adults with Type 2 Diabetes: A Systematic Review of Controlled Trials. Journal of Diabetes Research. 2016;2016:6979370. doi:10.1155/2016/6979370.
47. Kerr D, Gillam E, Ryder J, Trowbridge S, et al. An Eastern art form for a Western disease: randomised controlled trial of yoga in patients with poorly controlled insulin-treated diabetes. Pract Diabetes Intern. 2002; 19:164–6.
48. Bock BC, Fava JL, Gaskins R, et al. Yoga as a complementary treatment for smoking cessation in women. J Womens Health (Larchmt) 2012;21(2):240–248.
49. L Carim Todd, S Mitchell, B Oken. Does yoga improve smoking cessation outcomes? A systematic review of the literature. BMC Complement Altern Med. 2012; 12(Suppl 1): P389. Published online 2012 Jun 12.
50. Shahab L, Sarkar BK, West R. The acute effects of yogic breathing exercises on craving and withdrawal symptoms in abstaining smokers. Psychopharmacology (Berl). 2013 Feb;225(4):875-82.
51. Klinsophon T, Thaveeratitham P, Sitthipornvorakul E, Janwantanakul P. Effect of exercise type on smoking cessation: a meta-analysis of randomized controlled trials. BMC Research Notes. 2017;10:442. doi:10.1186/s13104-017-2762-y.
52. Dick H. J. Thijssen,Andrew J. Maiorana, et al. Impact of inactivity and exercise on the vasculature in humans. Eur J Appl Physiol. 2010 Mar; 108(5): 845–875.
53. Chastin SFM, Palarea-Albaladejo J, et al. (2015) Combined Effects of Time Spent in Physical Activity, Sedentary Behaviors and Sleep on Obesity and Cardio-Metabolic Health Markers: A Novel Compositional Data Analysis Approach. PLoS ONE 10(10): e0139984.
54. Long R. Scientific keys volume I: the key muscles of hatha yoga. 3. Bandha: Yoga; 2006.

55. McCall T. Yoga as medicine: The yogic prescription for health and healing. 1. New York: Bantam Dell; 2007.
56. Ray US, Pathak A, Tomer OS. Hatha yoga practices: Energy expenditure, respiratory changes and intensity of exercise. Evid Based Complement Alternat Med. 2011; 2011:241294.
57. Sovová E, Čajka V, Pastucha D, et al. Positive effect of yoga on cardiorespiratory fitness: A pilot study. Int J Yoga. 2015 Jul-Dec;8(2):134-8.
58. Vijayaraghava A, Doreswamy V, Narasipur OS, Kunnavil R, Srinivasamurthy N. Effect of Yoga Practice on Levels of Inflammatory Markers After Moderate and Strenuous Exercise. Journal of Clinical and Diagnostic Research : JCDR. 2015;9(6):CC08-CC12. doi:10.7860/JCDR/2015/12851.6021.
59. Kiecolt-Glaser JK, Christian L, Preston H, et al. Stress, Inflammation, and Yoga Practice. Psychosomatic medicine. 2010;72(2):113. doi:10.1097/PSY.0b013e3181cb9377.
60. Thirthalli J, Naveen GH, Rao MG, Varambally S, Christopher R, Gangadhar BN. Cortisol and antidepressant effects of yoga. Indian Journal of Psychiatry. 2013;55(Suppl 3):S405-S408. doi:10.4103/0019-5545.116315.
61. Yadav RK, Magan D, Mehta N, Sharma R, Mahapatra SC. Efficacy of a short-term yoga-based lifestyle intervention in reducing stress and inflammation: preliminary results. J Altern Complement Med. 2012 Jul;18(7):662-7. doi: 10.1089/acm.2011.0265.
62. Lau HL, Kwong JS, Yeung F, et al. Yoga for secondary prevention of coronary heart disease. Cochrane Database Syst Rev. 2012 Dec 12;12:CD009506.
63. Yadav A, Singh S, Singh KP. Role of Pranayama breathing exercises in rehabilitation of CAD patients - A pilot study. Indian J Tradit Knowledge. 2009;8:455–8.
64. Yadav A, Singh S, Singh K, Pai P. Effect of yoga regimen on lung functions including diffusion capacity in coronary artery disease patients: A randomized controlled study. International Journal of Yoga. 2015;8(1):62-67. doi:10.4103/0973-6131.146067.
65. Yogendra J, Yogendra H, Ambardekar S, et al. Beneficial effects of yoga lifestyle on reversibility of ischaemic heart disease: Caring Heart Project of International Board of Yoga. JAPI. 2004; 52:283.
66. Ramamurthy G, Trejo E, Faraone SV. Depression Treatment in Patients with Coronary Artery Disease: A Systematic Review. The Primary Care Companion for CNS Disorders. 2013;15(5):PCC.13r01509. doi:10.4088/PCC.13r01509.
67. Parswani MJ, Sharma MP, Iyengar S. Mindfulness-based stress reduction program in coronary heart disease: A randomized control trial. International Journal of Yoga. 2013;6(2):111-117. doi:10.4103/0973-6131.113405.
68. O'Connor GT, JE Buring, S Yusuf, et al. An overview of randomized trials of rehabilitation with exercise after myocardial infarction. Circulation 1989;80;234-244.
69. Raghuram N, Parachuri VR, Swarnagowri MV, et al. Yoga based cardiac rehabilitation after coronary artery bypass surgery: One-year results on LVEF, lipid profile and psychological states – A randomized controlled study. Indian Heart Journal. 2014;66(5):490-502. doi:10.1016/j.ihj.2014.08.007.

Diet

1. Nettleton JA, Polak JF, Tracy R, Burke GL, Jacobs DR., Jr Dietary patterns and incident cardiovascular disease in the Multi-Ethnic Study of Atherosclerosis. Am J Clin Nutr. 2009;90:647–654.
2. Babio N, Sorli M, Bullo M, Basora J, Ibarrola-Jurado N, Fernandez-Ballart J, Martinez-Gonzalez MA, Serra-Majem L, Gonzalez-Perez R, Salas-Salvado J, Nureta PI. Association between red meat consumption and metabolic syndrome in a Mediterranean population at high cardiovascular risk: cross-sectional and 1-year follow-up assessment. Nutr Metab Cardiovasc Dis. 2012;22:200–207.
3. World Cancer Research Fund/American Institute for Cancer Research. Food, Nutrition, Physical Activity, and the Prevention of Cancer: A Global Perspective. Washington, DC: AICR; 2007.
4. Huxley RR, Ansary-Moghaddam A, Clifton P, Czernichow S, Parr CL, Woodward M. The impact of dietary and lifestyle risk factors on risk of colorectal cancer: a quantitative

overview of the epidemiological evidence. Int J Cancer. 2009;125(1):171–80. 10.1002/ijc.24343.
5. Bernstein AM, Song M, Zhang X, et al. Processed and Unprocessed Red Meat and Risk of Colorectal Cancer: Analysis by Tumor Location and Modification by Time. PLoS One. 2015;10(8):e0135959. Published 2015 Aug 25. doi:10.1371/journal.pone.0135959.
6. Kim SY, Wie GA, Cho YA, et al. The Role of Red Meat and Flavonoid Consumption on Cancer Prevention: The Korean Cancer Screening Examination Cohort. Nutrients. 2017;9(9):938. Published 2017 Aug 25. doi:10.3390/nu9090938.
7. Vang A, Singh PN, Lee JW, Haddad EH, Brinegar CH. Meats, processed meats, obesity, weight gain and occurrence of diabetes among adults: findings from Adventist Health Studies. Ann Nutr Metab. 2008;52:96–104.
8. Fung TT, Schulze M, Manson JE, Willett WC, Hu FB. Dietary patterns, meat intake, and the risk of type 2 diabetes in women. Arch Intern Med. 2004;164:2235–2240.
9. Talaei M, Wang YL, Yuan JM, Pan A, Koh WP. Meat, Dietary Heme Iron, and Risk of Type 2 Diabetes Mellitus: The Singapore Chinese Health Study. Am J Epidemiol. 2017;186(7):824-833.
10. Pan A, Sun Q, Bernstein AM, et al. Red meat consumption and mortality: results from 2 prospective cohort studies. Arch Intern Med. 2012;172(7):555-63.
11. Rohrmann S., Overvad K., Bas Bueno-de-Mesquita H., Jakobsen M.U., Egeberg R., Tjønneland A., Nailler L., Boutron-Ruault M.-C., Clavel-Chapelon F., Krogh V., et al. Meat consumption and mortality—Results from the European Prospective Investigation into Cancer and Nutrition. BMC Med. 2013;11:63. doi: 10.1186/1741-7015-11-63.
12. Abete I, Romaguera D, Vieira AR, Lopez de Munain A, Norat T. Association between total, processed, red and white meat consumption and all-cause, CVD and IHD mortality: a meta-analysis of cohort studies. Br J Nutr. 2014 Sep 14;112(5):762-75. doi: 10.1017/S000711451400124X. Epub 2014 Jun 16.
13. Lajous M, Bijon A, Fagherazzi G, et al. Processed and unprocessed red meat consumption and hypertension in women. Am J Clin Nutr. 2014 Sep;100(3):948-52. doi: 10.3945/ajcn.113.080598. Epub 2014 Jul 30.
14. Micha R, Michas G, Mozaffarian D. Unprocessed red and processed meats and risk of coronary artery disease and type 2 diabetes--an updated review of the evidence. Curr Atheroscler Rep. 2012;14(6):515-24.
15. Kaluza J, Åkesson A, Wolk A. Processed and unprocessed red meat consumption and risk of heart failure: prospective study of men. Circ Heart Fail. 2014;7:552–557.
16. Kaluza J, Åkesson A, Wolk A. Long-term processed and unprocessed red meat consumption and risk of heart failure: A prospective cohort study of women. Int J Cardiol. 2015 Aug 15;193:42-6.
17. Chen GC, Lv DB, Pang Z et al, Red and processed meat consumption and risk of stroke: a meta-analysis of prospective cohort studies. European Journal of Clinical Nutrition (2013) 67, 91–95.
18. Kim K, Hyeon J, Lee SA, et al. Role of Total, Red, Processed, and White Meat Consumption in Stroke Incidence and Mortality: A Systematic Review and Meta-Analysis of Prospective Cohort Studies. J Am Heart Assoc. 2017;6(9):e005983. Published 2017 Aug 30. doi:10.1161/JAHA.117.005983.
19. Pan A, Sun Q, Bernstein AM, Schulze MB, Manson JE, Stampfer MJ, Willett WC, Hu FB. Red meat consumption and mortality: results from 2 prospective cohort studies. Arch Intern Med. 2012;172:555–563.
20. Haring B, Wang W, Fretts A, et al. Red meat consumption and cardiovascular target organ damage (from the Strong Heart Study). J Hypertens. 2017;35(9):1794-1800.
21. Mensink RP, Zock PL, Kester AD, Katan MB. Effects of dietary fatty acids and carbohydrates on the ratio of serum total to HDL cholesterol and on serum lipids and apolipoproteins: a meta-analysis of 60 controlled trials. Am J Clin Nutr. 2003;77:1146–1155.
22. Mensink RP, Katan MB. Effect of dietary trans fatty acids on high-density and low-density lipoprotein cholesterol levels in healthy subjects. N Engl J Med. 1990;323:439–445.

23. Shepherd J, Packard CJ, Grundy SM, Yeshurun D, Gotto A, Taunton O. Effects of saturated and polyunsaturated fat diets on the chemical composition and metabolism of low density lipoproteins in man. J Lipid Res. 1980;21:91–99.
24. Carlsen CU, Møller JK, Skibsted LH. Heme-iron in lipid oxidation. Coord Chem Rev. 2005;249:485–498.
25. Alderman MH. Evidence relating dietary sodium to cardiovascular disease. J Am Coll Nutr. 2006;25:256S–261S)
26. Honikel KO. The use and control of nitrate and nitrite for the processing of meat products. Meat Sci. 2008;78:68–76.
27. He FJ, MacGregor GA. Salt reduction lowers cardiovascular risk: meta-analysis of outcome trials. Lancet. 2011;378:380–2.
28. Heart Failure Society of America Executive summary: HFSA 2010 comprehensive heart failure practice guideline. J Card Fail. 2010;16(6):475–539.
29. Kleinbongard P, Dejam A, Lauer T, et al. Plasma nitrite concentrations reflect the degree of endothelial dysfunction in humans. Free Radic Biol Med. 2006;40(2):295–302.
30. ArturNowińskiM.D.MarcinUfnalM.D., Ph.D. Trimethylamine N-oxide: A harmful, protective or diagnostic marker in lifestyle diseases? Nutrition. Volume 46, February 2018, Pages 7-12.
31. Cheng TO. Effects of fast foods, rising blood pressure and increasing serum cholesterol on cardiovascular disease in China. Am J Cardiol. 2006;97:1676–1678.
32. Mozaffarian D, Willett WC. Trans fatty acids and cardiovascular risk: a unique cardiometabolic imprint? Curr Atheroscler Rep. 2007 Dec;9(6):486-93.
33. Rosenheck R. Fast food consumption and increased caloric intake: a systematic review of a trajectory towards weight gain and obesity risk. Obes Rev. 2008 Nov;9(6):535-47.
34. Rosenheck R. Fast food consumption and increased caloric intake: a systematic review of a trajectory towards weight gain and obesity risk. Obes Rev. 2008 Nov;9(6):535-47.
35. Micha R, Wallace SK, Mozaffarian D. Red and processed meat consumption and risk of incident coronary heart disease, stroke, and diabetes mellitus: a systematic review and meta-analysis. Circulation. 2010;121:2271–2283.
36. Andrew O. Odegaard, Woon Puay Koh, Jian-Min Yuan, Myron D. Gross, and Mark A. Pereira. Western-Style Fast Food Intake and Cardio-Metabolic Risk in an Eastern Country. Circulation, July 2, 2012.
37. Malik VS, Popkin BM, Bray GA, Despres JP, Hu FB. Sugar-sweetened beverages, obesity, type 2 diabetes mellitus, and cardiovascular disease risk. Circulation 2010;121:1356–64.
38. de Koning L, Malik VS, Rimm EB, Willett WC, Hu FB. Sugar-sweetened and artificially sweetened beverage consumption and risk of type 2 diabetes in men. Am J Clin Nutr 2011;93:1321–7.
39. Fung TT, Malik V, Rexrode KM, Manson JE, Willett WC, Hu FB. Sweetened beverage consumption and risk of coronary heart disease in women. Am J Clin Nutr 2009;89:1037 – 42.
40. Bernstein AM, De Koning L, Flint AJ, Rexrode KM, Willett WC. Soda consumption and the risk of stroke in men and women. Am J Clin Nutr 2012;95:1190–9.
41. de Koning L, Malik VS, Rimm EB, Willett WC, Hu FB. Sugar-sweetened and artificially sweetened beverage consumption and risk of type 2 diabetes in men. Am J Clin Nutr 2011;93:1321–7.
42. Fung TT, Malik V, Rexrode KM, Manson JE, Willett WC, Hu FB. Sweetened beverage consumption and risk of coronary heart disease in women. Am J Clin Nutr 2009;89:1037 – 42.
43. US Department of Agriculture US dietary guidelines for Americans, 2010. Available from: http://www.cnpp.usda.gov/dietaryguidelines.htm.
44. Vasanti S. Malik , Yanping Li , An Pan , Lawrence De Koning , Eva Schernhammer , Walter C. Willett , and Frank B. Hu. Long-Term Consumption of Sugar-Sweetened and Artificially Sweetened Beverages and Risk of Mortality in US Adults.18 Mar 2019https://doi.org/10.1161/CIRCULATIONAHA.118.037401Circulation. 2019;0.

45. Alsunni AA, Badar A. Energy drinks consumption pattern, perceived benefits and associated adverse effects amongst students of University of Dammam, Saudi Arabia. J Ayub Med Coll Abbottabad. 2011 Jul-Sep;23(3):3–9.
46. Bell DG, Bordeleau JMR, Jacobs I. Blood pressure and heart rate after caffeine and ephedrine ingestion. Can J Appl Physiol. 1999;24(5):426.
47. Moreno MA, Furtner F, Frederick PR. Sugary drinks and childhood obesity. Arch Pediatr Adolesc Med. 2009;163(4):400.
48. Di Rocco JR, During A, Morelli PJ, Heyden M, Biancaniello TA. Atrial fibrillation in healthy adolescents after highly caffeinated beverage consumption: two case reports. J Med Case Reports. 2011;5(1):18.
49. Pommerening MJ, Cardenas JC, Radwan ZA, Wade CE, Holcomb JB, Cotton BA. Hypercoagulability after energy drink consumption. Journal of Surgical Research. 2015.
50. González W, Altieri P, Alvarado E, Banchs H, Colón E, Escobales N, et al. Celiac trunk and branches dissection due to energy drink consumption and heavy resistance exercise: case report and review of literature. Boletin de la Asociacion Medica de Puerto Rico. 2014;107(1):38–40.
51. Appleton KM, Hemingway A, Saulais L, et al. Increasing vegetable intakes: rationale and systematic review of published interventions. European Journal of Nutrition. 2016;55:869-896.
52. Appleby PN, Key TJ. The long-term health of vegetarians and vegans. Proc Nutr Soc. 2016 Aug;75(3):287-93. doi: 10.1017/S0029665115004334. Epub 2015 Dec 28.
53. Satija A, Bhupathiraju SN, Rimm EB, et al. Plant-Based Dietary Patterns and Incidence of Type 2 Diabetes in US Men and Women: Results from Three Prospective Cohort Studies. PLoS Med. 2016;13(6):e1002039. Published 2016 Jun 14. doi:10.1371/journal.pmed.1002039.
54. Lee Y, Park K. Adherence to a Vegetarian Diet and Diabetes Risk: A Systematic Review and Meta-Analysis of Observational Studies. Nutrients. 2017;9(6):603. Published 2017 Jun 14. doi:10.3390/nu9060603.
55. Hughes TF, Andel R, Small BJ, et al. Midlife fruit and vegetable consumption and risk of dementia in later life in Swedish twins. Am J Geriatr Psychiatry. 2010;18(5):413-20.
56. Van't Veer P., Kampman E. Food, Nutrition, Physical Activity, and the Prevention of Cancer: A Global Perspective. Volume 1 World Cancer Research Fund/American Institute for Cancer Research; Washington, DC, USA: 2007.
57. Leenders M, Sluijs I, Ros MM, Boshuizen HC, et al. Fruit and vegetable consumption and mortality: European prospective investigation into cancer and nutrition. Am J Epidemiol. 2013 Aug 15;178(4):590-602.
58. Bazzano LA, He J, Ogden LG, Loria CM, Vupputuri S, Myers L, et al. Fruit and vegetable intake and risk of cardiovascular disease in US adults: the first National Health and Nutrition Examination Survey Epidemiologic Follow-up Study. Am J Clin Nutr. 2002;76.1:93–9.
59. Tuso PJ, Ismail MH, Ha BJ, Bartolotto C. Nutritional update for physicians: plant-based diets. Perm J. 2013 Spring;17(2):61–6. DOI: http://dx.doi.org/10.7812/TPP/12-085.
60. Hartley L, Igbinedion E, Holmes J, et al. Increased consumption of fruit and vegetables for the primary prevention of cardiovascular diseases. Cochrane Database Syst Rev. 2013;6:CD009874.
61. Bazzano LA, Serdula MK, Liu S. Dietary intake of fruits and vegetables and risk of cardiovascular disease. Curr Atheroscler Rep. 2003;5:492–9.
62. Appel LJ, Moore TJ, Obarzanek E, Vollmer WM, Svetkey LP, Sacks FM, Bray GA, Vogt TM, Cutler JA, Windhauser MM, et al. A clinical trial of the effects of dietary patterns on blood pressure. DASH Collaborative Research Group. N Engl J Med. 1997;336:1117–24.
63. Carter P, Gray LJ, Troughton J, Khunti K, Davies MJ. Fruit and vegetable intake and incidence of type 2 diabetes mellitus: systematic review and meta-analysis. BMJ. 2010;341:c4229.
64. Ornish D, Scherwitz LW, Billings JH, et al. Intensive lifestyle changes for reversal of coronary heart disease. JAMA. 1998 Dec 16;280(23):2001–7.

65. Yang SY, Zhang HJ, Sun SY, et al. Relationship of carotid intima-media thickness and duration of vegetarian diet in Chinese male vegetarians. Nutr Metab (Lond) 2011 Sep 19;8(1):63. DOI: http://dx.doi.org/10.1186/1743-7075-8-63.
66. Sebeková K, Boor P, Valachovicová M, et al. Association of metabolic syndrome risk factors with selected markers of oxidative status and microinflammation in healthy omnivores and vegetarians. Mol Nutr Food Res. 2006 Sep;50(9):858–68. DOI: http://dx.doi.org/10.1002/mnfr.200500170.
67. Liu RH. Health benefits of fruit and vegetables are from additive and synergistic combinations of phytochemicals. Am J Clin Nutr. 2003;78(Suppl):517S–20S.
68. Fu L., Xu B.T., Xu X.R., et al. Antioxidant capacities and total phenolic contents of 62 fruits. Food Chem. 2011;129:345–350.
69. Assefa AD, Ko EY, Moon SH, Keum Y-S. Antioxidant and antiplatelet activities of flavonoid-rich fractions of three citrus fruits from Korea. 3 Biotech. 2016;6(1):109.
70. Esselstyn CB., Jr Resolving the coronary artery disease epidemic through plant-based nutrition. Prev Cardiol. 2001 Autumn;4(4):171–7. DOI: http://dx.doi.org/10.1111/j.1520-037X.2001.00538.x.
71. Ornish D, Scherwitz LW, Billings JH, et al. Intensive lifestyle changes for reversal of coronary heart disease. JAMA. 1998 Dec 16;280(23):2001–7.
72. Oude Griep LM, Geleijnse JM, Kromhout D, Ocké MC, Verschuren WMM. Raw and Processed Fruit and Vegetable Consumption and 10-Year Coronary Heart Disease Incidence in a Population-Based Cohort Study in the Netherlands. Tomé D, ed. PLoS ONE. 2010;5(10):e13609.
73. Du H, Li L, Bennett D, et al. Fresh Fruit Consumption and Major Cardiovascular Disease in China. The New England journal of medicine. 2016;374(14):1332-1343.
74. He FJ, Nowson CA, Lucas M, MacGregor GA. Increased consumption of fruit and vegetables is related to a reduced risk of coronary heart disease: meta-analysis of cohort studies. J Hum Hypertens. 2007;21:717–728.
75. Wang X, Ouyang Y, Liu J, Zhu M, Zhao G, Bao W, et al. Fruit and vegetable consumption and mortality from all causes, cardiovascular disease, and cancer: systematic review and dose–response meta-analysis of prospective cohort studies. BMJ. 2014;349: g4490.
76. He FJ, Nowson CA, MacGregor GA. Fruit and vegetable consumption and stroke: meta-analysis of cohort studies. Lancet. 2006;367:320–326.
77. Basu A, Rhone M, Lyons TJ. Berries: emerging impact on cardiovascular health. Nutrition reviews. 2010;68(3):168-177.
78. de Souza VR, Pereira PA, da Silva TL, de Oliveira Lima LC, Pio R, Queiroz F. Determination of the bioactive compounds, antioxidant activity and chemical composition of Brazilian blackberry, red raspberry, strawberry, blueberry and sweet cherry fruits. Food Chem. 2014 Aug 1; 156:362-8.
79. Sala-Vila A, Estruch R, Ros E. New insights into the role of nutrition in CVD prevention. Curr Cardiol Rep. 2015;17:26.
80. Mellen PB, Walsh TF, Herrington DM. Whole grain intake and cardiovascular disease: a meta-analysis. Nutr Metab Cardiovasc Dis 2008;18:283–90.
81. Jacobs DR Jr, Meyer KA, Kushi LH, Folsom AR. Whole-grain intake may reduce the risk of ischemic heart disease death in postmenopausal women: the Iowa Women's Health Study. Am J Clin Nutr 1998;68:248–57.
82. Wu H, Flint AJ, Qi Q, van Dam RM, Sampson LA, Rimm EB, Holmes MD, Willett WC, Hu FB, Sun Q. Association between dietary whole grain intake and risk of mortality: two large prospective studies in US men and women. JAMA Intern Med 2015;175:373–84.
83. Fraser GE, Sabate J, Beeson WL, Strahan TM. A possible protective effect of nut consumption on risk of coronary heart disease. The Adventist Health Study. Arch Intern Med. 1992, 152, 1416-24.
84. O'Neil CE, Keast DR, Nicklas TA, Fulgoni VL 3rd. Nut consumption is associated with decreased health risk factors for cardiovascular disease and metabolic syndrome in U.S. adults: NHANES 1999-2004. J Am Coll Nutr. 2011, 30(6), 502-10.

85. Slavin, J.L. Position of the American Dietetic Association: health implications of dietary fiber. J Am Diet Assoc. 2008; 108: 1716–1731.
86. Whelton PK, He J, Cutler JA, Brancati FL, Appel LJ, Follmann D, Klag MJ. Effects of oral potassium on blood pressure. Meta-analysis of randomized controlled clinical trials. JAMA. 1997 May 28; 277(20):1624-32.
87. D'Elia L, Barba G, Cappuccio FP, Strazzullo P. Potassium intake, stroke, and cardiovascular disease. A meta-analysis of prospective studies. J Am Coll Cardiol. 2011;57:1210–9.
88. Rosanoff A, Dai Q, Shapses SA. Essential Nutrient Interactions: Does Low or Suboptimal Magnesium Status Interact with Vitamin D and/or Calcium Status?. Adv Nutr. 2016;7(1):25-43. Published 2016 Jan 7. doi:10.3945/an.115.008631.
89. Mattioli AV, Francesca C, Mario M, Alberto F. Fruit and vegetables in hypertensive women with asymptomatic peripheral arterial disease. Clin Nutr ESPEN. 2018 Oct;27:110-112. doi: 10.1016/j.clnesp.2018.05.010. Epub 2018 Jun 12.
90. Heffron SP, Rockman CB, Adelman MA, et al. Greater Frequency of Fruit and Vegetable Consumption Is Associated With Lower Prevalence of Peripheral Artery Disease. Arterioscler Thromb Vasc Biol. 2017;37(6):1234-1240.
91. Cramer H, Sibbritt D, Park CL, Adams J, Lauche R. Is the practice of yoga or meditation associated with a healthy lifestyle? Results of a national cross-sectional survey of 28,695 Australian women. J Psychosom Res. 2017 Oct;101:104-109. doi: 10.1016/j.jpsychores.2017.07.013. Epub 2017 Jul 27.
92. Ross A, Friedmann E, Bevans M, Thomas S. National survey of yoga practitioners: mental and physical health benefits. Complement Ther Med. 2013;21(4):313-23.

Drug Abuse/Addiction

1. https://www.drugabuse.gov/publications/drugs-brains-behavior-science-addiction/addiction-health.
2. https://www.asam.org/; https://www.aaap.org/.
3. Oyefeso A, Ghodse H, Clancy C, Corkery J, Goldfinch R. Drug abuse-related mortality: a study of teenage addicts over a 20-year period. Soc Psychiatry Psychiatr Epidemiol. 1999 Aug; 34(8):437-41.
4. Ghuran A, van der Wieken LR, Nolan J. Cardiovascular complications of recreational drugs: Are an important cause of morbidity and mortality. BMJ: British Medical Journal. 2001;323(7311):464-466.
5. Ghodse H, Oyefeso A, Hunt M, Pollard M, Mehta R, Corkery J. Drug related deaths as reported by the coroners in England and Wales Annual Review 1999. London: Centre for Addiction Studies, St. George's Hospital Medical School; 2000.
6. Chang LR, Lin YH, Kuo TB, Ho YC, Chen SH, Wu Chang HC, et al. Cardiac autonomic modulation during methadone therapy among heroin users: a pilot study. Prog Neuropsychopharmacol Biol Psychiatry. 2012;37:188–193. doi: 10.1016/j.pnpbp.2012.01.006.
7. Osterwalder JJ. Patients intoxicated with heroin or heroin mixtures: how long should they be monitored? Eur J Emerg Med. 1995 Jun; 2(2):97-101.
8. Mouhaffet A, Madu EC, Satmary W, Fraker TD. Cardiovascular complication of cocaine. Chest. 1995;107:1426–1434.
9. Vongpatanasin W, Mnsour Y, Chavoshan B, Arbique D, Victor RG. Cocaine stimulates the human cardiovascular system via a central mechanism of action. Circulation. 1999 Aug 3; 100(5):497-502.
10. Ghuran A, Nolan J. Recreational drug misuse: issues for the cardiologist. Heart. 2000 Jun; 83(6):627-33.
11. Osawa M, Mitsukuni Y, Saito T, Yukawa N, Matoba R, Takeichi S. Sudden death of a cocaine abuser. Tokai J Exp Clin Med. 1994 Dec;19(3-6):115-9.
12. Ghuran A, Nolan J. The cardiac complications of recreational drug use. Western Journal of Medicine. 2000;173(6):412-415.
13. Yogi Bhajan, Kundalini Yoga: The Flow of Eternal Power, p. 104.

14. Khanna S, Greeson JM. A narrative review of yoga and mindfulness as complementary therapies for addiction. Complementary Therapies in Medicine. 2013;21(3):244–252.
15. Pascoe MC, Thompson DR, Ski CF. Yoga, mindfulness-based stress reduction and stress-related physiological measures: A meta-analysis. Psychoneuroendocrinology. 2017 Dec;86:152-168. doi: 10.1016/j.psyneuen.2017.08.008. Epub 2017 Aug 30.
16. Carim-Todd L, Mitchell SH, Oken BS. Mind–body practices: An alternative, drug-free treatment for smoking cessation? A systematic review of the literature. Drug and Alcohol Dependence. 2013;132(3):399–410.
17. Prathikanti S, Rivera R, Cochran A, Tungol JG, Fayazmanesh N, Weinmann E. Treating major depression with yoga: A prospective, randomized, controlled pilot trial. PLoS One. 2017;12(3):e0173869. Published 2017 Mar 16. doi:10.1371/journal.pone.0173869.
18. Lohman R. Yoga techniques applicable within drug and alcohol rehabilitation programmes. Therapeutic Communities-London-Association of Therapeutic Communiities. 1999;20:61–72.
19. Deepeshwar S, Nagendra HR, Rana BB. Evolution from four mental states to the highest state of consciousness: A neurophysiological basis of meditation as defined in yoga texts. Prog Brain Res. 2019;244:31-83. doi: 10.1016/bs.pbr.2018.10.029. Epub 2019 Jan 3.
20. Chiesa A, Serretti A. Are mindfulness-based interventions effective for substance use disorders? A systematic review of the evidence. Substance Use and Misuse. 2014;49(5):492–512.
21. Patel NK, Nivethitha L, Mooventhan A. Effect of a Yoga Based Meditation Technique on Emotional Regulation, Self-compassion and Mindfulness in College Students. Explore (NY). 2018 Nov;14(6):443-447. doi: 10.1016/j.explore.2018.06.008. Epub 2018 Aug 2.
22. Samuelson M, Carmody J, Kabat-Zinn J, Bratt MA. Mindfulness-based stress reduction in Massachusetts correctional facilities. The Prison Journal. 2007;87:254–268.
23. Kissen M, Kissen-Kohn DA. Reducing addictions via the self-soothing effects of yoga. Bulletin of the Menninger Clinic. 2009;73(1):34.
24. Golec de Zavala A, Lantos D, Bowden D. Yoga Poses Increase Subjective Energy and State Self-Esteem in Comparison to 'Power Poses'. Front Psychol. 2017 May 11;8:752. doi: 10.3389/fpsyg.2017.00752. eCollection 2017.
25. Behere RV, Muralidharan K, Benegal V. Complementary and alternative medicine in the treatment of substance use disorders—a review of the evidence. Drug Alcohol Rev 2009;28:292–300.
26. Reddy S, Dick AM, Gerber MR, Mitchell K. The effect of a yoga intervention on alcohol and drug abuse risk in veteran and civilian women with posttraumatic stress disorder. J Altern Complement Med. 2014;20(10):750-6.
27. Butzer B, LoRusso A, Shin SH, Khalsa SB. Evaluation of Yoga for Preventing Adolescent Substance Use Risk Factors in a Middle School Setting: A Preliminary Group-Randomized Controlled Trial. J Youth Adolesc. 2016;46(3):603-632.
28. Bowen S, Chawla N, Collins SE, Witkiewitz K, Hsu S, Grow J, Marlatt A. Mindfulness-based relapse prevention for substance use disorders: A pilot efficacy trial. Substance Abuse. 2009;30:295–305.
29. Ricchuito AD. Yoga as adjunct therapy for substance use. Social Work Today. 2012;12:8.
30. Kuppili PP, Parmar A, Gupta A, Balhara YPS. Role of Yoga in Management of Substance-use Disorders: A Narrative Review. J Neurosci Rural Pract. 2018;9(1):117-122.

Erectile Dysfunction

1. Ponholzer A, Temml C, Mock K, Marszalek M, Obermayr R, Madersbacher S. Prevalence and risk factors for erectile dysfunction in 2869 men using a validated questionnaire. Eur Urol. 2005;47:80–5. discussion 85-6.
2. Feldman HA, Goldstein I, Hatzichristou DG, Krane RJ, McKinlay JB. Impotence and its medical and psychosocial correlates: results of the Massachusetts Male Aging Study. J Urol. 1994;151:54–61.

3. Nunes KP, Labazi H, Webb RC. New insights into hypertension-associated erectile dysfunction. Current Opinion in Nephrology and Hypertension. 2012;21(2):163–170.
4. Ayta IA, McKinlay JB, Krane RJ. The likely worldwide increase in erectile dysfunction between 1995 and 2025 and some possible policy consequences. BJU Int. 1999;84:50–56.
5. Sullivan ME, Keoghane SR, Miller MA. Vascular risk factors and erectile dysfunction. BJU Int. 2001;87:838–845.
6. Barrett-Connor E. Cardiovascular risk stratification and cardiovascular risk factors associated with erectile dysfunction: assessing cardiovascular risk in men with erectile dysfunction. Clin Cardiol. 2004;27:I8–13.
7. Gades NM, Nehra A, Jacobson DJ, McGree ME, Girman CJ, Rhodes T, Roberts RO, Lieber MM, Jacobsen SJ. Association between smoking and erectile dysfunction: a population-based study. Am J Epidemiol. 2005;161:346–51.
8. Kaiser FE, Korenman SG. Impotence in diabetic men. Am J Med. 1988;85:147–52.
9. Brackett NL, Lynne CM, Ibrahim E, Ohl DA, Sonksen J. Treatment of infertility in men with spinal cord injury. Nat Rev Urol. 2010;7:162–172.
10. Francis ME, Kusek JW, Nyberg LM, Eggers PW. The contribution of common medical conditions and drug exposures to erectile dysfunction in adult males. J Urol. 2007;178:591–596.
11. Tal R, et al. Persistent erectile dysfunction following radical prostatectomy: the association between nerve-sparing status and the prevalence and chronology of venous leak. J Sex Med. 2009;6:2813–2819.
12. Isidori AM, et al. A critical analysis of the role of testosterone in erectile function: from pathophysiology to treatment — a systematic review. Eur Urol. 2014;65:99–112.
13. McCabe MP, Althof SE. A systematic review of the psychosocial outcomes associated with erectile dysfunction: does the impact of erectile dysfunction extend beyond a man's inability to have sex? J Sex Med. 2014;11:347–363.
14. Shabsigh R, et al. Increased incidence of depressive symptoms in men with erectile dysfunction. Urology. 1998;52:848–852.
15. Hedon F. Anxiety and erectile dysfunction: a global approach to ED enhances results and quality of life. Int J Impot Res. 2003;15:S16–S19.
16. Uslu N, Gorgulu S, Alper AT, Eren M, Nurkalem Z, Yildirim A, Ozer O. Erectile dysfunction as a generalized vascular dysfunction. J Am Soc Echocardiogr 2006; 19:341–346.
17. Solomon H, Man J, Jackson G (2003) Erectile dysfunction and the cardiovascular patient: endothelial dysfunction is the common denominator. Heart 89: 251–253.
18. Bonetti PO, Lerman LO, Lerman A. Endothelial dysfunction: A marker of atherosclerotic risk. Arterioscler Thromb Vasc Biol. 2003;23:168–175.
19. Reriani MK, Lerman LO, Lerman A. Endothelial function as a functional expression of cardiovascular risk factors. Biomark Med. 2010;4:351–360.
20. Thompson IM, Tangen CM, Goodman PJ, Probstfield JL, Moinpour CM, et al. (2005) Erectile dysfunction and subsequent cardiovascular disease. JAMA 294: 2996–3002.
21. King A (2010) Erectile dysfunction and CVD. Nat Rev Cardiol 7: 241.
22. Reriani MK, Lerman LO, Lerman A. Endothelial function as a functional expression of cardiovascular risk factors. Biomark Med. 2010;4:351–360.
23. Dong JY, Zhang YH, Qin LQ. Erectile dysfunction and risk of cardiovascular disease: Meta-analysis of prospective cohort studies. J Am Coll Cardiol. 2011;58:1378–1385.
24. Jackson G. Erectile dysfunction and coronary disease: Evaluating the link. Maturitas. 2012;72:263–264.
25. Banks E, Joshy G, Abhayaratna WP, et al. Erectile dysfunction severity as a risk marker for cardiovascular disease hospitalisation and all-cause mortality: a prospective cohort study. PLoS Med. 2013;10(1):e1001372.
26. Hodges LD, Kirby M, Solanki J, O'Donnell J, Brodie DA. The temporal relationship between erectile dysfunction and cardiovascular disease. Int J Clin Pract. 2007;61:2019–2025.
27. Inman BA, Sauver JL, Jacobson DJ, McGree ME, Nehra A, Lieber MM, Roger VL, Jacobsen SJ. A population-based, longitudinal study of erectile dysfunction and future coronary artery disease. Mayo Clin Proc. 2009;84:108–113.

28. Jackson G, Boon N, Eardley I, Kirby M, Dean J, Hackett G, Montorsi P, Montorsi F, Vlachopoulos C, Kloner R, Sharlip I, Miner M. Erectile dysfunction and coronary artery disease prediction: Evidence-based guidance and consensus. Int J Clin Pract. 2010;64:848–857.
29. Banks E, Joshy G, Abhayaratna WP, et al. Erectile dysfunction severity as a risk marker for cardiovascular disease hospitalisation and all-cause mortality: a prospective cohort study. PLoS Med. 2013;10(1):e1001372.
30. Vlachopoulos CV, Terentes-Printzios DG, Ioakeimidis NK, Aznaouridis KA, Stefanadis CI. Prediction of cardiovascular events and all-cause mortality with erectile dysfunction: A systematic review and meta-analysis of cohort studies. Circ Cardiovasc Qual Outcomes. 2013;6:99–109.
31. Broderick GA, Arger P. Duplex Doppler ultrasonography: noninvasive assessment of penile anatomy and function. Semin Roentgenol. 1993;28(1):43–56.
32. Esposito K, Giugliano F, Di Palo C, Giugliano G, Marfella R, D'Andrea F, D'Armiento M, Giugliano D. Effect of lifestyle changes on erectile dysfunction in obese men: a randomized controlled trial. Jama. 2004;291:2978–84.
33. Pastuszak AW. Current Diagnosis and Management of Erectile Dysfunction. Curr Sex Health Rep. 2014;6(3):164-176.
34. Singh M., Kumar A. (2017) Yoga and Sexual Health. In: Kumar A., Sharma M. (eds) Basics of Human Andrology. Springer, Singapore.
35. Lori A. Brotto, Lisa Mehak & Cassandra Kit (2009) Yoga and Sexual Functioning: A Review, Journal of Sex & Marital Therapy, 35:5, 378-390, DOI: 10.1080/00926230903065955.
36. Rakshith, K. R., Sinha, K., Shivakumar., & Vijeth Kumar, L. A. (2017). Yogic Intervention in Sexual Dysfunction – A Review. Journal of Ayurveda and Integrated Medical Sciences, 2(4), 243–250.; July-Aug 2017.
37. Dhikav V, Karmarkar G, Verma M, Gupta R, Gupta S, Mittal D, and Anand K. Yoga in male sexual functioning: A noncompararive pilot study. J Sex Med 2010;7:3460–3466.
38. Dhikav, Vikas et al. Yoga in Premature Ejaculation: A Comparative Trial with Fluoxetine. The Journal of Sexual Medicine, 2007. Volume 4, Issue 6, 1726 – 1732.
39. Kalaitzidou, I., Venetikou, M. S., Konstadinidis, K., Artemiadis, A. K., Chrousos, G., & Darviri, C. (2014, August). Stress management and erectile dysfunction: A pilot comparative study [Abstract]. Andrologia, 46(6), 698–702.
40. Malathi, A. Damodaran. Stress Due To Exams In Medical Students - Role Of Yoga. Indian J Physiol Pharmacol 1999; 43 (2) : 218-224.
41. Richard P. Brown and Patricia L. Gerbarg. Sudarshan Kriya Yogic Breathing in the Treatment of Stress, Anxiety, and Depression: Part I—Neurophysiologic Model. The Journal of Alternative and Complementary Medicine 2005 11:1, 189-201.

Exercise

1. Agarwal SK. Cardiovascular benefits of exercise. International Journal of General Medicine. 2012;5:541-545.
2. Booth FW, Roberts CK, Laye MJ. Lack of exercise is a major cause of chronic diseases. Compr Physiol. 2012;2(2):1143-211.
3. Kelley DE, Goodpaster BH. Effects of exercise on glucose homeostasis in Type 2 diabetes mellitus. Med Sci Sports Exerc 2001; 33 Suppl 6: S495–501.
4. Rejeski WJ, Ettinger WH Jr, Martin K, Morgan T. Treating disability in knee osteoarthritis with exercise therapy: a central role for self-efficacy and pain. Arthritis Care Res 1998; 11: 94–101.
5. Komatireddy GR, Leitch RW, Cella K, Browning G, Minor M. Efficacy of low load resistive muscle training in patients with rheumatoid arthritis functional class II and III. J Rheumatol 1997; 24: 1531–9.
6. https://www.cancer.org/latest-news/exercise-linked-with-lower-risk-of-13-types-of-cancer.html.

7. Thune I, Furberg AS. Physical activity and cancer risk: dose-response and cancer, all sites and site-specific. [discussion S609-10]. Med Sci Sports Exerc 2001; 33: S530-50.
8. Ostman C, Smart NA, Morcos D, Duller A, Ridley W, Jewiss D. The effect of exercise training on clinical outcomes in patients with the metabolic syndrome: a systematic review and meta-analysis. Cardiovasc Diabetol. 2017;16(1):110. Published 2017 Aug 30. doi:10.1186/s12933-017-0590-y.
9. Willis LH, Slentz CA, Bateman LA, et al. Effects of aerobic and/or resistance training on body mass and fat mass in overweight or obese adults. J Appl Physiol (1985). 2012;113(12):1831-7.
10. Marson EC, Delevatti RS, Prado AK, Netto N, Kruel LF. Effects of aerobic, resistance, and combined exercise training on insulin resistance markers in overweight or obese children and adolescents: A systematic review and meta-analysis. Prev Med. 2016 Dec;93:211-218. doi: 10.1016/j.ypmed.2016.10.020. Epub 2016 Oct 20.
11. Rowan CP, Riddell MC, Gledhill N, Jamnik VK. Aerobic Exercise Training Modalities and Prediabetes Risk Reduction. Med Sci Sports Exerc. 2017 Mar;49(3):403-412. doi: 10.1249/MSS.0000000000001135.
12. Grace A, Chan E, Giallauria F, Graham PL, Smart NA. Clinical outcomes and glycaemic responses to different aerobic exercise training intensities in type II diabetes: a systematic review and meta-analysis. Cardiovasc Diabetol. 2017;16(1):37. doi: 10.1186/s12933-017-0518-6.
13. Hashida R, Kawaguchi T, Bekki M, et al. Aerobic vs. resistance exercise in non-alcoholic fatty liver disease: A systematic review. J Hepatol. 2017 Jan;66(1):142-152. doi: 10.1016/j.jhep.2016.08.023. Epub 2016 Sep 14.
14. Herting MM, Chu X. Exercise, cognition, and the adolescent brain. Birth Defects Res. 2017;109(20):1672-1679.
15. Gourgouvelis J, Yielder P, Clarke ST, Behbahani H, Murphy BA. Exercise Leads to Better Clinical Outcomes in Those Receiving Medication Plus Cognitive Behavioral Therapy for Major Depressive Disorder. Front Psychiatry. 2018;9:37. Published 2018 Mar 6. doi:10.3389/fpsyt.2018.00037.
16. Stonerock GL, Hoffman BM, Smith PJ, Blumenthal JA. Exercise as Treatment for Anxiety: Systematic Review and Analysis. Ann Behav Med. 2015;49(4):542-56.
17. Cosman F, de Beur SJ, LeBoff MS, et al. Clinician's Guide to Prevention and Treatment of Osteoporosis. Osteoporos Int. 2014;25(10):2359-81.
18. Golightly YM, Allen KD, Caine DJ. A comprehensive review of the effectiveness of different exercise programs for patients with osteoarthritis. Phys Sportsmed. 2012;40(4):52-65.
19. Howe TE, Rochester L, Neil F, Skelton DA, Ballinger C. Exercise for improving balance in older people. Cochrane Database Syst Rev. 2011 Nov 9;(11):CD004963. doi: 10.1002/14651858.CD004963.pub3.
20. Sherrington C, Whitney JC, Lord SR, Herbert RD, Cumming RG, Close JC. Effective exercise for the prevention of falls: a systematic review and meta-analysis. J Am Geriatr Soc. 2008;56:2234–43. doi: 10.1111/j.1532-5415.2008.02014.x.
21. Sherrington C, Tiedemann A, Fairhall N, Close JC, Lord SR. Exercise to prevent falls in older adults: an updated meta-analysis and best practice recommendations. N S W Public Health Bull. 2011;22:78–83. doi: 10.1071/NB10056.
22. Veldhuijzen van Zanten JJ, Rouse PC, Hale ED, et al. Perceived Barriers, Facilitators and Benefits for Regular Physical Activity and Exercise in Patients with Rheumatoid Arthritis: A Review of the Literature. Sports Med. 2015;45(10):1401-12.
23. Je Y, Jeon JY, Giovannucci EL, Meyerhardt JA. Association between physical activity and mortality in colorectal cancer: a meta-analysis of prospective cohort studies. International Journal of Cancer. 2013;133:1905–1913.
24. Patterson RE, Cadmus LA, Emond JA, Pierce JP. Physical activity, diet, adiposity and female breast cancer prognosis: a review of the epidemiologic literature. Maturitas. 2010;66:5–15.
25. Dieli-Conwright CM, Ma H, Lacey JV, et al. Long-term and baseline recreational physical activity and risk of endometrial cancer: the California Teachers Study. Br J Cancer. 2013;109(3):761-8.

26. Aune D, Sen A, Henriksen T, Saugstad OD, Tonstad S. Physical activity and the risk of gestational diabetes mellitus: a systematic review and dose-response meta-analysis of epidemiological studies. Eur J Epidemiol. 2016;31(10):967-997.
27. The American Congress of Obstetricians Gynecologist (ACOG) Physical activity and exercise during pregnancy and the postpartum period. n. 650, dec.2015. Obstet Gynecol. 2015;6:135–142.
28. Kite C, Lahart IM, Afzal I, et al. Exercise, or exercise and diet for the management of polycystic ovary syndrome: a systematic review and meta-analysis. Syst Rev. 2019;8(1):51. Published 2019 Feb 12. doi:10.1186/s13643-019-0962-3.
29. Bement MKH & Sluka KA (2016). Exercise-induced analgesia: an evidence-based review In Mechanisms and Management of Pain for the Physical Therapist, 2nd edn, ed. Sluka KA, editor. , Ch. 10. pp. 177–201. Wolters Kuwer, IASP Press, Seattle.
30. Strate LL, Liu YL, Aldoori WH, Giovannucci EL. Physical activity decreases diverticular complications. Am J Gastroenterol. 2009;104(5):1221-30.
31. Dukas L, Willett WC, Giovannucci EL (2003) Association between physical activity, fiber intake, and other lifestyle variables and constipation in a study of women. American Journal of Gastroenterology 98: 1790–6.
32. Williams PT. Effects of diet, physical activity and performance and body weight on incident gout in ostensibly healthy, vigorously active men. Am J Clin Nutr. 2008;87:1485–93.
33. Li C, Mikus C, Ahmed A, et al. A cross-sectional study of cardiorespiratory fitness and gallbladder disease. Ann Epidemiol. 2016;27(4):269-273.e3.
34. Anton SD, Hida A, Mankowski R, Layne A, Solberg LM, Mainous AG, Buford T. Nutrition and Exercise in Sarcopenia. Curr Protein Pept Sci. 2018;19(7):649-667. doi: 10.2174/1389203717666161227144349.
35. Gries KJ, Raue U, Perkins RK, Lavin KM, Overstreet BS, D'Acquisto LJ, Graham B, Finch WH, Kaminsky LA, Trappe TA, Trappe S. Cardiovascular and skeletal muscle health with lifelong exercise. J Appl Physiol (1985). 2018 Nov 1;125(5):1636-1645. doi: 10.1152/japplphysiol.00174.2018. Epub 2018 Aug 30.
36. Song D, Yu DSF. Effects of a moderate-intensity aerobic exercise programme on the cognitive function and quality of life of community-dwelling elderly people with mild cognitive impairment: A randomised controlled trial. Int J Nurs Stud. 2019 Mar 5;93:97-105. doi: 10.1016/j.ijnurstu.2019.02.019.
37. Mora JC, Valencia WM. Exercise and Older Adults. Clin Geriatr Med. 2018 Feb;34(1):145-162. doi: 10.1016/j.cger.2017.08.007. Epub 2017 Oct 10.
38. Warburton Darren E R, Nicol CW, Bredin Shannon S D. Health benefits of physical activity: the evidence. CMAJ. 2006 Mar 14;174(6):801–9. doi: 10.1503/cmaj.051351.
39. Lavie CJ, Arena R, Swift DL, et al. Exercise and the cardiovascular system: clinical science and cardiovascular outcomes. Circ Res. 2015;117(2):207-19.
40. Berlin JA, Colditz GA. A meta-analysis of physical activity in the prevention of coronary heart disease. Am J Epidemiol1990; 132: 612–28.
41. Wannamethee SG, Shaper AG, Walker M, Ebrahim S. Lifestyle and 15-year survival free of heart attack, stroke, and diabetes in middle-aged British men. Arch Intern Med 1998; 158: 2433–40.
42. S. Goya Wannamethee, A. Gerald Shaper. Physical Activity and Cardiovascular Disease. Seminars in Vascular Medicine 2002; 02(3): 257-266.
43. Cornelissen VA, Fagard RH, Coeckelberghs E, et al. Impact of resistance training on blood pressure and other cardiovascular risk factors: a meta-analysis of randomized, controlled trials. Hypertension. 2011;58(5):950–958.
44. Drenowatz C, Sui X, Fritz S, et al. The association between resistance exercise and cardiovascular disease risk in women. Journal of science and medicine in sport / Sports Medicine Australia. 2015;18(6):632-636.
45. American College of Sports Medicine Position Stand (ACSM). Quantity and quality of exercise for developing and maintain cardiorespiratory, musculoskeletal, and neuromotor fitness in apparently healthy adults: Guidance for prescribing exercise. Med Sci Sport Exerc. 2011;43:1334-1359.

46. Laukkanen KS, Salonen R, Rauramaa R, Salonen JT. The predictive value of cardiorespiratory fitness for cardiovascular events in men with various risk profiles: a prospective population-based cohort study. Eur Heart J 2004; 25: 1428–1437.
47. Ekelung LG, Haskell WL, Johnson JL, Whaley FS, Criqui MH, Sheps DS. Physical fitness as a predictor of cardiovascular mortality in asymptomatic North American men. The Lipid Research Clinics Mortality Follow-up Study. N Engl J Med 1988; 319: 1379–1384.
48. Blair SN, Goodyear NN, Gibbons LW, et al. Physical fitness and incidence of hypertension in healthy normotensive men and women. JAMA 1984;252:487-90.
49. Cornelissen VA, Fagard RH, Coeckelberghs E, et al. Impact of resistance training on blood pressure and other cardiovascular risk factors: a meta-analysis of randomized, controlled trials. Hypertension. 2011;58(5):950–958.
50. Paffenbarger RS Jr, Jung DL, Leung RW, et al. Physical activity and hypertension: an epidemiological view. Ann Med 1991;23:319-27.
51. Berg A, Halle M, Franz I, et al. Physical activity and lipoprotein metabolism: epidemiological evidence and clinical trials. Eur J Med Res 1997;2:259-64.
52. Prabhakaran B, Dowling EA, Branch JD, Swain DP, Leutholtz BC. Effect of 14 weeks of resistance training on lipid profile and body fat percentage in premenopausal women. Br J Sports Med.1999;33:190-195.
53. Halle M, Berg A, von Stein T, et al. Lipoprotein(a) in endurance athletes, power athletes, and sedentary controls. Med Sci Sports Exerc 1996;28:962-6.
54. Wallberg-Henriksson H, Rincon J, Zierath JR. Exercise in the management of non-insulin-dependent diabetes mellitus. Sports Med 1998;25:25-35.
55. Poehlman ET, Melby C. Resistance training and energy balance. Int J Sport Nutr.1998;8:143-159. Tremblay A, Despres JP, Leblanc C, et al. Effect of intensity of physical activity on body fatness and fat distribution. Am J Clin Nutr 1990;51:153-7.
56. Wallberg-Henriksson H, Rincon J, Zierath JR. Exercise in the management of non-insulin-dependent diabetes mellitus. Sports Med 1998;25:25-35.
57. Poehlman ET, Dvorak RV, DeNino WF, Brochu M, Ades PA. Effects of resistance training and endurance training on insulin sensitivity in nonobese, young women. J Clin Endocrinol Metab.2000;85:2463-2468.
58. Jurca R, Lamonte MJ, Barlow CE, et al. Association of muscular strength with incidence of metabolic syndrome in men. Med Sci Sports Exerc. 2005;37(11):1849–1855.
59. Adamopoulos S, Parissis J, Kroupis C, et al. Physical training reduces peripheral markers of inflammation in patients with chronic heart failure. Eur Heart J 2001;22:791-7.
60. Nicklas BJ, You T, Pahor M. Behavioural treatments for chronic systemic inflammation: effects of dietary weight loss and exercise training [review]. CMAJ 2005;172(9): 1199-209.
61. Tiukinhoy S, Beohar N, Hsie M. Improvement in heart rate recovery after cardiac rehabilitation. J Cardiopulm Rehabil 2003;23:84-7.
62. Farinatti PT, Brandão C, Soares PP, Duarte AF. Acute effects of stretching exercise on the heart rate variability in subjects with low flexibility levels. J Strength Cond Res. 2011 Jun;25(6):1579-85.
63. Rauramaa R, Salonen JT, Seppanen K, et al. Inhibition of platelet aggregability by moderate-intensity physical exercise: a randomized clinical trial in overweight men. Circulation 1986;74:939-44.
64. Gokce N, Vita JA, Bader DS, et al. Effect of exercise on upper and lower extremity endothelial function in patients with coronary artery disease. Am J Cardiol 2002;90:124-7.
65. Kenta Yamamoto, Hiroshi Kawano, Yuko Gando, et al. Poor trunk flexibility is associated with arterial stiffening. American Journal of Physiology - Heart and Circulatory Physiology Published 1 October 2009 Vol. 297 no. 4, H1314-H1318.
66. Vaitkevicius PV, Fleg JL, Engel JH, et al. Effects of age and aerobic capacity on arterial stiffness in healthy adults. Circulation 88: 1456–1462, 1993.
67. Laurent S, Boutouyrie P, Asmar R, Gautier I, Laloux B, Guize L, Ducimetiere P, Benetos A. Aortic stiffness is an independent predictor of all-cause and cardiovascular mortality in hypertensive patients. Hypertension 37: 1236–1241, 2001.

68. Hambrecht R, Wolf A, Gielen S, et al. Effect of exercise on coronary endothelial function in patients with coronary artery disease. N Engl J Med 2000;342:454-60.
69. Warburton DE, Haykowsky MJ, Quinney HA, et al. Blood volume expansion and cardiorespiratory function: effects of training modality. Med Sci Sports Exerc 2004;36:991-1000.
70. Dunn AL, Trivedi MH, O'Neal HA. Physical activity dose–response effects on outcomes of depression and anxiety. Med Sci Sports Exerc 2001;33:S587-97.
71. http://www.heart.org/HEARTORG/HealthyLiving/PhysicalActivity/FitnessBasics/Strength-and-Resistance-Training-Exercise_UCM_462357_Article.jsp#.WP-16tLys1I.
72. Kai Y, Nagamatsu T, Kitabatake Y, Sensui H. Effects of stretching on menopausal and depressive symptoms in middle-aged women: a randomized controlled trial. Menopause. 2016 Aug;23(8):827-32.
73. Williams PT (2010) Reductions in incident coronary heart disease risk above guideline physical activity levels in men. Atherosclerosis. 209: 524–7.
74. Petersen CB, Gronbaek M, Helge JW, Thygesen LC, Schnohr P, Tolstrup JS. Changes in physical activity in leisure time and the risk of myocardial infarction, ischemic heart disease, and all-cause mortality. Eur J Epidemiol. 2012;27(2):91–99.
75. Jolliffe JA, Rees K, Taylor RS, Thompson D, Oldridge N, Ebrahim S. Exercise-based rehabilitation for coronary heart disease. Cochrane Database Syst Rev. 2001;(1):CD001800.
76. Blair SN, Kohl HW, III, Barlow CE, Paffenbarger RS, Jr, Gibbons LW, Macera CA. Changes in physical fitness and all-cause mortality. A prospective study of healthy and unhealthy men. JAMA. 1995;273(14):1093–1098.
77. Kraigher-Krainer E, Lyass A, Massaro JM, Lee DS, Ho JE, Levy D, Kannel WB, Vasan RS. Association of physical activity and heart failure with preserved vs. reduced ejection fraction in the elderly: the Framingham Heart Study. Eur J Heart Fail 2013; 15: 742–746.
78. Berry JD, Pandey A, Gao A, Leonard D, Farzaneh-Far R, Ayers C, DeFina L, Willis B. Physical fitness and risk for heart failure and coronary artery disease. Circ Heart Fail 2013; 6: 627–634.
79. Intwala S, Balady GJ. Physical activity in the prevention of heart failure. Another step forward. Circulation 2015; 132: 1777–1779.
80. Pandey A, LaMonte M, Klein L, Ayers C, Psaty BM, Eaton CB, Allen NB, de Lemos JA, Carnethon M, Greenland P, Berry JD. Relationship between physical activity, body mass index and risk of heart failure. JACC 2017; 69: 1129–1142.
81. Haykowsky MJ, Liang Y, Pechter D, Jones LW, McAlister FA, Clark AM. A meta-analysis of the effect of exercise training on left ventricular remodeling in heart failure: the benefit depends on the type of training performed. J Am Coll Cardiol 2007; 49: 2329–2336.
82. Hambrecht R, Gielen S, Linke A, Fiehn E, Yu J, Walther C, Schoene N, Schuler G. Effects of exercise training on left ventricular function and peripheral resistance in patients with chronic heart failure: a randomized trial. JAMA 2000; 283: 3095–3101.
83. Mozaffarian D, Furberg CD, Psaty BM, Siscovick D (2008) Physical activity and incidence of atrial fibrillation in older adults: the Cardiovascular Health Study. Circulation. 19 118: 800–7.
84. Williams PT. Reduction in incident stroke risk with vigorous physical activity during 7.7-year follow-up of the National Runners' Health Study. Stroke. 2009;40:1921–3.
85. Kim Y, Sharp S, Hwang S, et al Exercise and incidence of myocardial infarction, stroke, hypertension, type 2 diabetes and site-specific cancers: prospective cohort study of 257 854 adults in South Korea BMJ Open 2019;9:e025590. doi: 10.1136/bmjopen-2018-025590.
86. Han P, Zhang W, Kang L, et al. Clinical Evidence of Exercise Benefits for Stroke. Adv Exp Med Biol. 2017;1000:131-151. doi: 10.1007/978-981-10-4304-8_9.
87. Wiener J, McIntyre A, Janssen S, Chow JT, Batey C, Teasell R. Effectiveness of High-Intensity Interval Training for Fitness and Mobility Post Stroke: A Systematic Review. PM R. 2019 Mar 12. doi: 10.1002/pmrj.12154.
88. Sesso HD et al. Physical activity and coronary heart disease in men. Circulation 2000; 102: 975–980.

89. Tanasescu M, Leitzmann MF, Rimm EB, Willett WC, Stampfer MJ, Hu FB. Exercise Type and Intensity in Relation to Coronary Heart Disease in Men. JAMA. 2002;288(16):1994-2000.
90. Lee IM, Rexrode KM, Cook NR, Manson JE, Buring JE. Physical activity and coronary heart disease in women: Is "no pain, no gain" passé? JAMA 2001; 285: 1447–1454.
91. S. Goya Wannamethee, A. Gerald Shaper. Physical Activity and Cardiovascular Disease. Seminars in Vascular Medicine 2002; 02(3): 257-266.
92. Li TY, Rana JS, Manson JE, Willett WC, Stampfer MJ, Colditz GA, et al. Obesity as compared with physical activity in predicting risk of coronary heart disease in women. Circulation 2006; 113: 499–506.
93. Hu G, Jousilahti P, Borodulin K, Barengo NC, Lakka TA, Nissinen A, et al. Occupational, commuting and leisure-time physical activity in relation to coronary heart disease among middle-aged Finnish men and women. Atherosclerosis 2007; 194: 490–497.
94. Sofi F, Capalbo A, Cesari F, Abbate R, Gensini GF. Physical activity during leisure time and primary prevention of coronary heart disease: An updated meta-analysis of cohort studies. Eur J Cardiovasc Prev Rehabil 2008; 15: 247–257.
95. Li J, Siegrist J. Physical activity and risk of cardiovascular disease: A meta-analysis of prospective cohort studies. Int J Environ Res Public Health 2012; 9: 391–407.
96. Sattelmair J, et al. Dose response between physical activity and risk of coronary heart disease: a meta-analysis. Circulation. 2011;124(7):789-95.
97. Leon AS, Connett J, Jacobs DR Jr., et al. Leisure-time physical activity levels and risk of coronary heart disease and death. The Multiple Risk Factor Intervention Trial. JAMA 1987;258:2388-95.
98. Hakim AA, Curb JD, Petrovitch H, et al. Effects of walking on coronary heart disease in elderly men: the Honolulu Heart Program. Circulation. 1999. 100 (1):9-13.
99. Berry JD, Willis B, Gupta S, Barlow CE, Lakoski SG, Khera A, et al. Lifetime risks for cardiovascular disease mortality by cardiorespiratory fitness levels measured at ages 45, 55, and 65 years in Menthe Cooper Center Longitudinal Study. J Am Coll Cardiol 2011; 57:1604–1610.
100. Katzmarzyk PT, Church TS, Blair SN. Cardiorespiratory fitness attenuates the effects of the metabolic syndrome on all-cause and cardiovascular disease mortality in men. Arch Intern Med 2004; 164: 1092–1097.
101. Leon AS, Myers MJ, Connett J. Leisure time physical activity and the 16-year risks of mortality from coronary heart disease and all-causes in the MRFIT. Int J Sports Med. 1997 Jul;18: S208–S215.
102. Kodama S, Saito K, Tanaka S, Maki M, Yachi Y, Asumi M, et al.Cardiorespiratory fitness as a quantitative predictor of all-cause mortality and cardiovascular events in healthy men and women. JAMA 2009; 301: 2024–2035.
103. D. Lee, R.R. Pate, C.J. Lavie, X. Sui, T.S. Church, S.N. Blair Leisure-time running reduces all-cause and cardiovascular mortality risk. J Am Coll Cardiol, 64 (2014), pp. 472-481.
104. C.P. Wen, J.P. Wai, M.K. Tsai, et al. Minimum amount of physical activity for reduced mortality and extended life expectancy: a prospective cohort study. Lancet, 378 (2011), pp. 1244-1253.
105. http://www.heart.org/HEARTORG/HealthyLiving/PhysicalActivity/FitnessBasics/American-Heart-Association-Recommendations-for-Physical-Activity-in-Adults_UCM_307976_Article.jsp#.WRKU2uXys1I (Accessed May 8, 2017).
106. Garber CE, Blissmer B, Deschenes MR, Franklin BA, Lamonte MJ, Lee IM, Nieman DC, Swain DP. American College of Sports Medicine position stand. Quantity and quality of exercise for developing and maintaining cardiorespiratory, musculoskeletal, and neuromotor fitness in apparently healthy adults: guidance for prescribing exercise. Med Sci Sports Exerc. 2011 Jul;43(7):1334-59. doi: 10.1249/MSS.0b013e318213fefb.
107. Fakhry F, van de Luijtgaarden KM, Bax L, et al. Supervised walking therapy in patients with intermittent claudication. J Vasc Surg. 2012;56(4):1132–1142.
108. McDermott MM, Liu K, Guralnik JM, et al. Home-based walking exercise intervention in peripheral artery disease: a randomized clinical trial. JAMA. 2013;310(1):57-65.

109. Nicolosi A, Glasser DB, Moreira ED, Villa M. Prevalence of erectile dysfunction and associated factors among men without concomitant disease: a population study. Int J Impot Res. 2003;15:253–257.
110. Bacon CG, Mittleman MA, Kawachi I, Giovannucci E, Glasser DB, Rimm EB. Sexual function in men older than 50 years of age: results from the health Professionals' follow-up study. Ann Intern Med. 2003;139:161–168.
111. Maio G, Saraed S, Marchiori A. Physical activity and PDE5 inhibitors in the treatment of erectile dysfunction: results of a randomized controlled study. Journal of Sex Med. 2010;7(6):2201–2208.
112. Lamina S, Agbanusi E, Nwacha RC. Effects of aerobic exercise in the management of erectile dysfunction: a meta analysis study on randomized controlled trials. Ethiop J Health Sci. 2011;21(3):195-201.
113. Esposito K, Giugliano F, DiPalo C, Giugliano G, Marfella R, D'Andrea F, et al. Effect of lifestyle changes on erectile dysfunction in obese men: a randomized controlled trial. JAMA. 2004;291(24):2978–2984. 23.
114. Lamina S, Okoye CG, Dagogo TT. Therapeutic effect of an interval exercise training program in the management of erectile dysfunction in hypertensive patients. J Clinical Hypertension. 2008;11(3):125–129.
115. Gothe NP, McAuley E. Yoga Is as Good as Stretching-Strengthening Exercises in Improving Functional Fitness Outcomes: Results From a Randomized Controlled Trial. J Gerontol A Biol Sci Med Sci. 2015;71(3):406-11.
116. Larson-Meyer DE. A Systematic Review of the Energy Cost and Metabolic Intensity of Yoga. Med Sci Sports Exerc. 2016 Aug;48(8):1558-69.
117. Long R. Scientific keys volume I: the key muscles of hatha yoga. 3. Bandha: Yoga; 2006.
118. McCall T. Yoga as medicine: The yogic prescription for health and healing. 1. New York: Bantam Dell; 2007.
119. Ray US, Pathak A, Tomer OS. Hatha yoga practices: Energy expenditure, respiratory changes and intensity of exercise. Evid Based Complement Alternat Med. 2011; 2011:241294.
120. Sovová E, Čajka V, Pastucha D, et al. Positive effect of yoga on cardiorespiratory fitness: A pilot study. Int J Yoga. 2015 Jul-Dec;8(2):134-8.
121. Sherman SA, Rogers RJ, Davis KK, Minster RL, Creasy SA, Mullarkey NC, O'Dell M, Donahue P, Jakicic JM. Energy Expenditure in Vinyasa Yoga Versus Walking. J Phys Act Health. 2017 Aug;14(8):597-605. doi: 10.1123/jpah.2016-0548. Epub 2017 Apr 19.
122. Watts AW, Rydell SA, Eisenberg ME, Laska MN, Neumark-Sztainer D. Yoga's potential for promoting healthy eating and physical activity behaviors among young adults: a mixed-methods study. Int J Behav Nutr Phys Act. 2018;15(1):42. Published 2018 May 2. doi:10.1186/s12966-018-0674-4.
123. Bhavesh Surendra Mody. Acute effects of Surya Namaskar on the cardiovascular & metabolic system. Journal of Bodywork and Movement Therapies. Volume 15, Issue 3, July 2011, Pages 343-347

Heart Rate

1. Richard CV Tyser et al, Calcium handling precedes cardiac differentiation to initiate the first heartbeat. eLife 2016;5:e17113 DOI: 10.7554/eLife.17113.
2. Bauman Adrian E, Blair Steven N. Everyone could enjoy the "survival advantage" of elite athletes BMJ 2012; 345 :e8338.
3. Wang A, Chen S, Wang C, et al. Resting heart rate and risk of cardiovascular diseases and all-cause death: the Kailuan study. PLoS One. 2014;9(10):e110985. Published 2014 Oct 24.
4. Lonn EM, Rambihar S, Gao P, Custodis FF, Sliwa K, et al. (2014) Heart rate is associated with increased risk of major cardiovascular events, cardiovascular and all-cause death in patients with stable chronic cardiovascular disease: an analysis of ONTARGET/TRANSCEND. Clin Res Cardiol 103: 149–159.
5. Bohm M. et al. . Heart rate as a risk factor in chronic heart failure (SHIFT): the association between heart rate and outcomes in a randomised placebo-controlled trial. Lancet 376, 886–894 (2010).

6. Ferrari R, Censi S, Mastrorilli F, Boraso A. Prognostic benefits of heart rate reduction in cardiovascular disease. Eur Heart J Suppl. 2003;5(Suppl G):G10–G14.
7. Kannel W. B., Kannel C., Paffenbarger R. S., Cupples P. H. & Cupples L. A. Heart rate and cardiovascular mortality: the Framingham study. Am. Heart J. 113, 1489–1494 (1987).
8. Jouven X., Zureik M., Desnos M., Guerot C., Ducimetiere P. Resting heart rate as a predictive risk factor for sudden death in middle-aged men. Cardiovasc Res. 2001;50:373–378.
9. Cheng YJ, Macera CA, Church TS, Blair SN. Heart rate reserve as a predictor of cardiovascular and all-cause mortality in men. Med Sci Sports Exerc. 2002 Dec;34(12):1873-8.
10. Cooney M.T., Vartiainen E., Laatikainen T. Elevated resting heart rate is an independent risk factor for cardiovascular disease in healthy men and women. Am Heart J. 2010;159(4):612–619.
11. Koskela JK, Tahvanainen A, Haring A, et al. Association of resting heart rate with cardiovascular function: a cross-sectional study in 522 Finnish subjects. BMC Cardiovasc Disord. 2013;13:102. Published 2013 Nov 15. doi:10.1186/1471-2261-13-102.
12. Van der Ploeg CP, Dankelman J, Spaan JA. Heart rate affects the dependency of myocardial oxygen consumption on flow in goats. Heart Vessels. 1995;10(5):258-65.
13. Caetano J, Delgado Alves J. Heart rate and cardiovascular protection. Eur J Intern Med. 2015 May;26(4):217-22. doi: 10.1016/j.ejim.2015.02.009. Epub 2015 Feb 20.; Tardif JC. Heart rate as a treatable cardiovascular risk factor. Br Med Bull. 2009;90:71-84. doi: 10.1093/bmb/ldp016. Epub 2009 May 27.
14. Sivasankaran S., Pollard-Quintner S., Sachdeva R., Pugeda J., Hoq S. M., Zarich S. W. The effect of a six-week program of yoga and meditation on brachial artery reactivity: do psychosocial interventions affect vascular tone? Clinical Cardiology. 2006;29(9):393–398. doi: 10.1002/clc.4960290905.
15. Veerabhadrappa SG, Baljoshi VS, Khanapure S, et al. Effect of yogic bellows on cardiovascular autonomic reactivity. J Cardiovasc Dis Res. 2011;2:223–7.
16. Ankad RB, Herur A, Patil S, Shashikala GV, Chinagudi S. Effect of Short-Term Pranayama and Meditation on Cardiovascular Functions in Healthy Individuals. Heart Views. 2011;12:58–62.
17. Devasena I., Narhare P. Effect of yoga on heart rate and blood pressure and its clinical significance. International Journal of Biological & Medical Research. 2011;2:750–753.
18. Larson-Meyer DE. A Systematic Review of the Energy Cost and Metabolic Intensity of Yoga. Med Sci Sports Exerc. 2016 Aug. 48 (8): 1558-69.
19. Elshazly A, Khorshid H, Hanna H, Ali A. Effect of exercise training on heart rate recovery in patients post anterior myocardial infarction. Egypt Heart J. 2018;70(4):283-285.
20. Jerath RJ, Edry VA, Barnes VA, Jerath V. Physiology of long pranayamic breathing: Neural respiratory elements may provide a mechanism that explains how slow breathing shifts the autonomic nervous system. Med Hypotheses. 2006;67:566–71.
21. Wallace RK, Benson H, Wilson AF. A wakeful hypo-metabolic physiological state. Am J Physiol. 1971;221:795–9.

Heart Rate Variability

1. American Society of Pacing and Electrophysiology (1996). Heart rate variability: standards of measurement, physiological interpretation, and clinical use. Circulation 93, 1043–1065.
2. Bigger J. T., Jr. (1997). The predictive value of RR variability and baroreflex sensitivity in coronary heart disease. Card. Electrophysiol. Rev. 1, 198–20410.1023/A:1009902022073.
3. De Jong M. J., Randall D. C. (2005). Heart rate variability analysis in the assessment of autonomic function in heart failure. J. Cardiovasc. Nurs. 20, 186–19510.1111/j.0889-7204.2005.04605.x.
4. Thayler J. F., Yamamoto S. S., Brosschot J. F. (2010). The relationship of autonomic imbalance, heart rate variability and cardiovascular disease risk factors. Int. J. Cardiol. 141, 122–13110.1016/j.ijcard.2009.09.543.
5. Schroeder E. B. et al. . Diabetes, glucose, insulin, and heart rate variability. Diabet. Care 28, 668–674 (2005).
6. Brotman D. J. et al. . Heart rate variability predicts ESRD and CKD-related hospitalization.

J. Am. Soc. Nephrol. 21, 1560–1570 (2010).
7. Alvares GA, Quintana DS, Kemp AH, et al. Reduced heart rate variability in social anxiety disorder: associations with gender and symptom severity. PLoS One. 2013;8:7.
8. Schroeder EB, Liao D, Chambless LE, et al. Hypertension, blood pressure, and heart rate variability: the Atherosclerosis Risk in Communities (ARIC) study. Hypertension. 2003;42:1106–11.
9. T. H, Venditti Jr FJ, Manders ES, et al. Reduced heart rate variability and mortality risk in an elderly cohort. The Framingham Heart Study. Circulation 1994;90:878–83.
10. Ryan C, Hollenberg M, Harvey DB, Gwynn R. Impaired parasympathetic responses in patients after myocardial infarction. Am J Cardiol. 1976;37:1013–1018.
11. Kristal-Boneh E, Raifel M, Froom P, Ribak J. Heart rate variability in health and disease. Scand J Work Environ Health. 1995;21:85–95.
12. Kleiger RE, Miller JP, Bigger JT, Moss AJ. Decreased heart rate variability and its association with increased mortality after acute myocardial infarction. Am J Cardiol. 1987;59:256-262.
13. Wolk R. Central origin of decreased heart rate variability in patients with cardiovascular diseases. Med Hypotheses. 1996;46:479–481.
14. Tapanainen JM, Thomsem PEB, Køber L, Torp-Pedersen C, Mäkikallio TH, Still A-M, Lindgren KS, Huikuri HV. Fractal analysis of heart rate variability and mortality after an acute myocardial infarction. Am J Cardiol. 2002;90:347–352.)
15. Liao D, Cai J, Barnes RW, Tyroler HA, Rautaharju P, Holme I, Heiss G. Association of cardiac autonomic function and the development of hypertension: the ARIC study. Am J Hypertens. 1996 Dec;9(12 Pt 1):1147-56.
16. Goit R. K. & Ansari A. H. Reduced parasympathetic tone in newly diagnosed essential hypertension. Indian Heart J. 68, 153–157 (2016).
17. Carthy ER. Autonomic dysfunction in essential hypertension: A systematic review. Ann Med Surg (Lond). 2013;3(1):2-7. Published 2013 Dec 11. doi:10.1016/j.amsu.2013.11.002.
18. Stefanie Hillebrand, Karin B. Gast, Renée de Mutsert, Cees A. Swenne, J. Wouter Jukema, Saskia Middeldorp, Frits R. Rosendaal, Olaf M. Dekkers; Heart rate variability and first cardiovascular event in populations without known cardiovascular disease: meta-analysis and dose–response meta-regression, EP Europace, Volume 15, Issue 5, 1 May 2013, Pages 742–749.
19. Hisako Tsuji, MD; Martin G. Larson, ScD; Ferdinand J. Venditti, Jr, MD; Emily S. Manders, BS; Jane C. Evans, MPH; Charles L. Feldman, ScD; Daniel Levy, MD. Impact of Reduced Heart Rate Variability on Risk for Cardiac Events The Framingham Heart Study. Circulation. 1996;94:2850-2855.
20. Liao D. et al. . Cardiac autonomic function and incident coronary heart disease: a population-based case-cohort study. The ARIC Study. Atherosclerosis Risk in Communities Study. Am. J. Epidemiol. 145, 696–706 (1997).
21. Musialik-Lydka A, Sredniawa B, Pasyk S. Heart rate variability in heart failure. Kardiol Pol. 2003 Jan;58(1):10-6.
22. Kleiger, Robert E. et al. Decreased heart rate variability and its association with increased mortality after acute myocardial infarction. American Journal of Cardiology , Volume 59 , Issue 4 , 256 - 262.
23. R.J Myerburg, A Interian, R.M Mitrani, K.M Kessler, A CastellanosFrequency of sudden cardiac death and profiles of risk. Am J Cardiol, 80 (1997), pp. 10F-19F.
24. Makikallio TH, Huikuri HV, Mäkikallio A, Sourander LB, Mitrani RD, Castellanos A, et al. Prediction of sudden cardiac death by fractal analysis of heart rate variability in elderly subjects. J Am Coll Cardiol. 2001;37:1395–402.
25. Tyagi A, Cohen M. Yoga and heart rate variability: A comprehensive review of the literature. Int J Yoga. 2016;9(2):97-113.
26. Khattab K, Khattab AA, Ortak J, Richardt G, Bonnemeier H. Iyengar yoga increases cardiac parasympathetic nervous modulation among healthy yoga practitioners. Evid Based Complement Alternat Med. 2007;4:511–17.
27. Cheema BS, Marshall PW, Chang D, Colagiuri B, Machliss B. Effect of an office worksite-based yoga program on heart rate variability: A randomized controlled trial. BMC Public Health. 2011;11:578.
28. Vinay AV, Venkatesh D, Ambarish V. Impact of short-term practice of yoga on heart rate variability. Int J Yoga. 2016;9(1):62-6.

29. Telles S, et al. Blood pressure and heart rate variability during yoga-based alternate nostril breathing practice and breath awareness. Med Sci Monit Basic Res. 2014 Nov 19;20:184-93. doi: 10.12659/MSMBR.892063.
30. Muralikrishnan K, Balakrishnan B, Balasubramanian K, Visnegarawla F. Measurement of the effect of Isha Yoga on cardiac autonomic nervous system using short-term heart rate variability. J Ayurveda Integr Med. 2012;3:91–6.
31. Markil N et al. Yoga Nidra relaxation increases heart rate variability and is unaffected by a prior bout of Hatha yoga. J Altern Complement Med. 2012 Oct;18(10):953-8. doi: 10.1089/acm.2011.0331. Epub 2012 Aug 6.
32. Telles S, Mahapatra RS, Naveen KV. Heart rate variability spectrum during Vipassana mindfulness meditation. J Indian Psychol. 2005;23:1–5.
33. Dolgoff-Kaspar R, Baldwin A, Johnson MS, Edling N, Sethi GK. Effect of laughter yoga on mood and heart rate variability in patients awaiting organ transplantation: A pilot study. Altern Ther Health Med. 2012;18:61–6.
34. Poscoe MC et al. Yoga, mindfulness-based stress reduction and stress-related physiological measures: A meta-analysis. Psychoneuroendocrinology. 2017 Dec;86:152-168.

Lipids

1. Stary HC, Chandler AB, Glagov S, et al. A definition of initial, fatty streak, and intermediate lesions of atherosclerosis. A report from the Committee on Vascular Lesions of the Council on Arteriosclerosis, American Heart Association. Circulation. 1994; 89:2462–2478.
2. Mallika V, Goswami B, Rajappa M. Atherosclerosis pathophysiology and the role of novel risk factors: a clinicobiochemical perspective. Angiology 2007;58:513-22.
3. Verschuren Wmm, Jacobs DR, Bloemberg Bpm, Kromhout D, Menotti A, Aravanis C, et al. Serum total cholesterol and long-term coronary heart disease mortality in different cultures. Twenty-five-year follow-up of the Seven Countries Study. JAMA 1995; 274: 131 6.
4. Houterman, S. , Verschuren, W. M., Hofman, A. and Witteman, J. C. (1999), Serum cholesterol is a risk factor for myocardial infarction in elderly men and women: the Rotterdam Study. Journal of Internal Medicine, 246: 25-33. doi:10.1046/j.1365-2796.1999.00525.x.
5. Klag MJ, Ford DE, Mead LA, He J, Whelton PK, Liang K-Y, Levine DM. Serum cholesterol in young men and subsequent cardiovascular disease. N Engl J Med. 1993; 328:313–318.
6. Su-Min Jeong, Seulggie Choi, Kyuwoong Kim, et al. Effect of Change in Total Cholesterol Levels on Cardiovascular Disease Among Young Adults. JAHA, June 19, 2018,Vol 7, Issue 12.
7. -Prospective Studies Collaboration, Lewington S, Whitlock G, Clarke R, Sherliker P, Emberson J, Halsey J, Qizilbash N, Peto R, Collins R.Blood cholesterol and vascular mortality by age, sex, and blood pressure: a meta-analysis of individual data from 61 prospective studies with 55,000 vascular deaths. Lancet 2007;370:1829–1839.
8. Sanne A.E. Peters, Yankuba Singhateh, Diana Mackay, Rachel R. Huxley, Mark Woodward. Total cholesterol as a risk factor for coronary heart disease and stroke in women compared with men: A systematic review and meta-analysis. Atherosclerosis. Volume 248, May 2016, Pages 123-131.
9. Keaven M. Anderson, William P. Castelli, Daniel Levy. Cholesterol and Mortality. 30 Years of Follow-up from the Framingham Study. JAMA. 1987;257(16):2176-2180. doi:10.1001/jama.1987.03390160062027.
10. W. M. Monique Verschuren and D. Kromhout. Total cholesterol concentration and mortality at a relatively young age: do men and women differ? BMJ. 1995 Sep 23; 311(7008): 779–783.
11. https://www.ahajournals.org/doi/pdf/10.1161/01.CIR.82.6.1916.
12. Pignone MP, Phillips CJ, Lannon CM, Mulrow CD, Teutsch SM, Lohr KN, Whitener BL. Screening for Lipid Disorders. Rockville (MD): Agency for Healthcare Research and Quality (US); 2001 Apr. Report No.: 01-S004.
13. Baigent C, Keech A, Kearney PM, Blackwell L, Buck G, Pollicino C, Kirby A, Sourjina T, Peto R, Collins R, Simes R; Cholesterol Treatment Trialists' (CTT) Collaborators.Efficacy and safety of cholesterol-lowering treatment: prospective meta-analysis of data from 90 056 participants in 14 randomised trials of statins. Lancet. 2005; 366:1267–1278.
14. Descamps OS, Bruniaux M, Guilmot PF, Tonglet R, Heller FR. Lipoprotein concentrations in newborns are associated with allelic variations in their mothers. Atherosclerosis

2004;172:287–298.
15. Expert panel on integrated guidelines for cardiovascular health and risk reduction in children and adolescents: summary report. Pediatrics. 2011;128 (Suppl 5):S213–256.
16. Goldstein JL, Brown MS. A century of cholesterol and coronaries: from plaques to genes to statins. Cell 2015;161:161–172.
17. Yancy C.W. ACCF/AHA guideline for the management of heart failure: executive summary: a report of the American College of Cardiology Foundation/American Heart Association Task Force on practice guidelines. Circulation. 2013;128(16):1810–1852.
18. Brian A. Ference Henry N. Ginsberg Ian Graham et al. Low-density lipoproteins cause atherosclerotic cardiovascular disease. 1. Evidence from genetic, epidemiologic, and clinical studies. A consensus statement from the European Atherosclerosis Society Consensus Panel. European Heart Journal, Volume 38, Issue 32, 21 August 2017, Pages 2459–2472, https://doi.org/10.1093/eurheartj/ehx144
19. Emerging Risk Factors C, Di Angelantonio E, Gao P, Pennells L, et al. Lipid-related markers and cardiovascular disease prediction. JAMA 2012;307:2499–2506.
20. Goldstein JL, Brown MS. A century of cholesterol and coronaries: from plaques to genes to statins. Cell. 2015;161(1):161-172.
21. Scandinavian Simvastatin Survival Study Group Randomised trial of cholesterol lowering in 4444 patients with coronary heart disease: the Scandinavian Simvastatin Survival Study (4S). Lancet. 1994;344:1383–1389.
22. Heart Protection Collaborative Group, MRC/BHF Heart Protection Study of cholesterol lowering with simvastatin in 20 536 high-risk individuals: a randomised placebo-controlled trial, Lancet (2002);360: pp. 7-22.
23. Shepherd J, Blauw GJ, Murphy MB et al., on behalf of the PROSPER study group, Pravastatin in elderly individuals at risk of vascular disease (PROSPER): a randomised controlled trial. Prospective Study of Pravastatin in the Elderly at Risk, Lancet (2002);360: pp. 1,623-1,630.
24. ALLHAT Officers and Coordinators for the ALLHAT Collaborative Research Group, The Antihypertensive and Lipid- Lowering Treatment to Prevent Heart Attack Trial. Major outcomes in moderately hypercholesterolemic, hypertensive patients randomized to pravastatin vs usual care: the Antihypertensive and Lipid-Lowering Treatment to Prevent Heart Attack Trial (ALLHAT-LLT), JAMA (2002);288: pp. 2,998-3,007.
25. Sever P S, Dahl ├Âf B, Poulter N R et al., for the ASCOT investigators, Prevention of coronary and stroke events with atorvastatin in hypertensive patients who have average or lower-than-average cholesterol concentrations, in the Anglo- Scandinavian Cardiac Outcomes Trial - Lipid Lowering Arm (ASCOT-LLA): a multicentre randomised controlled trial, Lancet (2003);361: pp. 1,149-1,158.
26. Silverman MG. Ference BA, Im K, Wiviott SD, Giugliano RP, Grundy SM, Braunwald E, Sabatine MS. Association Between Lowering LDL-C and Cardiovascular Risk Reduction Among Different Therapeutic Interventions: A Systematic Review and Meta-analysis. JAMA. 2016 Sep 27;316(12):1289-97. doi: 10.1001/jama.2016.13985.
27. Cholesterol Treatment Trialists' (CTT) Collaboration, Baigent C, Blackwell L, et al. Efficacy and safety of more intensive lowering of LDL cholesterol: a meta-analysis of data from 170,000 participants in 26 randomised trials. Lancet. 2010;376(9753):1670-81.
28. Gordon T, Castelli WP, Hjortland MC, Kannel WB, Dawber TR. High density lipoprotein as a protective factor against coronary heart disease. The Framingham Study. Am J Med. 1977;62:707–714.
29. Ibanez B., Vilahur G., Cimmino G., Speidl W.S., Pinero A., Choi B.G., Zafar M.U., Santos-Gallego C.G., Krause B., Badimon L., et al. Rapid change in plaque size, composition, and molecular footprint after recombinant apolipoprotein A-I Milano (ETC-216) administration: Magnetic resonance imaging study in an experimental model of atherosclerosis. J. Am. Coll. Cardiol. 2008;51:1104–1109. doi: 10.1016/j.jacc.2007.09.071.
30. Goff D.C., Lloyd-Jones D.M., Bennett G., Coady S., D'Agostino R.B., Gibbons R., Greenland P., Lackland D.T., Levy D., O'Donnell C.J., et al. American College of Cardiology/American Heart Association Task Force on Practice Guidelines 2013 ACC/AHA guideline on the assessment of cardiovascular risk: A report of the American College of Cardiology/American Heart Association Task Force on Practice Guidelines. J. Am. Coll. Cardiol. 2014;63:2935–2959. doi: 10.1016/j.jacc.2013.11.005.
31. Wilson PW, Abbott RD, Castelli WP. High density lipoprotein cholesterol and mortality. The

Framingham Heart Study. Arteriosclerosis. 1988;8:737–741.
32. Wilson PW, D'Agostino RB, Levy D, Belanger AM, Silbershatz H, Kannel WB. (1998) Prediction of coronary heart disease using risk factor categories. Circulation; 97(18):1837-47.
33. Gordon DJ, Probstfield JL, Garrison RJ, Neaton JD, Castelli WP, Knoke JD, et al. High-density lipoprotein cholesterol and cardiovascular disease. Four prospective American studies. Circulation. 1989;79:8–15.
34. Gordon DJ, Probstfield JL, Garrison RJ, et al. High-density lipoprotein cholesterol and cardiovascular disease: four prospective American studies. Circulation 1989;79:8-15.
35. Estrada-Luna D, Ortiz-Rodriguez MA, Medina-Briseño L, et al. Current Therapies Focused on High-Density Lipoproteins Associated with Cardiovascular Disease. Molecules. 2018;23(11):2730. Published 2018 Oct 23. doi:10.3390/molecules23112730.
36. Olivero-David R., Ruiz-Roso M.B., Caporaso N., Perez-Olleros L., De Las Heras N., Lahera V., Ruiz-Roso B. In vivo bioavailability of polyphenols from grape by-product extracts, and effect on lipemia of normocholesterolemic Wistar rats. J. Sci. Food Agric. 2018 doi: 10.1002/jsfa.9100.
37. Sarwar N, Danesh J, Eiriksdottir G, et al. Triglycerides and the risk of coronary heart disease: 10,158 incident cases among 262,525 participants in 29 Western prospective studies. Circulation. 2007;115(4):450–458.
38. Freiberg JJ, Tybjaerg-Hansen A, Jensen JS, Nordestgaard BG. Nonfasting triglycerides and risk of ischemic stroke in the general population. JAMA. 2008;300(18):2142–2152.
39. Austin MA, Hokanson JE, Edwards KL. Hypertriglyceridemia as a cardiovascular risk factor. Am J Cardiol. 1998 Feb 26;81(4A):7B-12B.
40. Hokanson J.E., Austin M.A. Plasma triglyceride level is a risk factor for cardiovascular disease independent of high-density lipoprotein cholesterol level: A meta-analysis of population-based prospective studies. J. Cardiovasc. Risk. 1996;3:213–219. doi: 10.1097/00043798-199604000-00014.
41. Austin MA, Hokanson JE, Edwards KL. Hypertriglyceridemia as a cardiovascular risk factor. Am J Cardiol. 1998;81(4A):7B–12B. doi: 10.1016/S0002-9149(98)00031-9.
42. Hokanson JE. Hypertriglyceridemia and risk of coronary heart disease. Curr Cardiol Rep. 2002;4(6):488–493. doi: 10.1007/s11886-002-0112-7.
43. I Stensvold, A Tverdal, P Urdal, and S Graff-Iversen. Non-fasting serum triglyceride concentration and mortality from coronary heart disease and any cause in middle aged Norwegian women. BMJ. 1993 Nov 20; 307(6915): 1318–1322.
44. Jun M, Foote C, Lv J, et al. Effects of fibrates on cardiovascularoutcomes: a systematic review and meta-analysis. Lancet 2010; 375: 1875–84.
45. Carlson LA, Rosenhamer G. Reduction of mortality in the Stockholm Ischaemic Heart Disease Secondary Prevention Study by combined treatment with clofibrate and nicotinic acid. Acta Med Scand 1988; 223: 405–18.
46. Daskalopoulou SS, Daskalopoulos ME, Mikhailidis DP, Liapis CD. Lipid management and peripheral arterial disease. Curr Drug Targets. 2007 Apr;8(4):561-70.
47. Glynn RJ, Danielson E, Fonseca FA, et al. A randomized trial of rosuvastatin in the prevention of venous thromboembolism. N Engl J Med. 2009;360(18):1851–1861. doi: 10.1056/NEJMoa0900241.
48. Ramcharan AS, Van Stralen KJ, Snoep JD, et al. HMG-CoA reductase inhibitors, other lipid-lowering medication, antiplatelet therapy, and the risk of venous thrombosis. J Thromb Haemost. 2009;7(4):514–520. doi: 10.1111/j.1538-7836.2008.03235.x.
49. Rahimi K, Bhala N, Kamphuisen P, et al. Effect of statins on venous thromboembolic events: a meta-analysis of published and unpublished evidence from randomised controlled trials. PLoS Med. 2012;9(9):e1001310. doi: 10.1371/journal.pmed.1001310.
50. Chamberlain AM, Folsom AR, Heckbert SR, et al. High-density lipoprotein cholesterol and venous thromboembolism in the Longitudinal Investigation of Thromboembolism Etiology (LITE) Blood. 2008;112(7):2675–2680. doi: 10.1182/blood-2008-05-157412.
51. Everett BM, Glynn RJ, Buring JE, et al. Lipid biomarkers, hormone therapy and the risk of venous thromboembolism in women. J Thromb Haemost. 2009;7(4):588–596. doi: 10.1111/j.1538-7836.2009.03302.x.
52. Quist-Paulsen P, Naess IA, Cannegieter SC, et al. Arterial cardiovascular risk factors and venous thrombosis: results from a population-based, prospective study (the HUNT 2) Haematologica. 2010;95(1):119–125. doi: 10.3324/haematol.2009.011866.
53. Delluc A, Malécot JM, Kerspern H, et al. Lipid parameters, lipid lowering drugs and the risk

of venous thromboembolism. Atherosclerosis. 2012;220(1):184–188. doi: 10.1016/j.atherosclerosis.2011.10.007.
54. Acharya B K, Upadhyay A K, Upadhyay RT, Kumar A. Effect of Pranayama (voluntary regulated breathing) and Yogasana (yoga postures) on lipid profile in normal healthy junior footballers. Int J Yoga 2010;3:70.
55. Chen N, Xia X, Qin L, et al. Effects of 8-Week Hatha Yoga Training on Metabolic and Inflammatory Markers in Healthy, Female Chinese Subjects: A Randomized Clinical Trial. Biomed Res Int. 2016;2016:5387258.
56. Cramer H, Lauche R, Haller H, Steckhan N, Michalsen A, Dobos G. Effects of yoga on cardiovascular disease risk factors: a systematic review and meta-analysis. Int J Cardiol 2014;173:170–183.
57. Chu P, Gotink RA, Yeh GY, Goldie SJ, Hunink MG. The effectiveness of yoga in modifying risk factors for cardiovascular disease and metabolic syndrome: A systematic review and meta-analysis of randomized controlled trials. Eur J Prev Cardiol. 2016 Feb;23(3):291-307. doi: 10.1177/2047487314562741. Epub 2014 Dec 15.
58. American Heart Association. Cardiovascular disease & diabetes. 2015 http://www.heart.org/HEARTORG/Conditions/More/Diabetes/WhyDiabetesMatters/Cardiovascular-Disease-Diabetes_UCM_313865_Article.jsp/#.Wh_-eNKg_RY. Accessed 30 Nov 2017.
59. Taskinen M.R. Diabetic dyslipidemia. Atheroscler Suppl. 2002;3(1):47–51.
60. Innes KE, Selfe TK. Yoga for Adults with Type 2 Diabetes: A Systematic Review of Controlled Trials. Journal of Diabetes Research. 2016;2016:6979370. doi:10.1155/2016/6979370.
61. Thind H, Lantini R, Balletto BL, et al. The effects of yoga among adults with type 2 diabetes: A systematic review and meta-analysis. Prev Med. 2017;105:116-126.
62. Cui J, Yan JH, Yan LM, Pan L, Le JJ, Guo YZ. Effects of yoga in adults with type 2 diabetes mellitus: A meta-analysis. J Diabetes Investig. 2016;8(2):201-209.
63. Krentz AJ. Lipoprotein abnormalities and their consequences for patients with type 2 diabetes. Diabetes Obes Metab. 2003 Nov;5 Suppl 1:S19-27.

Lymphedema

1. Grabb and Smith's Plastic Surgery. Thorne CH, editor. Wolters Kluwer Health. (7th edition) 2013; Chapter 97:980–988. Lymphedema: Diagnosis and treatment.
2. Grada AA, Phillips TJ. Lymphedema: Pathophysiology and clinical manifestations. J Am Acad Dermatol. 2017 Dec;77(6):1009-1020. doi: 10.1016/j.jaad.2017.03.022.
3. Smeltzer D M, Stickler G B, Schirger A. Primary lymphedema in children and adolescents: a follow-up study and review. Pediatrics. 1985;76(02):206–218.
4. Schook C C, Mulliken J B, Fishman S J, Grant F D, Zurakowski D, Greene A K. Primary lymphedema: clinical features and management in 138 pediatric patients. Plast Reconstr Surg. 2011;127(06):2419–2431.
5. World Health Organization. Progress report 2000–2009 and strategic plan 2010–2020 of the global programme to eliminate lymphatic filariasis: halfway towards eliminating lymphatic filariasis WHO Library Catalogue; 2010.
6. Tahan G, Johnson R, Mager L, Soran A. The role of occupational upper extremity use in breast cancer related upper extremity lymphedema. J Cancer Surviv. 2010;4:15–19. 3.
7. Armer JM, Stewart BR. Post-breast cancer lymphedema: incidence increases from 12 to 30 to 60 months. Lymphology. 2010;43:118–127.
8. Ramaiah KD, Ottesen EA. Progress and impact of 13 years of the global programme to eliminate lymphatic filariasis on reducing the burden of filarial disease. PLoS Negl Trop Dis. 2014;8(11):e3319 10.1371/journal.pntd.0003319.
9. Williams AF, Franks PJ, Moffatt CJ. Lymphoedema: estimating the size of the problem. Palliative Medicine. 2005;19(4):300–13.
10. Rockson SG, Rivera KK. Estimating the population burden of lymphedema. Ann N Y Acad Sci. 2008;1131:147–154.
11. Basta MN, Gao LL, Wu LC. Operative treatment of peripheral lymphedema: a systematic meta-analysis of the efficacy and safety of lymphovenous microsurgery and tissue transplantation. Plast Reconstr Surg. 2014;133:905–913.

12. Brorson H, Svensson H. Liposuction combined with controlled compression therapy reduces arm lymphedema more effectively than controlled compression therapy alone Plast Reconstr Surg 1998102041058–1067., discussion 1068.
13. Brorson H, Ohlin K, Olsson G, Karlsson M K. Breast cancer-related chronic arm lymphedema is associated with excess adipose and muscle tissue. Lymphat Res Biol. 2009;7(01):3–10.
14. International Society of Lymphology.The diagnosis and treatment of peripheral lymphedema: 2013 Consensus Document of the International Society of Lymphology Lymphology 201346011–11.
15. Chachaj A, Malyszczak K, Pyszel K, Lukas J, Tarkowski R, Pudelko M, Szuba A. Physical and psychological impairments of women with upper limb lymphedema following breast cancer treatment. Psychooncology. 2010;19(3):299–305. doi:10.1002/pon.1573.
16. Vignes S. [Lymphedema: From diagnosis to treatment]. Rev Med Interne. 2017 Feb;38(2):97-105. doi: 10.1016/j.revmed.2016.07.005. Epub 2016 Aug 31.
17. Ridner SH. The psycho-social impact of lymphedema. Lymphatic research and biology. 2009;7(2):109–112. doi: 10.1089/lrb.2009.0004.
18. Keeley V, Sue C, Locke J, Veigas D, Riches K. R H: A quality of life measure for limb lymphoedema (LYMQOL). Journal of Lymphoedema. 2010;5(1).
19. World Health Organization. Lymphatic filariasis: managing morbidity and preventing disability: an aide-mémoire for national programme managers. WHO Library Catalogue; 2013.
20. Wijesinghe RS, Wickremasinghe AR, Ekanayake S, Perera MSA. Efficacy of a limb-care regime in preventing acute adenolymphangitis in patients with lymphoedema caused by bancroftian filariasis, in Colombo, Sri Lanka. Ann Trop Med Parasitol. 2007;101(6):487–97.
21. Lawenda BD, Mondry TE, Johnstone PAS. Lymphedema: A primer on the identification and management of a chronic condition in oncologic treatment. CA Cancer Journal for Clinicians. 2009;59(1):8–24. 10.3322/caac.20001.
22. Narahari SR, Ryan TJ, Mahadevan PE, Bose KS, Prasanna KS. Integrated management of filarial lymphedema for rural communities. Lymphology. 2007;40:3–13.
23. Loudon A, Barnett T, Piller N, Williams A, Immink M. Using yoga in breast cancer-related lymphoedema. J Lymphoedema. 2012;7:27–36.
24. Aggithaya MG, Narahari SR, Ryan TJ. Yoga for correction of lymphedema's impairment of gait as an adjunct to lymphatic drainage: A pilot observational study. International Journal of Yoga. 2015;8(1):54-61. doi:10.4103/0973-6131.146063.
25. Loudon A, Barnett T, Piller N, Immink MA, Williams AD. Yoga management of breast cancer-related lymphoedema: A randomised controlled pilot-trial. BMC Complement Altern Med. 2014;14:214.
26. Fisher M, Donahoe-Fillmore B, Leach L, O'Malley C, Paeplow C, Prescott T, Merriman H. Effects of yoga on arm volume among women with breast cancer related lymphedema: A pilot study. J Bodyw Mov Ther. 2014 Oct;18(4):559-65. doi: 10.1016/j.jbmt.2014.02.006.

Metabolic Syndrome

1. Balkau B, Charles MA. Comment on the provisional report from the WHO consultation. European Group for the Study of Insulin Resistance (EGIR) Diabet Med. 1999;16:442–443.
2. Srikanthan K, Feyh A, Visweshwar H, Shapiro JI, Sodhi K. Systematic Review of Metabolic Syndrome Biomarkers: A Panel for Early Detection, Management, and Risk Stratification in the West Virginian Population. International Journal of Medical Sciences. 2016;13(1):25-38. doi:10.7150/ijms.13800.
3. Scott M. Grundy, James I. Cleeman, Stephen R. Daniels, Karen A. Donato, Robert H. Eckel, Barry A. Franklin, David J. Gordon, Ronald M. Krauss, Peter J. Savage, Sidney C. Smith, John A. Spertus, Fernando Costa. Diagnosis and Management of the Metabolic Syndrome. An American Heart Association/National Heart, Lung, and Blood Institute Scientific Statement. Circulation. 2005;112:2735-2752.

4. Alberti KG, Eckel RH, Grundy SM et al. Harmonizing the metabolic syndrome: a joint interim statement of the International Diabetes Federation Task Force on Epidemiology and Prevention; National Heart, Lung, and Blood Institute; American Heart Association; World Heart Federation; International Atherosclerosis Society; and International Association for the Study of Obesity. Circulation. 2009;120:1640–1645.
5. Aguilar M, Bhuket T, Torres S, Liu B, Wong RJ. Prevalence of the metabolic syndrome in the United States, 2003-2012. Jama. 2015;313:1973–4.
6. Alberti KGMM, Eckel RH, Grundy SM, et al. Harmonizing the metabolic syndrome: a joint interim statement of the international diabetes federation task force on epidemiology and prevention; National heart, lung, and blood institute; American heart association; World heart federation; International atherosclerosis society; And international association for the study of obesity. Circulation. 2009;120(16):1640–1645.
7. Pérez-Martínez P, Mikhailidis DP, Athyros VG, et al. Lifestyle recommendations for the prevention and management of metabolic syndrome: an international panel recommendation. Nutr Rev. 2017;75(5):307-326.
8. Lakka HM, Laaksonen DE, Lakka TA, Niskanen LK, Kumpusalo E, Tuomilehto J, Salonen JT. The metabolic syndrome and total and cardiovascular disease mortality in middle-aged men. JAMA. 2002;288:2709–2716.
9. Wu SH, Liu Z, Ho SC. Metabolic syndrome and all-cause mortality: a meta-analysis of prospective cohort studies. Eur J Epidemiol 2010;25:375–84.
10. Ju SY, Lee JY, Kim DH. Association of metabolic syndrome and its components with all-cause and cardiovascular mortality in the elderly: A meta-analysis of prospective cohort studies. Medicine (Baltimore). 2017;96(45):e8491.
11. Grundy SM. Metabolic syndrome pandemic. Arteriosclerosis, Thrombosis, and Vascular Biology. 2008;28(4):629–636.
12. Wilson PWF, Kannel WB, Silbershatz H, D'Agostino RB. Clustering of metabolic factors and coronary heart disease. Archives of Internal Medicine. 1999;159(10):1104–1109.
13. Suzuki T, Hirata K, Elkind MSV, et al. Metabolic syndrome, endothelial dysfunction, and risk of cardiovascular events: the Northern Manhattan study (NOMAS) American Heart Journal. 2008;156(2):405–410.
14. Isomaa B, Almgren P, Tuomi T, Forsen B, Lahti K, Nissen M, Taskinen MR, Groop L. Cardiovascular morbidity and mortality associated with the metabolic syndrome. Diabetes Care. 2001;24:683–689.
15. Sperling LS, Mechanick JI, Neeland IJ, Herrick CJ, Despres JP, Ndumele CE, et al. The CardioMetabolic Health Alliance: Working Toward a New Care Model for the Metabolic Syndrome. J Am Coll Cardiol. 2015;66(9):1050–67.
16. O'Neill S, O'Driscoll L. Metabolic syndrome: a closer look at the growing epidemic and its associated pathologies. Obes Rev. 2015;16(1):1–12.
17. Assmann G, Schulte H, Seedorf U. Cardiovascular risk assessment in the metabolic syndrome: results from the Prospective Cardiovascular Munster (PROCAM) study. International Journal of Obesity. 2008;32(supplement 2):S11–S16.
18. Ford ES. The metabolic syndrome and mortality from cardiovascular disease and all-causes: findings from the National Health and Nutrition Examination Survey II Mortality Study. Atherosclerosis. 2004;173:309–14.
19. Ju SY, Lee JY, Kim DH. Association of metabolic syndrome and its components with all-cause and cardiovascular mortality in the elderly: A meta-analysis of prospective cohort studies. Medicine (Baltimore). 2017;96(45):e8491.
20. Gami AS, Witt BJ, Howard DE, Erwin PJ, Gami LA, Somers VK, Montori VM. Metabolic syndrome and risk of incident cardiovascular events and death: a systematic review and meta-analysis of longitudinal studies. J Am Coll Cardiol. 2007;49:403–414.
21. Hess PL, Al-Khalidi HR, Friedman DJ, et al. The Metabolic Syndrome and Risk of Sudden Cardiac Death: The Atherosclerosis Risk in Communities Study. J Am Heart Assoc. 2017;6(8):e006103. Published 2017 Aug 23. doi:10.1161/JAHA.117.006103.
22. Carrie Armstrong. AHA and NHLBI Review Diagnosis and Management of the Metabolic Syndrome Am Fam Physician. 2006 Sep 15;74(6):1039-1047.

23. Wagh A, Stone NJ. Treatment of metabolic syndrome. Expert Rev Cardiovasc Ther. 2004 Mar;2(2):213-28.
24. Deedwania PC, Gupta R. Management issues in the metabolic syndrome. J Assoc Physicians India. 2006 Oct;54:797-810.
25. Graf BL, Raskin I, Cefalu WT, Ribnicky DM. Plant-derived therapeutics for the treatment of metabolic syndrome. Current opinion in investigational drugs (London, England : 2000). 2010;11(10):1107-1115.
26. Jang S, Jang B-H, Ko Y, et al. Herbal Medicines for Treating Metabolic Syndrome: A Systematic Review of Randomized Controlled Trials. Evidence-based Complementary and Alternative Medicine : eCAM. 2016;2016:5936402. doi:10.1155/2016/5936402.
27. Garg PK, Biggs ML, Carnethon M, et al. Metabolic syndrome and risk of incident peripheral artery disease: the cardiovascular health study. Hypertension. 2013;63(2):413-9.
28. Carlos Lahoz, Ignacio Vicente, Fernando Laguna, et al, Metabolic Syndrome and Asymptomatic Peripheral Artery Disease in Subjects Over 60 Years of Age. Diabetes Care 2006 Jan; 29(1): 148-150.
29. Brevetti, Gregorio et al. Metabolic syndrome in peripheral arterial disease: Relationship with severity of peripheral circulatory insufficiency, inflammatory status, and cardiovascular comorbidity. Journal of Vascular Surgery , Volume 44 , Issue 1 , 101 – 107.
30. Heidler S, Temml C, Broessner C, et al. Is the metabolic syndrome an independent risk factor for erectile dysfunction? Journal of Urology. 2007;177(2):651–654.
31. Arrabal-Polo MÁ, Arias-Santiago S, López-Carmona Pintado F, et al. Metabolic syndrome, hormone levels, and inflammation in patients with erectile dysfunction. ScientificWorldJournal. 2012;2012:272769.
32. Chaya M, Kurpad A, Nagendra H, Nagarathna R: The effect of long term combined yoga practice on the basal metabolic rate of healthy adults. BMC Complement Altern Med. 2006, 6 (1): 28-10.1186/1472-6882-6-28.
33. Cohen BE, Chang AA, Grady D, Kanaya AM. Restorative yoga in adults with metabolic syndrome: a randomized, controlled pilot trial. Metab Syndr Relat Disord. 2008;6:223–9. doi: 10.1089/met.2008.0016.
34. Chaya M, Nagendra H: Long-term effect of yogic practices on diurnal metabolic rates of healthy subjects. Int J Yoga. 2008, 1 (1): 27-10.4103/0973-6131.36761.
35. Swathi Gowda, Sriloy Mohanty, Apar Saoji, Raghuram Nagarathna. Integrated Yoga and Naturopathy module in management of Metabolic Syndrome: A case report. J Ayurveda Integr Med. 2017 Jan-Mar; 8(1): 45–48. Published online 2017 Mar 16. doi: 10.1016/j.jaim.2016.10.006.
36. Khatri D, Mathur KC, Gahlot S, Jain S, Agrawal RP. Effects of yoga and meditation on clinical and biochemical parameters of metabolic syndrome. Diabetes Res Clin Pract. 2007;78:e9–10. doi: 10.1016/j.diabres.2007.05.002.
37. Tyagi A, Cohen M, Reece J, Telles S. An explorative study of metabolic responses to mental stress and yoga practices in yoga practitioners, non-yoga practitioners and individuals with metabolic syndrome. BMC Complement Altern Med. 2014;14:445. Published 2014 Nov 15. doi:10.1186/1472-6882-14-445.
38. Parco M Siu, Angus P Yu, Iris F Benzie, Jean Woo. Effects of 1-year yoga on cardiovascular risk factors in middle-aged and older adults with metabolic syndrome: a randomized trial. Diabetol Metab Syndr. 2015; 7: 40. Published online 2015 Apr 30. doi: 10.1186/s13098-015-0034-3.
39. Lau C, Yu R, Woo J. Effects of a 12-Week Hatha Yoga Intervention on Metabolic Risk and Quality of Life in Hong Kong Chinese Adults with and without Metabolic Syndrome. PLoS One. 2015;10(6):e0130731. Published 2015 Jun 25. doi:10.1371/journal.pone.0130731.
40. Stephanie J. Sohl, Kenneth A. Wallston, Keiana Watkins, Gurjeet S. Birdee. Yoga for Risk Reduction of Metabolic Syndrome: Patient-Reported Outcomes from a Randomized Controlled Pilot Study. Evid Based Complement Alternat Med. 2016; 2016: 3094589.
41. Paul-Labrador M, Polk D, Dwyer JH, et al. Effects of a randomized controlled trial of transcendental meditation on components of the metabolic syndrome in subjects with coronary heart disease. Archives of Internal Medicine. 2006;166(11):1218–1224.

42. Corey SM, Epel E, Schembri M, et al. Effect of restorative yoga vs. stretching on diurnal cortisol dynamics and psychosocial outcomes in individuals with the metabolic syndrome: the PRYSMS randomized controlled trial. Psychoneuroendocrinology. 2014;49:260-271. doi:10.1016/j.psyneuen.2014.07.012.

Negative Emotions

1. Hershfield HE, Scheibe S, Sims TL, Carstensen LL. When Feeling Bad Can Be Good: Mixed Emotions Benefit Physical Health Across Adulthood. Soc Psychol Personal Sci. 2013;4(1):54–61.
2. Penninx BWJH, Guralnik JM, Pahor M, Ferrucci L, Cerhan JR, Wallace RB, Havlik RJ. Chronically depressed mood and cancer risk in older persons. J Natl Cancer Inst. 1998;90:1888–1893.
3. Everson SA, Kauhanen J, Kaplan GA, Goldberg DE, Julkunen J, Tuomilehto J, Salonen JT. Hostility and increased risk of mortality and acute myocardial infarction: the mediating role of behavioral risk factors. Am. J. Epidemiol. 1997;146:142–152.
4. Wilson RS, Krueger KR, Gu L, Bienias JL, Mendes de Leon CF, Evans DA. Neuroticism, extraversion, and mortality in a defined population of older persons. Psychosomatic Medicine. 2005;67:841–845.
5. Kubzansky LD, Kawachi I. Going to the heart of the matter: do negative emotions cause coronary heart disease? J Psychosom Res. 2000;48:323–337.
6. Steptoe A, Brydon L, Kunz-Ebrecht S. Changes in financial strain over three years, ambulatory blood pressure, and cortisol responses to awakening. Psychosom Med. 2005;67:281–287.
7. Yan LL, Liu K, Matthews KA, et al. Psychosocial factors and risk of hypertension: the Coronary Artery Risk Development in Young Adults (CARDIA) study. JAMA. 2003;290:2138–2148.
8. Moseley JV, Linden W. Predicting blood pressure and heart rate change with cardiovascular reactivity and recovery: results from 3-year and 10-year follow up. Psychosom Med. 2006;68:833–843.
9. Kubzansky LD, Kawachi I. Going to the heart of the matter: do negative emotions cause coronary heart disease? J Psychosom Res. 2000 Apr-May;48(4-5):323-37.; Sirois BC, Burg MM. Negative emotion and coronary heart disease. A review. Behav Modif. 2003 Jan;27(1):83-102.
10. Todaro JF, Shen BJ, Niaura R, Spiro A 3rd, Ward KD. Effect of negative emotions on frequency of coronary heart disease (The Normative Aging Study) Am J Cardiol. 2003 Oct 15;92(8):901-6.
11. Rosengren A, Hawken S, Ounpuu S, et al. Association of psychosocial risk factors with risk of acute myocardial infarction in 11119 cases and 13648 controls from 52 countries (INTERHEART study): case-control study. Lancet. 2004;364:953–962.
12. May M. Does psychological distress predict the risk of ischemic stroke and transient ischemic attack? The Caerphilly Study. Stroke. 2002;33:7–12.
13. Joseph NT, Kamarck TW, Muldoon MF, Manuck SB. Daily Marital Interaction Quality and Carotid Artery Intima Medial Thickness in Healthy Middle Aged Adults. Psychosomatic medicine. 2014;76(5):347-354.
14. Williams JE, Paton CC, Siegler IC, Eigenbrodt ML, Nieto FJ, Tyroler HA. Anger proneness predicts coronary heart disease risk: prospective analysis from the atherosclerosis risk in communities (ARIC) study. Circulation. 2000 May 2;101(17):2034-9.
15. Hering D, Lachowska K, Schlaich M. Role of the Sympathetic Nervous System in Stress-Mediated Cardiovascular Disease. Curr Hypertens Rep. 2015 Oct;17(10):80. doi: 10.1007/s11906-015-0594-5.
16. Miyamoto Y, Boylan JM, Coe CL, et al. Negative Emotions Predict Elevated Interleukin-6 in the United States but not in Japan. Brain, behavior, and immunity. 2013; 34:10.1016/j.bbi.2013.07.173.

17. Ridker PM, Rifai N, Stampfer MJ, Hennekens CH. Plasma concentration of interleukin-6 and the risk of future myocardial infarction among apparently healthy men. Circulation. 2000;101:1767–1772.
18. Joseph NT, Kamarck TW, Muldoon MF, Manuck SB. Daily Marital Interaction Quality and Carotid Artery Intima Medial Thickness in Healthy Middle Aged Adults. Psychosomatic medicine. 2014;76(5):347-354.
19. van den Oord SCH, Sijbrands EJG, ten Kate GL, van Klaveren D, van Domburg RT, van der Steen AFW, et al. Carotid intima-media thickness for cardiovascular risk assessment: systematic review and meta-analysis. Atherosclerosis. 2013;228:1–11.
20. Monroe SM, Slavich GM, Torres LD, et al. Severe life events predict specific patterns of change in cognitive biases in major depression. Psychol Med. 2007;37(6):863–871. ;24.
21. Monroe SM, Slavich GM, Torres LD, et al. Major life events and major chronic difficulties are differentially associated with history of major depressive episodes. J Abnorm Psychol. 2007;116(1):116–124.
22. Van Dooren FEP, Nefs G, Schram MT, Verhey FRJ, Denollet J, Pouwer F. Depression and Risk of Mortality in People with Diabetes Mellitus: A Systematic Review and Meta-Analysis. Berthold HK, ed. PLoS ONE. 2013;8(3): e57058.
23. Boltwood MD, Taylor CB, Boutte Burke M, Grogin H, Giacomini J. Anger report predicts coronary artery vasomotor response to mental stress in atherosclerotic segments. Am J Cardiol. 1993;72:1361-1365.
24. Verrier RL, Hagestad EL, Lown B. Delayed myocardial ischemia induced by anger. Circulation. 1987;75:249-254.
25. Thomas Buckley, Soon Y Soo Hoo, Judith Fethney et al. Triggering of acute coronary occlusion by episodes of anger. European Heart Journal: Acute Cardiovascular Care. Vol 4, Issue 6, 2015, page(s): 493-498.
26. Haynes SG, Feinleib M, Kannel WB. The relationship of psychosocial factors to coronary heart disease in the Framingham study, III: Eight-year incidence of coronary heart disease. Am J Epidemiol. 1980 Jan;111(1):37-58.
27. Koskenvuo M, Kaprio J, Rose RJ, Kesaniemi A, Sarna S, Heikkila K, Langinvainio H. Hostility as a risk factor for mortality and ischemic heart disease in men. Psychosom Med. 1988;50:153-164.
28. Dembroski TM, MacDougall JM, Costa PT Jr, Grandits GA. Components of hostility as predictors of sudden death and myocardial infarction in the Multiple Risk Factor Intervention Trial. Psychosom Med. 1989;51:514-522.
29. Dembroski TM, MacDougall JM, Costa PT Jr, Grandits GA. Components of Mittleman MA, Maclure M, Sherwood JB, et al. Triggering of acute myocardial infarction onset by episodes of anger. Circulation. 1995;92:1720-1725.
30. Kawachi I, Sparrow D, Spiro A III, Vokonas P, Weiss ST. A prospective study of anger and coronary heart disease: the Normative Aging Study. Circulation. 1996;94:2090–2095.
31. Miller TQ, Smith TW, Turner CW, Guijarro ML, Hallet AJ. A meta-analytic review of research on hostility and physical health. Psychological Bulletin. 1996;119:322–348.
32. McLaughlin KA, Green JG, Hwang I, Sampson NA, Zaslavsky AM, Kessler RC. Intermittent explosive disorder in the National Comorbidity Survey Replication Adolescent Supplement. Arch Gen Psychiatry. 2012;69(11):1131-9.
33. Siegman AW, Dembroski TM, Ringel N. Components of hostility and the severity of coronary artery disease. Psychosom Med. 1987;49:127–135.
34. Brosschot JF, Thayer JF. Anger inhibition, cardiovascular recovery, and vagal function:a model of the link between hostility and cardiovascular disease. Ann Behav Med. 1998;20:326–332.
35. Siegman AW, Townsend ST, Civelek AC, Blumenthal RS. Antagonistic behavior,dominance,hostility,and coronary heart disease. Psychosom Med. 2000;62:248–257.
36. Brydon L, Strike PC, Bhattacharyya MR, et al. Hostility and physiological responses to laboratory stress in acute coronary syndrome patients. J Psychosom Res. 2010;68:109–116.

37. Chida Y, Steptoe A. The association of anger and hostility with future coronary heart disease:a meta-analytic review of prospective evidence. J Am Coll Cardiol. 2009;53:936–946.
38. Miller TQ, Smith TW, Turner CW et al. A meta-analytic review of research on hostility and physical health. Psychol Bull. 1996 Mar;119(2):322-48.
39. Everson SA, Kauhanen J, Kaplan GA, Goldberg DE, Julkunen J, Tuomilehto J, Salonen JT. Hostility and increased risk of mortality and acute myocardial infarction: the mediating role of behavioral risk factors. Am. J. Epidemiol. 1997;146:142–152.
40. Wattanakit K, Williams JE, Schreiner PJ, Hirsch AT, Folsom AR. Association of anger proneness, depression and low social support with peripheral arterial disease: the Atherosclerosis Risk in Communities Study. Vasc Med. 2005 Aug;10(3):199-206.
41. Yoshihara K, Hiramoto T, Sudo N, Kubo C. Profile of mood states and stress-related biochemical indices in long-term yoga practitioners. Biopsychosocial Medicine. 2011;5:6. doi:10.1186/1751-0759-5-6.
42. Dwivedi U, Kumari S, Akhilesh KB, Nagendra HR. Well-being at workplace through mindfulness: Influence of Yoga practice on positive affect and aggression. Ayu. 2015;36(4):375-379. doi:10.4103/0974-8520.190693.
43. Felver JC, Butzer B, Olson KJ, Smith IM, Khalsa SB. Yoga in public school improves adolescent mood and affect. Contemp Sch Psychol. 2014;19(3):184-192.
44. Dwivedi U, Kumari S, Akhilesh KB, Nagendra HR. Well-being at workplace through mindfulness: Influence of Yoga practice on positive affect and aggression. Ayu. 2015;36(4):375-379.
45. Bilderbeck AC, Farias M, Brazil IA, Jakobowitz S, Wikholm C. Participation in a 10-week course of yoga improves behavioural control and decreases psychological distress in a prison population. J Psychiatr Res. 2013;47:1438–45.
46. Yoga in Correctional Settings: A Randomized Controlled Study. Front Psychiatry. 2017;8:204. Published 2017 Oct 16. doi:10.3389/fpsyt.2017.00204.
47. Bryant C, Jackson H, Ames D. Depression and anxiety in medically unwell older adults: prevalence and short-term course. Int Psychogeriatr. 2009;21(4):754–763.
48. Baxter A, Scott K, Vos T, Whiteford H. Global prevalence of anxiety disorders: a systematic review and meta-regression. Psychol Med. 2013;43(5):897–910.
49. Kogan JN, Edelstein BA, McKee DR. Assessment of anxiety in older adults: current status. J Anxiety Disord. 2000;14(2):109–132.
50. Fagundes CP, Jaremka LM, Glaser R, et al. Attachment anxiety is related to Epstein-Barr virus latency. Brain Behav Immun. 2014;41:232–238. doi:10.1016/j.bbi.2014.04.002.
51. Cohen S, Tyrell DA, Smith AP. Psychological stress and susceptibility to the common cold. N Engl J Med. 1991;325:606–612.
52. Leserman J, Petitto JM, Gu H, et al. Progression to AIDS, a clinical AIDS con-dition and mortality: psychosocial and physiological predictors.Psychol Med. 2002;32(6):1059-1073.
53. Sadeh A, Keinan G, Daon K. Effects of stress on sleep: the moderating role of coping style. Health Psychology: Official Journal of the Division of Health Psychology. 2004;23:542–545. doi: 10.1037/0278-6133.23.5.542.
54. Schneiderman N, Ironson G, Siegel SD. Stress and health: psychological, behavioral, and biological determinants. Annual Review of Clinical Psychology. 2005;1:607–628. doi: 10.1146/annurev.clinpsy.1.102803.144141.
55. Cohen S et al. "Psychological Stress and Disease." JAMA 2007; 298(14): 1685-1687.; Pinquart M, Duberstein PR. Depression and cancer mortality: a meta-analysis. Psychol Med. 2010;40:1979–1810.
56. Vasunilashorn S, Glei DA, Weinstein M, Goldman N. Perceived Stress and Mortality in a Taiwanese Older Adult Population. Stress (Amsterdam, Netherlands). 2013;16(6):600-606. doi:10.3109/10253890.2013.823943.
57. Rosengren A, Orth-Gomér K, Wedel H, Wilhelmsen L. Stressful life events, social support, and mortality in men born in 1933. Br Med J. 1993;307:1102–1105.

58. van Hout HP, Beekman AT, de Beurs E, Comijs H, van Marwijk H, de Haan M, van Tilburg W, Deeg DJ. Anxiety and the risk of death in older men and women. Br J Psychiatry. 2004 Nov;185:399-404.
59. Mineka S, Watson D, Clark LA. Comorbidity of anxiety and unipolar mood disorders. Annu Rev Psychol. 1998;49:377–412.
60. Cairney J, Corna LM, Veldhuizen S, Herrmann N, Streiner DL. Comorbid depression and anxiety in later life: patterns of association, subjective well-being, and impairment. Am J Geriatr Psychiatry. 2008;16(3):201–208.
61. Bentley KH, Franklin JC, Ribeiro JD, Kleiman EM, Fox KR, Nock MK. Anxiety and its disorders as risk factors for suicidal thoughts and behaviors: A meta-analytic review. Clin Psychol Rev. 2015;43:30-46.
62. Health Quality Ontario . Psychotherapy for Major Depressive Disorder and Generalized Anxiety Disorder: A Health Technology Assessment. Ont Health Technol Assess Ser. 2017;17(15):1–167. Published 2017 Nov 13.
63. Katzman MA, Bleau P, Blier P, et al. Canadian clinical practice guidelines for the management of anxiety, posttraumatic stress and obsessive-compulsive disorders. BMC Psychiatry. 2014;14 Suppl 1(Suppl 1):S1. doi:10.1186/1471-244X-14-S1-S1.
64. Williams T, Hattingh CJ, Kariuki CM, et al. Pharmacotherapy for social anxiety disorder (SAnD). Cochrane Database Syst Rev. 2017;10(10):CD001206. Published 2017 Oct 19. doi:10.1002/14651858.CD001206.pub3.
65. Swedish Council on Health Technology Assessment. Treatment of Anxiety Disorders: A Systematic Review (Summary and conclusions) [Internet]. Stockholm: Swedish Council on Health Technology Assessment (SBU); 2005 Nov. SBU Yellow Report No. 171/1+2. Available from: https://www.ncbi.nlm.nih.gov/books/NBK447974/
66. Cohen BE, Edmondson D, Kronish IM. State of the Art Review: Depression, Stress, Anxiety, and Cardiovascular Disease. American Journal of Hypertension. 2015;28(11):1295-1302.
67. Janszky I, Ahnve S, Lundberg I et al. Early-onset depression, anxiety, and risk of subsequent coronary heart disease: 37-year follow-up of 49,321 young Swedish men. J Am Coll Cardiol 2010;56:31–7. 10.1016/j.jacc.2010.03.033.
68. Roest AM, Martens EJ, de Jonge P et al. Anxiety and risk of incident coronary heart disease: a meta-analysis. J Am Coll Cardiol 2010;56:38–46. 10.1016/j.jacc.2010.03.034.
69. Berge LI, Skogen JC, Sulo G, et al. Health anxiety and risk of ischaemic heart disease: a prospective cohort study linking the Hordaland Health Study (HUSK) with the Cardiovascular Diseases in Norway (CVDNOR) project. BMJ Open. 2016;6(11): e012914.
70. Janszky I, Ahnve S, Lundberg I, Hemmingsson T. Early-onset depression, anxiety, and risk of subsequent coronary heart disease: 37-year follow-up of 49,321 young Swedish men. J Am Coll Cardiol. 2010;56(1):31-37.
71. Chamberlain AM, Vickers KS, Colligan RC, et al. Associations of Preexisting Depression and Anxiety with Hospitalization in Patients with Cardiovascular Disease. Mayo Clinic Proceedings. 2011;86(11):1056-1062.
72. Edmondson D, Richardson S, Falzon L, et al. Posttraumatic stress disorder prevalence and risk of recurrence in acute coronary syndrome patients: a meta-analytic review. PLoS ONE. 2012;7:e38915.
73. Tully PJ, Cosh SM, Baumeister H. The anxious heart in whose mind? A systematic review and meta-regression of factors associated with anxiety disorder diagnosis, treatment and morbidity risk in coronary heart disease. J Psychosom Res. 2014;77:439–48.
74. Roest AM, Martens EJ, de Jonge P, Denollet J. Anxiety and risk of incident coronary heart disease: a meta-analysis. J Am Coll Cardiol. 2010;56(1): 38-46.
75. Celano CM, Millstein RA, Bedoya CA, Healy BC, Roest AM, Huffman JC. Association between anxiety and mortality in patients with coronary artery disease: A meta-analysis. Am Heart J. 2015;170(6):1105-15.
76. Aquarius AE, De Vries J, Henegouwen DP, Hamming JF. Clinical indicators and psychosocial aspects in peripheral arterial disease. Arch Surg. 2006 Feb;141(2):161-6; discussion 166.

77. Peterson LG, Pbert L. Effectiveness of a meditation-based stress reduction program in the treatment of anxiety disorders. Am J Psychiatry. 1992;149:936–943.
78. Malathi A., Damodaran A. Stress due to exams in medical students—role of yoga. Indian Journal of Physiology and Pharmacology. 1999;43(2):218–224.
79. Ospina MB, Bond K, Karkhaneh M, et al. Meditation practices for health: state of the research. Evidence Report/Technology Assessment. 2007;(155).
80. Chong CS, Tsunaka M, Tsang HW, Chan EP, Cheung WM. Effects of yoga on stress management in healthy adults: a systematic review. Alternative Therapies in Health and Medicine. 2011;17(1):32–38.
81. Huang FJ, Chien DK, Chung UL. Effects of Hatha yoga on stress in middle-aged women. J Nurs Res. 2013 Mar;21(1):59-66. doi: 10.1097/jnr.0b013e3182829d6d.
82. de Bruin EI, Formsma AR, Frijstein G, Bögels SM. Mindful2Work: Effects of Combined Physical Exercise, Yoga, and Mindfulness Meditations for Stress Relieve in Employees. A Proof of Concept Study. Mindfulness (N Y). 2016;8(1):204-217.
83. Kimbrough E, Magyari T, Langenberg P, Chesney M, Berman B. Mindfulness intervention for child abuse survivors. Journal of clinical psychology. 2010;66:17–33.
84. Niles BL, Klunk-Gillis J, Ryngala DJ, Silberbogen AK, Paysnick A, Wolf EJ. Comparing mindfulness and psychoeducation treatments for combat-related PTSD using a telehealth approach. Psychological Trauma: Theory, Research, Practice, and Policy. 2012;4:538.
85. Bilderbeck AC, Brazil IA, Farias M. Preliminary evidence that yoga practice progressively improves mood and decreases stress in a sample of UK prisoners. Evid Based Complement Alternat Med (2015) 2015:819183.10.1155/2015/819183.
86. Kessler R.C.and Bromet E.J. The epidemiology of depression across cultures. Annu Rev Public Health. 2013; 34: 119–138.
87. WHO, 2010: http://www.nimh.nih.gov/health/statistics/prevalence/major-depression-among-adults.shtml.
88. Hirschfeld RM. The epidemiology of depression and the evolution of treatment. J Clin Psychiatry. 2012;73(suppl 1):5–9.
89. Vos T, Flaxman AD, Naghavi M, et al. Years lived with disability (YLDs) for 1160 sequelae of 289 diseases and injuries 1990–2010: a systematic analysis for the Global Burden of Disease Study 2010. Lancet. 2012;380(9859):2163–2196.
90. Kessler RC, Birnbaum H, Bromet E, et al. Age differences in major depression: results from the National Comorbidity Survey Replication (NCS-R) Psychol Med. 2010;40(2):225–237.
91. Stafford RS, Ausiello JC, Misra B, et al. National patterns of depression treatment in primary care. Prim Care Companion J Clin Psychiatry. 2000;2(6):211–216.
92. Evans-Lacko S, Knapp M. Global patterns of workplace productivity for people with depression: absenteeism and presenteeism costs across eight diverse countries. Soc Psychiatry Psychiatr Epidemiol. 2016;51(11):1525–1537. doi:10.1007/s00127-016-1278-4.
93. Vakrat A, Apter-Levy Y, Feldman R. Fathering moderates the effects of maternal depression on the family process. Dev Psychopathol. 2018 Feb;30(1):27-38. doi: 10.1017/S095457941700044X. Epub 2017 Apr 19.
94. Pedrelli P, Borsari B, Lipson SK, Heinze JE, Eisenberg D. Gender Differences in the Relationships Among Major Depressive Disorder, Heavy Alcohol Use, and Mental Health Treatment Engagement Among College Students. J Stud Alcohol Drugs. 2016;77(4):620–628. doi:10.15288/jsad.2016.77.620.
95. Sreelakshmy, Krishnankutty, Velayudhan, Rajmohan, Kuriakose, Deepak, & Nair, Rema. (2017). Sexual dysfunction in females with depression: a cross-sectional study. Trends in Psychiatry and Psychotherapy, 39(2), 106-109. https://dx.doi.org/10.1590/2237-6089-2016-0072.
96. Arango-Lievano M, Kaplitt MG. [Depression and addiction comorbidity: towards a common molecular target?]. Med Sci (Paris). 2015 May;31(5):546-50. doi: 10.1051/medsci/20153105017. Epub 2015 Jun 9.
97. Fazel S, Wolf A, Chang Z et al. Depression and violence: a Swedish total population study. Lancet Psychiatry. 2015; 2: 224-232

98. Hawton K, Casañas I Comabella C, Haw C, Saunders K. Risk factors for suicide in individuals with depression: a systematic review. J Affect Disord. 2013 May;147(1-3):17-28. doi: 10.1016/j.jad.2013.01.004. Epub 2013 Feb 12.
99. Walker ER, McGee RE, Druss BG. Mortality in mental disorders and global disease burden implications: a systematic review and meta-analysis. JAMA Psychiatry 2015;72:334–41.
100. Gilman SE, Sucha E, Kingsbury M, Horton NJ, Murphy JM, Colman I. Depression and mortality in a longitudinal study: 1952-2011. CMAJ. 2017;189(42):E1304–E1310. doi:10.1503/cmaj.170125.
101. Saran RK, Puri A, Agarwal M. Depression and the heart. Indian Heart Journal. 2012;64(4):397-401.
102. Meng L, Chen D, Yang Y, Zheng Y, Hui R. Depression increases the risk of hypertension incidence: a meta-analysis of prospective cohort studies. J Hypertens. 2012 May; 30(5):842-51.
103. Nicholson A, Kuper H, Hemingway H. Depression as an aetiologic and prognostic factor in coronary heart disease: a meta-analysis of 6362 events among 146 538 participants in 54 observational studies. Eur Heart J. 2006 Dec; 27(23):2763-74.
104. Katon WJ, Lin EH, Russo J, Von Korff M, Ciechanowski P, Simon G, et al. Cardiac risk factors in patients with diabetes mellitus and major depression. J Gen Intern Med (2004) 19:1192–9.10.1111/j.1525-1497.2004.30405.x.
105. Glassman AH, Shapiro PA. Depression and the course of coronary artery disease. Am J Psychiatry. 1998;155:4–11.
106. Lane D, Carroll D, Ring C, Beevers DG, Lip GY. The prevalence and persistence of depression and anxiety following myocardial infarction. Br J Health Psychol 2002; 7:11–21.
107. Rutledge T, Reis VA, Linke SE, Greenberg BH, Mills PJ. Depression in heart failure a meta-analytic review of prevalence, intervention effects, and associations with clinical outcomes. J Am Coll Cardiol2006; 48:1527–1537.
108. Nicholson A, Kuper H, Hemingway H. Depression as an aetiologic and prognostic factor in coronary heart disease: a meta-analysis of 6362 events among 146 538 participants in 54 observational studies. Eur Heart J 2006; 27:2763–2774.
109. Jiang W, Alexander J, Christopher E, Kuchibhatla M, Gaulden LH, Cuffe MS, Blazing MA, Davenport C, Califf RM, Krishnan RR, O'Connor CM. Relationship of depression to increased risk of mortality and rehospitalization in patients with congestive heart failure. Arch Intern Med 2001; 161:1849–1856.
110. Barefoot JC, Helms MJ, Mark DB, Blumenthal JA, Califf RM, Haney TL, O'Connor CM, Siegler IC, Williams RB. Depression and long-term mortality risk in patients with coronary artery disease. Am J Cardiol. 1996;78:613–617.
111. Carney RM, Rich MW, Freedland KE, Saini J, teVelde A, Simeone C, Clark K. Major depressive disorder predicts cardiac events in patients with coronary artery disease. Psychosom Med. 1988a;50:627–633.
112. Nicholson A, Kuper H, Hemingway H. Depression as an aetiologic and prognostic factor in coronary heart disease: a meta-analysis of 6362 events among 146 538 participants in 54 observational studies. Eur Heart J (2006) 27:2763–74.10.1093/eurheartj/ehl338.
113. Lange-Asschenfeldt C, Lederbogen F. [Antidepressant therapy in coronary artery disease]. Nervenarzt (2011) 82:657–64.10.1007/s00115-010-3181-7.
114. Barefoot JC, Helms MJ, Mark DB, Blumenthal JA, Califf RM, Haney TL, O'Connor CM, Siegler IC, Williams RB. Depression and long-term mortality risk in patients with coronary artery disease. Am J Cardiol. 1996;78:613–617.
115. Pan A, Sun Q, Okereke OI, Rexrode KM, Hu FB. Depression and risk of stroke morbidity and mortality: a meta-analysis and systematic review. JAMA. 2011 Sep 21; 306(11):1241-9.
116. Hackett ML, Yapa C, Parag V, Anderson CS. Frequency of depression after stroke: a systematic review of observational studies. Stroke. 2005; 36:1330–1340.
117. Bartoli F, Lillia N, Lax A, Crocamo C, Mantero V, Carrà G, Agostoni E, Clerici M. Depression after stroke and risk of mortality: a systematic review and meta-analysis. Stroke Res Treat 2013; 2013:862978.

118. Cramer H, Lauche R, Langhorst J, Dobos G. Yoga for depression: a systematic review and meta-analysis. Depress Anxiety. 2013 Nov;30(11):1068-83. doi: 10.1002/da.22166. Epub 2013 Aug 6.
119. Pilkington K, Kirkwood G, Rampes H, Richardson J. Yoga for depression: The research evidence. J Affect Disord. 2005;89: 13–24. 10.1016/j.jad.2005.08.013.
120. Uebelacker LA, Broughton MK. Yoga for Depression and Anxiety: A Review of Published Research and Implications for Healthcare Providers. R I Med J (2013). 2016 Mar 1;99(3):20-2.
121. de Manincor M, Bensoussan A, Smith CA, et al. Individualized yoga for reducing depression and anxiety, and improving well-being: a randomized controlled trial. Depress Anxiety. 2016 Sep;33(9):816-28. doi: 10.1002/da.22502. Epub 2016 Mar 31.
122. Cramer H, Anheyer D, Lauche R, Dobos G. A systematic review of yoga for major depressive disorder. Affect Disord. 2017 Apr 15;213:70-77. doi: 10.1016/j.jad.2017.02.006. Epub 2017 Feb 7.
123. Streeter CC, Gerbarg PL, Whitfield TH, et al. Treatment of Major Depressive Disorder with Iyengar Yoga and Coherent Breathing: A Randomized Controlled Dosing Study. J Altern Complement Med. 2017;23(3):201-207.
124. Prathikanti S, Rivera R, Cochran A, Tungol JG, Fayazmanesh N, Weinmann E. Treating major depression with yoga: A prospective, randomized, controlled pilot trial. PLoS One. 2017;12(3):e0173869. Published 2017 Mar 16. doi:10.1371/journal.pone.0173869.
125. Streeter CC, Gerbarg PL, Saper RB, Ciraulo DA, Brown RP. Effects of yoga on the autonomic nervous system, gamma-aminobutyric-acid, and allostasis in epilepsy, depression, and post-traumatic stress disorder. Med Hypotheses. 2012 May;78(5):571-9. doi: 10.1016/j.mehy.2012.01.021. Epub 2012 Feb 24.
126. Lim SA, Cheong KJ, Regular Yoga Practice Improves Antioxidant Status, Immune Function, and Stress Hormone Releases in Young Healthy People: A Randomized, Double-Blind, Controlled Pilot Study. J Altern Complement Med 2015 Sep;21(9):530-8.
127. Kinser PA, Goehler LE, Taylor AG. How might yoga help depression? A neurobiological perspective. Explore (NY). 2012;8(2):118–126. doi:10.1016/j.explore.2011.12.005.
128. Tyagi A, Cohen M. Yoga and heart rate variability: A comprehensive review of the literature. Int J Yoga. 2016;9(2):97–113. doi:10.4103/0973-6131.183712.
129. Kamei T, Toriumi Y, Kimura H, Ohno S, Kumano H, Kimura K. Decrease in serum cortisol during yoga exercise is correlated with alpha wave activation. Percept Mot Skills. 2000 Jun;90(3 Pt 1):1027-32.
130. Schuver KJ, Lewis BA. Mindfulness-based yoga intervention for women with depression. Complement Ther Med. 2016;26: 85–91. 10.1016/j.ctim.2016.03.003.
131. Katzman M. A., Vermani M., Gerbarg P. L., Brown R. P., Iorio C., Davis M., et al. (2012). A multicomponent yoga-based, breath intervention program as an adjunctive treatment in patients suffering from Generalized Anxiety Disorder with or without comorbidities. Int. J. Yoga 5, 57–6510.4103/0973-6131.91716.
132. de Groot M, Anderson R, Freedland KE, Clouse RE, Lustman PJ. Association of depression and diabetes complications: A meta-analysis. Psychosom Med. 2001;63(4):619–630.
133. Boutoille D, Feraille A, Maulaz D, Krempf M. Quality of life with diabetes-associated foot complications: Comparison between lower-limb amputation and chronic foot ulceration. Foot Ankle Int. 2008;29(11):1074–1078.
134. Beydoun MA, Kuczmarski MT, Mason MA, Ling SM, Evans MK, Zonderman AB. Role of depressive symptoms in explaining socioeconomic status disparities in dietary quality and central adiposity among us adults: A structural equation modeling approach. Am J Clin Nutr. 2009;90(4):1084–1095.
135. Toker S, Shirom A, Melamed S. Depression and the metabolic syndrome: Gender-dependent associations. Depress Anxiety. 2008;25(8):661–669.
136. Giugliano G, Brevetti G, Laurenzano E, Brevetti L, Luciano R, et al. (2010) The prognostic impact of general and abdominal obesity in peripheral arterial disease. Int J Obes (Lond) 34: 280–286.

137. Golledge J, Cronin O, Iyer V, Bradshaw B, Moxon JV, et al. (2013) Body mass index is inversely associated with mortality in patients with peripheral vascular disease. Atherosclerosis 229 (2) 549–55.
138. Garg PK, Biggs ML, Carnethon M, et al. Metabolic syndrome and risk of incident peripheral artery disease: the cardiovascular health study. Hypertension. 2013;63(2):413–419. doi:10.1161/HYPERTENSIONAHA.113.01925.
139. Corona G, Ricca V, Bandini E, et al. Association between psychiatric symptoms and erectile dysfunction. J Sex Med 2008;5:458-68. 10.1111/j.1743-6109.2007.00663.x.
140. Atlantis E, Sullivan T. Bidirectional association between depression and sexual dysfunction: A systematic review and meta-analysis. J Sex Med 2012;9:1497-507. 10.1111/j.1743-6109.2012.02709.x.
141. Hale VE, Strassberg DS. The role of anxiety on sexual arousal. Arch Sex Behav 1990;19:569-81. 10.1007/BF01542466.
142. Beck JG, Barlow DH. The effects of anxiety and attentional focus on sexual responding — II: cognitive and affective patterns in erectile dysfunction. Behav Res Ther 1986;24:19-26. 10.1016/0005-7967(86)90145-2.

Obesity

1. Hruby A, Hu FB. The Epidemiology of Obesity: A Big Picture. PharmacoEconomics. 2015;33(7):673-689.
2. Marie Ng, Tom Fleming, BS, Margaret Robinson et al. Global, regional, and national prevalence of overweight and obesity in children and adults during 1980–2013: a systematic analysis for the Global Burden of Disease Study 2013. Lancet, 2014, Volume 384, No. 9945, p766–781.
3. Craig M. Hales, Margaret D. Carroll, Cheryl D. Fryar, and Cynthia L. Ogden, Ph.D. Prevalence of Obesity Among Adults and Youth: United States, 2015–2016. NCHS Data Brief. No. 288. October 2017.
4. https://www.cdc.gov/obesity/adult/defining.html.
5. Gopinath S, Ganesh BA, Manoj K, Rubiya. Comparision between body mass index and abdominal obesity for the screening for diabetes in healthy individuals. Indian Journal of Endocrinology and Metabolism. 2012;16 (Suppl 2): S441-S442.
6. Jensen MD. Health consequences of fat distribution. Horm Res. 1997;48 Suppl 5:88-92.
7. http://www.scielosp.org/pdf/rpsp/v10n2/5870.pdf (accessed May 6, 2017).
8. Despres J.P., Moorjani S., Lupien P.J., Tremblay A., Nadeau A., Bouchard C. Regional distribution of body fat, plasma lipoproteins, and cardiovascular disease. Arteriosclerosis. 1990;10:497–511. doi: 10.1161/01.ATV.10.4.497.
9. Jensen MD. Role of body fat distribution and the metabolic complications of obesity. J Am Coll Cardiol. 2008;93(11_supplement_1): s57–s63.
10. Browning, L., Hsieh, S., & Ashwell, M. (2010). A systematic review of waist-to-height ratio as a screening tool for the prediction of cardiovascular disease and diabetes: 0·5 could be a suitable global boundary value. Nutrition Research Reviews, 23(2), 247-269.
11. Must A, Spadano J, Coakley EH, Field AE, et al. The disease burden associated withoverweight and obesity. JAMA. 1999;282:1523-1529.
12. Hartemink N, Boshuizen HC, Nagelkerke NJ, et al. Combining risk estimates from observational studies with different exposure cutpoints: a meta-analysis on body mass index and diabetes type 2. Am J Epidemiol 2006;163:1042-52. 10.1093/aje/kwj141.
13. Mokhlesi B, Tulaimat A, Faibussowitsch I, et al. Obesity hypoventilation syndrome: prevalence and predictors in patients with obstructive sleep apnea. Sleep Breath 2007;11:117-24. 10.1007/s11325-006-0092-8.
14. Nowbar S, Burkart KM, Gonzales R, et al. Obesity-associated hypoventilation in hospitalized patients: prevalence, effects, and outcome. Am J Med 2004;116:1-7. 10.1016/j.amjmed.2003.08.022.

15. Prospective Studies Collaboration, Whitlock G, Lewington S, et al. Body-mass index and cause-specific mortality in 900 000 adults: collaborative analyses of 57 prospective studies. Lancet 2009;373:1083-96. 10.1016/S0140-6736(09)60318-4.
16. Machado M, Marques-Vidal P, Cortez-Pinto H. Hepatic histology in obese patients undergoing bariatric surgery. J Hepatol 2006;45:600-6. 10.1016/j.jhep.2006.06.013.
17. Pasquali R, Patton L, Gambineri A. Obesity and infertility. Curr Opin Endocrinol Diabetes Obes2007;14:482-7. 10.1097/MED.0b013e3282f1d6cb,; Gosman GG, King WC, Schrope B, et al. Reproductive health of women electing bariatric surgery.Fertil Steril 2010;94:1426-31. 10.1016/j.fertnstert.2009.08.028.
18. El-Serag HB, Ergun GA, Pandolfino J, et al. Obesity increases oesophageal acid exposure. Gut2007;56:749-55. 10.1136/gut.2006.100263.
19. Daphne P Guh, et al. The incidence of co-morbidities related to obesity and overweight: A systematic review and meta-analysis. BMC Public Health20099:88.
20. Feng J, Chen Q, Yu F, et al. Body mass index and risk of rheumatoid arthritis: a meta-analysis of observational stud-ies. Medicine (Baltimore). 2016;95(8):e2859. doi: 10.1097/MD.0000000000002859.
21. Calle EE, Rodriguez C, Walker-Thurmond K, Thun MJ. Overweight, obesity, and mortality from cancer in a prospectively studied cohort of US adults. N Engl J Med. 2003;348(17):1625-1638.
22. Kasen, Stephanie, et al. "Obesity and psychopathology in women: a three decade prospective study." International Journal of Obesity 32.3 (2008): 558-566.
23. Williams GA, Hudson DL, Whisenhunt BL, et al. An examination of body tracing among women with high body dissatisfaction. Body Image 2014;11:346-9. 10.1016/j.bodyim.2014.05.005.
24. Luppino, Floriana S., et al. "Overweight, obesity, and depression: a systematic review and meta-analysis of longitudinal studies." Archives of general psychiatry 67.3 (2010): 220-229.
25. Wadden TA, Sarwer DB, Fabricatore AN, et al. Psychosocial and behavioral status of patients undergoing bariatric surgery: what to expect before and after surgery. Med Clin North Am2007;91:451-69, xi-xii. 10.1016/j.mcna.2007.01.003.
26. Bardel A, Wallander MA, Svardsudd K. Reported current use of prescription drugs and some of its determinants among 35 to 65-year-old women in mid-Sweden: A population-based study. J Clin Epidemiol 2000;53:637-43. 10.1016/S0895-4356(99)00228-0.
27. Narbro K, Agren G, Jonsson E, et al. Pharmaceutical costs in obese individuals: comparison with a randomly selected population sample and long-term changes after conventional and surgical treatment: the SOS intervention study. Arch Intern Med 2002;162:2061-9. 10.1001/archinte.162.18.2061.
28. Whitlock G, Lewington S, Sherliker P, et al; Prospective Studies Collaboration. Body-mass index and cause-specific mortal-ity in 900 000 adults: collaborative analyses of 57 prospective studies. Lancet. 2009:373(9669);1083-1096. doi: 10.1016/S0140-6736(09)60318-4.
29. Berrington de Gonzalez A, Hartge P, Cerhan JR, et al. Body-mass index and mortality among 1.46 million white adults. N Engl J Med 2010;363:2211-9. 10.1056/NEJMoa1000367.
30. Kitahara CM, Flint AJ, Berrington de Gonzalez A, et al. Association between class III obesity (BMI of 40-59 kg/m2) and mortality: a pooled analysis of 20 prospective studies. PLoS Med. 2014;11(7):e1001673. doi: 10.1371/journal.pmed.1001673.;)
31. Haslam DW, James WP. Obesity. Lancet 2005;366:1197-209. 10.1016/S0140-6736(05)67483-1.
32. Flegal KM KB, Orpana H, Graubard BI. Association of all cause mortality with overweight and obesity using standard body mass index categories: a systematic review and metaanalysis. JAMA2013;309:71-82. 10.1001/jama.2012.113905.
33. Zalesin K.C., Franklin B.A., Miller W.M., et al. Impact of obesity on cardiovascular disease. Med. Clin. North Am. 2011;95:919–937.
34. Kotchen TA, Grim CE, Kotchen JM, et al. Altered relationship of blood pressure to adiposity in hypertension. Am J Hypertens 2008;21:284-9. 10.1038/ajh.2007.48.

35. Nakamura K, Fuster JJ, Walsh K. Adipokines: a link between obesity and cardiovascular disease. J Cardiol 2014;63:250-9. 10.1016/j.jjcc.2013.11.006.
36. Reis JP, Allen N, Gunderson EP, et al. Excess Body Mass Index- and Waist Circumference-Years and Incident Cardiovascular Disease: The CARDIA Study. Obesity (Silver Spring, Md). 2015;23(4):879-885.
37. Hartemink N, Boshuizen HC, Nagelkerke NJ, et al. Combining risk estimates from observational studies with different exposure cutpoints: a meta-analysis on body mass index and diabetes type 2. Am J Epidemiol 2006;163:1042-52. 10.1093/aje/kwj141.
38. Floriana S. Luppino, MD; Leonore M. de Wit, et al. Overweight, Obesity, and Depression. A Systematic Review and Meta-analysis of Longitudinal Studies. Arch Gen Psychiatry. 2010;67(3):220-229.
39. Stevens VJ, Obarzanek E, Cook NR, et al. Long-term weight loss and changes in blood pressure: results of the Trials of Hypertension Prevention, phase II. Ann Intern Med. 2001;134:1–11.
40. (G, Lewington S, Sherliker P, et al. Body-mass index and cause-specific mortality in 900 000 adults: collaborative analyses of 57 prospective studies. Lancet. 2009 Mar 28;373(9669):1083–1096.
41. Berrington de Gonzalez A, Hartge P, Cerhan JR, et al. Body-mass index and mortality among 1.46 million white adults. New Engl J Med. 2010 Dec 2;363(23):2211–2219.
42. Global Burden of Metabolic Risk Factors for Chronic Diseases Collaboration (BMI Mediated Effects), Lu Y, Hajifathalian K, et al. Metabolic mediators of the effects of body-mass index, overweight, and obesity on coronary heart disease and stroke: a pooled analysis of 97 prospective cohorts with 1·8 million participants. Lancet. 2014;383(9921):970-83.
43. Reilly JJ, Kelly J. Long-term impact of overweight and obesity in childhood and adolescence on morbidity and premature mortality in adulthood: systematic review. Int J Obes. 2011 Jul;35(7):891–8.
44. Grundy SM, Brewer HB, Jr, Cleeman JI, et al. Definition of metabolic syndrome: report of the National Heart, Lung, and Blood Institute/American Heart Association conference on scientific issues related to definition. Arterioscler Thromb Vasc Biol 2004;24:e13-8. 10.1161/01.ATV.0000111245.75752.C6.
45. Brassard P, Legault S, Garneau C, et al. Normalization of diastolic dysfunction in type 2 diabetics after exercise training. Med Sci Sports Exerc 2007;39:1896-901. 10.1249/mss.0b013e318145b642.
46. Lakhani M, Fein S. Effects of obesity and subsequent weight reduction on left ventricular function. Cardiol Rev 2011;19:1-4. 10.1097/CRD.0b013e3181f877d2.
47. Wanahita N, Messerli FH, Bangalore S, et al. Atrial fibrillation and obesity--results of a meta-analysis. Am Heart J 2008;155:310-5. 10.1016/j.ahj.2007.10.004.
48. Metropolitan Life Insurance Company. Build and pressure study 1959. Vol I, II. Chicago: Society of Actuaries, 1960.
49. Chen Y, Copeland WK, Vedanthan R, Grant E, Lee JE, Gu D, et al. Association between body mass index and cardiovascular disease mortality in east Asians and south Asians: pooled analysis of prospective data from the Asia Cohort Consortium. BMJ. 2013 Oct 1;347.
50. James R. Cerhan, Steven C. Moore, Eric J. Jacobs, et al. A Pooled Analysis of Waist Circumference and Mortality in 650,000 Adults. Mayo Clin Proc. 2014 March; 89(3): 335–345.
51. Peeters A, Barendregt JJ, Willekens F, Mackenbach JP, Al Mamun A, Bonneux L, et al. Obesity in adulthood and its consequences for life expectancy: a life-table analysis. Ann Intern Med. 2003 Jan 7;138(1):24–32.
52. Caitlin W. Hicks, Chao Yang, Chiadi E. Ndumelem et al. Associations of Obesity With Incident Hospitalization Related to Peripheral Artery Disease and Critical Limb Ischemia in the ARIC Study. JAHA. August 21, 2018. Vol 7, Issue 16.
53. Bacon CG, Mittleman MA, Kawachi I, Giovannucci E, Glasser DB, Rimm EB. Sexual function in men older than 50 years of age: results from the health Professionals' follow-up study. Ann Intern Med. 2003;139:161–168.

54. Skrypnik D, Bogdański P, Musialik K. Obesity--significant risk factor for erectile dysfunction in men].[Article in Polish]. Pol Merkur Lekarski. 2014 Feb;36(212):137-41.
55. Davies HO, Popplewell M, Singhal R, Smith N, Bradbury AW. Obesity and lower limb venous disease - The epidemic of phlebesity. Phlebology. 2017 May;32(4):227-233. doi: 10.1177/0268355516649333. Epub 2016 May 13.
56. van Rij, A.M. et al. Obesity and Impaired Venous Function. European Journal of Vascular and Endovascular Surgery , Volume 35 , Issue 6 , 739 – 744.
57. Horvath K, Jeitler K, Siering U, et al. Long-term effects of weight-reducing interventions in hypertensive patients: systematic review and meta-analysis. Arch Intern Med. 2008 Mar 24;168(6):571–580.
58. Anderson JW, Kendall CWC, Jenkins DJA. Importance of weight management in type 2 diabetes: review with meta-analysis of clinical studies. J Am Coll Nutr. 2003 Oct;22(5):331–339.
59. Malin SK, Niemi N, Solomon TP, et al. Exercise training with weight loss and either a high- or low-glycemic index diet reduces metabolic syndrome severity in older adults. Ann Nutr Metab. 2012;61(2):135–141.
60. Kelley GA, Kelley KS, Roberts S, Haskell W. Comparison of aerobic exercise, diet or both on lipids and lipoproteins in adults: a meta-analysis of randomized controlled trials. Clin Nutr. 2012 Apr;31(2):156–167.
61. Sierra-Johnson J, Romero-Corral A, Somers VK, et al. Prognostic importance of weight loss in patients with coronary heart disease regardless of initial body mass index. Eur J Cardiovasc Prev Rehabil. 2008 Jun;15(3):336–340.
62. Lavie CJ, Milani RV, Artham SM, Patel DA, Ventura HO. The obesity paradox, weight loss, and coronary disease. Am J Med. 2009 Dec;122(12):1106–1114.
63. Pack QR, Rodriguez-Escudero JP, Thomas RJ, et al. The prognostic importance of weight loss in coronary artery disease: a systematic review and meta-analysis. Mayo Clin Proc. 2014;89(10):1368-77.
64. Smith SC, Jr, Benjamin EJ, Bonow RO, et al. AHA/ACCF secondary prevention and risk reduction therapy for patients with coronary and other atherosclerotic vascular disease: 2011 update: a guideline from the American Heart Association and American College of Cardiology Foundation endorsed by the World Heart Federation and the Preventive Cardiovascular Nurses Association. J Am Coll Cardiol. 2011 Nov 29;58(23):2432–2446.
65. Mechanick JI, Youdim A, Jones DB, et al. Clinical practice guidelines for the perioperative nutritional, metabolic, and nonsurgical support of the bariatric surgery patient--2013 update: cosponsored by American Association of Clinical Endocrinologists, The Obesity Society, and American Society for Metabolic & Bariatric Surgery. Obesity (Silver Spring). 2013;21 Suppl 1(0 1):S1-27.
66. Lee JA, Kim JW, Kim DY. Effects of yoga exercise on serum adiponectin and metabolic syndrome factors in obese postmenopausal women. Menopause. 2012;19:296–301.
67. Rshikesan PB, Subramanya P, Nidhi R. Yoga Practice for Reducing the Male Obesity and Weight Related Psychological Difficulties-A Randomized Controlled Trial. J Clin Diagn Res. 2016;10(11):OC22-OC28.
68. Cramer H, Sushila Thoms M, Anheyer D, Lauche R, Dobos G. Yoga in Women With Abdominal Obesity— a Randomized Controlled Trial. Deutsches Ärzteblatt International. 2016;113(39):645-652. doi:10.3238/arztebl.2016.0645.
69. Siu PM, Yu AP, Benzie IF, Woo J. Effects of 1-year yoga on cardiovascular risk factors in middle-aged and older adults with metabolic syndrome: a randomized trial. Diabetol Metab Syndr. 2015;7:40. Published 2015 Apr 30. doi:10.1186/s13098-015-0034-3.
70. Olson K. L., Emery C. F. Mindfulness and weight loss: a systematic review. Psychosomatic Medicine. 2015;77(1):59-67.
71. Neumark-Sztainer D, MacLehose RF, Watts AW, Eisenberg ME, Laska MN, Larson N. How Is the Practice of Yoga Related to Weight Status? Population-Based Findings From Project EAT-IV. J Phys Act Health. 2017;14(12):905-912.

72. Kristal AR, Littman AJ, Benitez D, White E. Yoga practice is associated with attenuated weight gain in healthy, middle-aged men and women. Altern Ther Health Med. 2005;11:28–33.
73. Lauche R, Langhorst J, Lee MS, Dobos G, Cramer H. A systematic review and meta-analysis on the effects of yoga on weight-related outcomes. Prev Med. (2016) 87:213–32. 10.1016/j.ypmed.2016.03.013.
74. Hagins M, Moore W, Rundle A. Does practicing hatha yoga satisfy recommendations for intensity of physical activity which improves and maintains health and cardiovascular fitness? BMC Complement Altern Med. 2007;7.
75. Larson-Meyer DE. A Systematic Review of the Energy Cost and Metabolic Intensity of Yoga. Med Sci Sports Exerc. 2016 Aug;48(8):1558-69. doi: 10.1249/MSS.0000000000000922.
76. Watts AW, Rydell SA, Eisenberg ME, Laska MN, Neumark-Sztainer D. Yoga's potential for promoting healthy eating and physical activity behaviors among young adults: a mixed-methods study. Int J Behav Nutr Phys Act. 2018;15(1):42. Published 2018 May 2. doi:10.1186/s12966-018-0674-4.
77. Telles S, Sharma SK, Kala N, Pal S, Gupta RK, Balkrishna A. Twelve Weeks of Yoga or Nutritional Advice for Centrally Obese Adult Females. Front Endocrinol (Lausanne). 2018;9:466. Published 2018 Aug 17. doi:10.3389/fendo.2018.00466.
78. Watts AW, Rydell SA, Eisenberg ME, Laska MN, Neumark-Sztainer D. Yoga's potential for promoting healthy eating and physical activity behaviors among young adults: a mixed-methods study. Int J Behav Nutr Phys Act. 2018;15(1):42. Published 2018 May 2. doi:10.1186/s12966-018-0674-4.
79. Cramer H, Lauche R, Langhorst J, Dobos G. Yoga for depression: a systematic review and meta-analysis. Depress Anxiety. 2013;30:1068–1083.
80. Dallman MF, Pecoraro N, Akana SF, et al. Chronic stress and obesity: a new view of comfort food" Proc Natl Acad Sci USA. 2003;100:11696–11701.

Peripheral Artery Disease

1. Selvin E, Erlinger TP. Prevalence of and risk factors for peripheral arterial disease in the United States: results from the National Health and Nutrition Examination Survey, 1999-2000. Circulation 2004;110:738-43.
2. Fowkes FGR, Rudan D, Rudan I, et al. Comparison of global estimates of prevalence and risk factors for peripheral artery disease in 2000 and 2010: a systematic review and analysis. Lancet 2013; 382:1329-40.
3. Gregg EW, Sorlie P, Paulose-Ram R, et al. Prevalence of lower-extremity disease in the US adult population >=40 years of age with and without diabetes: 1999-2000 national health and nutrition examination survey. Diabetes Care 2004;27:1591-7.
4. Guijarro C, Mostaza JM, Hernández-Mijares A. [Lower limb arterial disease and renal artery stenosis] Clin Investig Arterioscler. 2013;25:218–223.
5. Ouriel K. Peripheral arterial disease. Lancet. 2001;358:1257–64.
6. Al-Delaimy WK, Merchant AT, Rimm EB, et al. Effect of type 2 diabetes and its duration on the risk of peripheral arterial disease among men. Am J Med. 2004;116:236–40.
7. Wang L, DU F, Mao H, Wang HX, Zhao S. Prevalence and related risk factors of peripheral arterial disease in elderly patients with type 2 diabetes in Wuhan, Central China. Chin Med J (Engl) 2011;124(24):4264–68.
8. Emdin CA, Anderson SG, Callender T, et al. Usual blood pressure, peripheral arterial disease, and vascular risk: cohort study of 4.2 million adults. BMJ. 2015;351:h4865. Published 2015 Sep 29. doi:10.1136/bmj.h4865.
9. Afaq A, Montgomery PS, Scott KJ, Blevins SM, Whitsett TL, Gardner AW. The effect of current cigarette smoking on calf muscle hemoglobin oxygen saturation in patients with intermittent claudication. Vasc Med. 2007;12:167–173.
10. Huang Y, Xu M, Xie L, et al. Obesity and peripheral arterial disease: A Mendelian Randomization analysis. Atherosclerosis. 2016 Apr;247:218-24. doi: 10.1016/j.atherosclerosis.2015.12.034. Epub 2015 Dec 29.

11. Norgren L, Hiatt WR, Dormandy JA, Nehler MR, Harris KA, Fowkes FGR. Inter-society consensus for the management of peripheral arterial disease (TASC II) J Vasc Surg. 2007;45:S5A–S67A.
12. Kullo IJ, Leeper NJ. The genetic basis of peripheral arterial disease: current knowledge, challenges, and future directions. Circ Res. 2015;116(9):1551-60.
13. Criqui MH. Peripheral arterial disease – epidemiological aspects. Vasc Med. 2001;6(Suppl 1):3–7.
14. Ankle Brachial Index Collaboration. Ankle brachial index combined with Framingham Risk Score to predict cardiovascular events and mortality: a meta-analysis. JAMA. 2008; 300:197-208.
15. Chhabra A, Aronow WS, Ahn C, et al. Incidence of new cardiovascular events in patients with and without peripheral arterial disease seen in a vascular surgery clinic. Med Sci Monit.2012;18(3):CR131–34.
16. Tekin N, Baskan M, Yesilkayali T, Karabay O. Prevalence of peripheral arterial disease and related risk factors in Turkish elders. BMC Fam Pract. 2011;12:96.
17. Ankle Brachial Index Collaboration. Ankle brachial index combined with Framingham Risk Score to predict cardiovascular events and mortality: a meta-analysis. JAMA. 2008; 300:197-208.
18. Dawson DL, Mills JL. Critical limb ischemia. Curr Treat Options Cardiovasc Med.2007;9:159–70.
19. Izquierdo-Porrera AM, Gardner AW, Bradham DD, et al. Relationship between objective measures of peripheral arterial disease severity to self-reported quality of life in older adults with intermittent claudication. J Vasc Surg. 2005;41:625–30.
20. Aboyans V, Criqui MH, Abraham P, Allison MA, Creager MA, Diehm C, Fowkes FG, Hiatt WR, Jönsson B, Lacroix P, et al. Measurement and interpretation of the ankle-brachial index: a scientific statement from the American Heart Association. Circulation. 2012;126:2890–2909.
21. Girolami B, Bernardi E, Prins MH, Ten Cate JW, Hettiarachchi R, Prandoni P, Girolami A, Buller HR. Treatment of intermittent claudication with physical training, smoking cessation, pentoxifylline, or nafronyl: a meta-analysis. Arch Int Med. 1999;159:337–345.
22. Rice TW, Lumsden AB. Optimal medical management of peripheral arterial disease. Vasc Endovasc Surg. 2006;40:312–327.
23. Hagins M, States R, Selfe T, et al. Effectiveness of Yoga for Hypertension: Systematic Review and Meta-Analysis Evidence-Based Complementary and Alternative Medicine. Volume 2013 (2013), Article ID 649836, 13 pages.
24. Chu P, Gotink RA, Yeh GY, Goldie SJ, Hunink MG. The effectiveness of yoga in modifying risk factors for cardiovascular disease and metabolic syndrome: A systematic review and meta-analysis of randomized controlled trials. Eur J Prev Cardiol. 2016 Feb;23(3):291-307. doi: 10.1177/2047487314562741. Epub 2014 Dec 15.
25. Innes KE, Bourguignon C, Taylor AG. Risk indices associated with the insulin resistance syndrome, cardiovascular disease and possible protection with yoga: a systematic review. J Am Board Fam Pract. 2005;18:491–519. doi: 10.3122/jabfm.18.6.491.
26. Lee JA, Kim JW, Kim DY. Effects of yoga exercise on serum adiponectin and metabolic syndrome factors in obese postmenopausal women. Menopause. 2012;19:296–301.
27. Olson K. L., Emery C. F. Mindfulness and weight loss: a systematic review. Psychosomatic Medicine. 2015;77(1):59-67.
28. Yogendra J, Yogendra HJ, Ambardekar S, Lele RD, Shetty S, Dave M, Husein N. Beneficial effects of yoga lifestyle on reversibility of ischaemic heart disease: caring heart project of International Board of Yoga. J Assoc Physicians India. 2004 Apr;52:283-9.
29. Manchanda SC, Mehrotra UC, Makhija A, Mohanty A, Dhawan S, et al. (2013) Reversal of Early Atherosclerosis in Metabolic Syndrome by Yoga – A Randomized Controlled Trial. J Yoga Phys Ther 3:132. doi: 10.4172/2157-7595.1000132.
30. Bock BC, Fava JL, Gaskins R, et al. Yoga as a complementary treatment for smoking cessation in women. J Womens Health (Larchmt) 2012;21(2):240–248.

31. L Carim Todd, S Mitchell, B Oken. Does yoga improve smoking cessation outcomes? A systematic review of the literature. BMC Complement Altern Med. 2012; 12(Suppl 1): P389. Published online 2012 Jun 12.

Positivity/Happiness/Laughter

1. Caprara GV, Alessandri G, Eisenberg N, et al. The positivity scale. Psychol Assess. 2012;24(3):701–712.
2. Caprara GV, Alessandri G, Eisenberg N, Kupfer A, Steca P, Caprara MG, et al. The Positivity Scale. Psychol Assess. 2012; 24: 701–712. doi: 10.1037/a0026681.
3. Caprara GV, Fagnani C, Alessandri G, et al. Human optimal functioning: the genetics of positive orientation towards self, life, and the future. Behav Genet. 2009;39(3):277–284.
4. Catalino LI, Algoe SB, Fredrickson BL. Prioritizing positivity: an effective approach to pursuing happiness?. Emotion. 2014;14(6):1155-61.
5. Diener E, Saptya JJ, Suh EM. Subjective well-being is essential to well-being. Psychological Inquiry. 1998;9:33–37. doi: 10.1207/s15327965pli0901_3.
6. De Neve J-E, Christakis NA, Fowler JH, Frey BS. Genes, Economics, and Happiness. Journal of neuroscience, psychology, and economics. 2012;5(4):10.1037/a0030292.
7. Galati D, Manzano M, Sotgiu I. The subjective components of happiness and their attainment: A cross-cultural comparison between Italy and Cuba . Social Science Information 2006, 45: 601–630.
8. Abdel-Khalek AM. Religiosity, health and happiness: significant relations in adolescents from Qatar. Int J Soc Psychiatry. 2014 Nov;60(7):656-61. doi: 10.1177/0020764013511792. Epub 2013 Dec 10.
9. Sotgiu I. Conceptions of Happiness and Unhappiness among Italian Psychology Undergraduates. PLoS One. 2016;11(12):e0167745. Published 2016 Dec 15. doi:10.1371/journal.pone.0167745.
10. Tan CS, Low SK, Viapude GN. Extraversion and happiness: The mediating role of social support and hope. Psych J. 2018 Sep;7(3):133-143. doi: 10.1002/pchj.220. Epub 2018 Jul 17.
11. Lyubomirsky S, King LA, Diener E. The benefits of frequent positive affect. Psychological Bulletin. 2005;131:803–855. doi: 10.1037/0033-2909.131.6.803.
12. Cohen S, Pressman SD. Positive affect and health. Current Directions in Psychological Science. 2006;15:122–125.; Veenhoven R. Healthy happiness: Effects of happiness on physical health and the consequences for preventive health care. Journal of Happiness Studies. 2008;9:449–469.
13. Ong AD. Pathways linking positive emotion and health in later life. Current Directions in Psychological Science. 2010;19:358–362.
14. Lyubomirsky S, King LA, Diener E. The benefits of frequent positive affect. Psychological Bulletin. 2005;131:803–855. doi: 10.1037/0033-2909.131.6.803.
15. Barak Y. The immune system and happiness. Autoimmunity Reviews. 2006; 5: 523–527. 10.1016/j.autrev.2006.02.010.
16. Grassi MC, Alessandri G, Pasquariello S, et al. Association between positivity and smoking cessation. Biomed Res Int. 2014;2014:780146.
17. Steptoe A, Dockray S, Wardle J. Positive affect and psycho-biological processes relevant to health. Journal of Personality. 2009;77:1747–1776. doi: 10.1111/j.1467-6494.2009.00599.x.
18. Chida Y, Steptoe A. Positive psychological well-being and mortality: a quantitative review of prospective observational studies. Psychosomatic Medicine. 2008; 70: 741–756. 10.1097/PSY.0b013e31818105ba.
19. Mojon-Azzi S, Sousa-Poza A. Hypertension and life satisfaction: an analysis using data from the Survey of Health, Ageing and Retirement in Europe. Applied Economics Letters. 2011; 18: 183–187. 10.1080/13504850903508291.
20. Blanchflower DG, Oswald AJ. Hypertension and happiness across nations. Journal of Health Economics. 2008; 27: 218–233. 10.1016/j.jhealeco.2007.06.002.
21. Nouri R, Okabe-Miyamoto K, Silke O, Waln B, Wen J, Boehm JK. Do happiness and optimism promote healthy and unhealthy food consumption in daily life? Student research

22. Steptoe A, Demakakos P, de Oliveira C, Wardle J. Distinctive biological correlates of positive psychological well-being in older men and women. Psychosomatic Medicine. 2012; 74: 501–508. 10.1097/PSY.0b013e31824f82c8.
23. El Shebini LS, Kazem YMI, Moaty MIA, El-Arabi NHA. (2011). Obesity in Relation to Cognitive Functions and Subjective Wellbeing among a Group of Adult Egyptian Females. Aus J Basic Appl Sci, 5(6): 69–76.
24. Katsaiti MS. Obesity and happiness. Applied Economics. 2012; 44: 4101–4114. 10.1080/00036846.2011.587779.
25. Shahab L, West R. Differences in happiness between smokers, ex-smokers and never smokers: cross-sectional findings from a national household survey. Drug Alcohol Depend. 2012 Feb 1;121(1-2):38-44. doi: 10.1016/j.drugalcdep.2011.08.011. Epub 2011 Sep 8.
26. Christopher W. Kahler, Nichea S. Spillane, Andrew M. Busch, Adam M. Leventhal; Time-Varying Smoking Abstinence Predicts Lower Depressive Symptoms Following Smoking Cessation Treatment, Nicotine & Tobacco Research, Volume 13, Issue 2, 1 February 2011, Pages 146–150, https://doi.org/10.1093/ntr/ntq213.
27. Nordestgaard BG, Varbo A. Triglycerides and cardiovascular disease. The Lancet. 2014; 384: 626–635. 10.1016/S0140-6736(14)61177-6.
28. David L. Hare, Samia R. Toukhsati, Peter Johansson, Tiny Jaarsma; Depression and cardiovascular disease: a clinical review, European Heart Journal, Volume 35, Issue 21, 1 June 2014, Pages 1365–1372, https://doi.org/10.1093/eurheartj/eht462.
29. Cohen BE, Edmondson D, Kronish IM. State of the Art Review: Depression, Stress, Anxiety, and Cardiovascular Disease. Am J Hypertens. 2015;28(11):1295-302.
30. Richard L.Verrier, Murray A.Mittleman. Life-threatening cardiovascular consequences of anger in patients with coronary heart disease. Cardiology Clinics. Volume 14, Issue 2, 1 May 1996, Pages 289-307.
31. Matthews KA, Gump BB, Harris KF, Haney TL, Barefoot JC. Hostile behaviors predict cardiovascular mortality among men enrolled in the Multiple Risk Factor Intervention Trial. Circulation. 2004 Jan 6;109(1):66-70. Epub 2003 Dec 8.
32. Lambert D'raven LT, Moliver N, Thompson D. Happiness intervention decreases pain and depression, boosts happiness among primary care patients. Prim Health Care Res Dev. 2015 Apr;16(2):114-26. doi: 10.1017/S146342361300056X. Epub 2014 Jan 22.
33. Sahoo S, Padhy SK, Padhee B, Singla N, Sarkar S. Role of personality in cardiovascular diseases: An issue that needs to be focused too! Indian Heart J. 2018 Dec;70 Suppl 3:S471-S477. doi: 10.1016/j.ihj.2018.11.003. Epub 2018 Nov 8.
34. Smith TW, MacKenzie J. Personality and risk of physical illness. Annu Rev Clin Psychol. 2006;2:435-67.
35. Julia K. Boehm and Laura D. Kubzansky. The Heart's Content: The Association Between Positive Psychological Well-Being and Cardiovascular Health. Psychological Bulletin. 2012, Vol. 138, No. 4, 655– 691.
36. Kubzansky LD, Thurston RC. Emotional vitality and incident coronary heart disease: Benefits of healthy psychological functioning. Archives of General Psychiatry. 2007;64:1393–1401.
37. Davidson KW, Mostofsky E, Whang W. Don't worry, be happy: positive affect and reduced 10-year incident coronary heart disease: the Canadian Nova Scotia Health Survey. Eur Heart J. 2010;31(9):1065-70.
38. Koizumi M, Ito H, Kaneko Y, Motohashi Y. Effect of Having a Sense of Purpose in Life on the Risk of Death from Cardiovascular Diseases. Journal of Epidemiology. 2008;18(5):191-196.
39. Mannell, R. C. & McMahon, L. (1982). 'Humour as play: Its relationship to psychological well-being during the course of a day'. Leisure Sciences 5, pp. 143–155.
40. Foley E, Matheis R, Schaefer C. Effect of forced laughter on mood. Psychol Rep. 2002;90(1):184. doi: 10.2466/pr0.2002.90.1.184. ; Neuhoff CC, Schaefer C. Effects of laughing, smiling, and howling on mood. Psychol Rep. 2002;91(3):1079. doi: 10.2466/pr0.2002.91.3f.1079.

41. Schwartz KD, Saunders JC. Laughter, Leininger, and home healthcare. Home Healthc Nurse. 2010;28(9):552–7. doi: 10.1097/NHH.0b013e3181f2f312.
42. Walter M, Hanni B, Haug M, Amrhein I, Krebs-Roubicek E, Muller-Spahn F, Savaskan E. Humour therapy in patients with late-life depression or Alzheimer's disease: a pilot study. Int J Geriatr Psychiatry. 2007;22(1):77–83. doi: 10.1002/gps.16582–4.
43. De La Fuente Mochales MB, Gonzalez Cascante ME. [Laughter therapy for chronic skeletal muscular pain] Rev Enferm. 2010;33(6):43–4.
44. Ko HJ, Youn CH. Effects of laughter therapy on depression, cognition and sleep among the community-dwelling elderly. Geriatr Gerontol Int. 2011;11(3):267–74. doi: 10.1111/j.1447-0594.2010.00680.x.
45. Shahidi M, Mojtahed A, Modabbernia A, Mojtahed M, Shafiabady A, Delavar A, Honari H. Laughter yoga versus group exercise program in elderly depressed women: a randomized controlled trial. Int J Geriatr Psychiatry. 2011;26(3):322–7. doi: 10.1002/gps.2545.
46. Mora-Ripoll R. Potential health benefits of simulated laughter: a narrative review of the literature and recommendations for future research. Complement Ther Med. 2011;19(3):170–7. doi: 10.1016/j.ctim.2011.05.003.
47. Broderick M. Laughter yoga. Alive: Canada's Natural Health & Wellness Magazine. 2012;355:39–71.
48. Yazdani M, Esmaeilzadeh M, Pahlavanzadeh S, Khaledi F. The effect of laughter yoga on general health among nursing students. Iran J Nurs Midwifery Res. 2014;19(1):36–40.].
49. Weinberg MK, Hammond TG, Cummins RA. The impact of laughter yoga on subjective wellbeing: a pilot study. Eur J Humour Res. 2014;1(4):25–34.
50. Sroufe LA, Waters E. The ontogenesis of smiling and laughter: a perspective on the organization of development in infancy. Psychol Rev. 1976, 83(3), 173-89.
51. Chaya MS, Kataria M, Nagendra R, et al. American Society of Hypertension 2008 Annual Meeting; May 14, 2008; New Orleans, LA.
52. Fry W. The respiratory components of mirthful laughter. J Biol Psychol. 1977, 19, 39-50.
53. Boone T, Hansen S, Erlandson A. Cardiovascular responses to laughter: a pilot project. Appl Nurs Res. 2000 Nov;13(4):204-8.
54. Miller M, Fry WF. The effect of mirthful laughter on the human cardiovascular system. Med Hypotheses, 2009, 73(5), 636-9.
55. Hirosaki M, Ohira T, Kajiura M, Kiyama M, Kitamura A, Sato S, Iso H. Effects of a laughter and exercise program on physiological and psychological health among communitydwelling elderly in Japan: randomized controlled trial. Geriatr Gerontol Int. 2013, 13(1), 152-60.
56. Leiber DB. Laughter and humor in critical care. Dimens Crit Care Nurs. 1976, 5, 162-70.
57. Berk LS, Tan SA, Fry WF, Napier BJ, Lee JW, Hubbard RW, Lewis JE, Eby WC. Neuroendocrine and stress hormone changes during mirthful laughter. Am J Med Sci. 1989, 298(6), 390-6.
58. Provine RR, Fischer KR. Laughing, smiling, and talking: Relation to sleeping and social context in humans. Ethology. 1989;83(4):295–305.; Provine RR, Emmorey K. Laughter among deaf signers. J Deaf Stud Deaf Educ. 2006 Fall;11(4):403–9.
59. Prasad L, Varrey A, Sisti G. Medical students' stress levels and sense of well-being after six weeks of yoga and meditation. Evid Based Complement Alternat Med. 2016;2016:9251849.
60. Hartfiel N, Havenhand J, Khalsa SB, et al. The effectiveness of yoga for the improvement of well-being and resilience to stress in the workplace. Scand J Work Environ Health. 2011;37:70–76.
61. Gupta RK, Singh S, Singh N. Does yoga influence happiness and mental balance: A comparison between yoga practitioners and non-yoga practitioners? OJMR. 2016;2:1–5.
62. Ross A, Friedmann E, Bevans M, Thomas S. National survey of yoga practitioners: mental and physical health benefits. Complement Ther Med. 2013;21(4):313-23.
63. MacDonald CM. A chuckle a day keeps the doctor away: therapeutic humor and laughter. J Psychosoc Nurs Ment Health Serv. 2004 Mar;42(3):18-25.
64. Law MM, Broadbent EA, Sollers JJ. A comparison of the cardiovascular effects of simulated and spontaneous laughter. Complement Ther Med. 2018 Apr;37:103-109. doi: 10.1016/j.ctim.2018.02.005. Epub 2018 Feb 21.

Sedentary Behavior/Sitting

1. Owen N, Leslie E, Salmon J, Fotheringham MJ. Environmental determinants of physical activity and sedentary behavior. Exer Sport Sci Rev. 2000;28(4):153–8.
2. Matthews CE, Chen KY, Freedson PS, Buchowski MS, Beech BM, Pate RR et al. Amount of time spent in sedentary behaviors in the United States, 2003–2004. Am J Epidemiol 2008; 167: 875–881.
3. Salmon J, Tremblay MS, Marshall SJ, Hume C. Health risks, correlates, and interventions to reduce sedentary behavior in young people. Am J Prev Med. 2011 Aug;41(2):197-206. doi: 10.1016/j.amepre.2011.05.001.
4. Owen N, Healy GN, Matthews CE, Dunstan DW. Too much sitting: the population health science of sedentary behavior. Exerc Sport Sci Rev. 2010;38(3):105–113. doi: 10.1097/JES.0b013e3181e373a2.
5. Warburton DE, Nicol CW, Bredin SS. Health benefits of physical activity: the evidence. CMAJ. 2006;174(6):801–809. doi:10.1503/cmaj.051351.
6. Dunstan DW, Howard B, Healy GN, Owen N. Too much sitting--a health hazard. Diabetes Res Clin Pract. 2012 Sep;97(3):368-76. doi: 10.1016/j.diabres.2012.05.020. Epub 2012 Jun 9.
7. Nourbakhsh MR, Moussavi SJ, Salavati M. Effects of lifestyle and work-related physical activity on the degree of lumbar lordosis and chronic low back pain in a Middle East population. J Spinal Disord Tech. 2001;14:283–92. doi: 10.1097/00002517-200108000-00002.
8. Friedenreich CM, Cook LS, Magliocco AM, Duggan MA, Courneya KS. Case-control study of lifetime total physical activity and endometrial cancer risk. Cancer Causes Control. 2010;21(7):1105–1116. doi:10.1007/s10552-010-9538-1.
9. Matthews CE, George SM, Moore SC, et al. Amount of time spent in sedentary behaviors and cause-specific mortality in US adults. Am J Clin Nutr. 2012;95(2):437–445.
10. Dr I-Min Lee, Eric J Shiroma, Felipe Lobelo, et al. Effect of physical inactivity on major non-communicable diseases worldwide: an analysis of burden of disease and life expectancy. Lancet. 380, 9838, P219-229, July 21, 2012.
11. Young DR, Hivert MF, Alhassan S, Camhi SM, Ferguson JF, Katzmarzyk PT, Lewis CE, Owen N, Perry CK, Siddique J, Yong CM; Physical Activity Committee of the Council on Lifestyle and Cardiometabolic Health; Council on Clinical Cardiology; Council on Epidemiology and Prevention; Council on Functional Genomics and Translational Biology; and Stroke Council. Sedentary Behavior and Cardiovascular Morbidity and Mortality: A Science Advisory From the American Heart Association.Circulation. 2016 Sep 27;134(13):e262-79. doi: 10.1161/CIR.0000000000000440. Epub 2016 Aug 15.
12. Wijndaele K, Healy GN, Dunstan DW, et al. Increased cardio-metabolic risk is associated with increased TV viewing time. Med Sci Sports Exerc. 2010;42:1511–1518. doi: 10.1249/MSS.0b013e3181d322ac.
13. Hu FB. Sedentary lifestyle and risk of obesity and type 2 diabetes. Lipids. 2003 Feb;38(2):103-8.
14. Knowler WC, Barrett-Connor E, Fowler SC, et al. Reduction in the incidence of type 2 diabetes with lifestyle intervention or metformin. N Engl J Med. 2002;346(6):393–403.
15. Isaac Debache, Audrey Bergouignan, Basile Chaix, Emiel M Sneekes, Frédérique Thomas and Cédric Sueur. Associations of Sensor-Derived Physical Behavior with Metabolic Health: A Compositional Analysis in the Record Multisensor Study. Int. J. Environ. Res. Public Health 2019, 16(5), 741; doi:10.3390/ijerph16050741.
16. Lee PH, Wong FK. The association between time spent in sedentary behaviors and blood pressure: a systematic review and meta-analysis. Sports Med. 2015;45(6):867–880.
17. Ford ES, Caspersen CJ. Sedentary behaviour and cardiovascular disease: a review of prospective studies. International journal of epidemiology. 2012;41(5):1338-1353.
18. Stamatakis E, Hamer M, Dunstan DW. Screen-based entertainment time, all-cause mortality, and cardiovascular events: population-based study with ongoing mortality and hospital events follow-up. J Am Coll Cardiol 2011;57:292–99.

19. Dunstan DW, Thorp AA, Healy GN. Prolonged sitting: is it a distinct coronary heart disease risk factor? Curr Opin Cardiol. 2011 Sep;26(5):412-9. doi: 10.1097/HCO.0b013e3283496605.
20. Wannamethee SG, Shaper AG, Alberti KG. Physical activity, metabolic factors, and the incidence of coronary heart disease and type 2 diabetes. Arch Intern Med. 2000 Jul 24;160(14):2108-16.
21. Kim Y, Wilkens LR, Park SY, Goodman MT, Monroe KR, Kolonel LN. Association between various sedentary behaviours and all-cause, cardiovascular disease and cancer mortality: the Multiethnic Cohort Study. Int J Epidemiol. 2013;42:1040–56.
22. Warren TY, Barry V, Hooker SP, Sui X, Church TS, Blair SN. Sedentary behaviors increase risk of cardiovascular disease mortality in men. Sci Sports Exerc. 2010 May;42(5):879-85. doi: 10.1249/MSS.0b013e3181c3aa7e.
23. Matthews CE, George SM, Moore SC, et al. Amount of time spent in sedentary behaviors and cause-specific mortality in US adults. Am J Clin Nutr. 2012;95:437– 445.
24. Healy GN, Dunstan DW, Salmon J, Cerin E, Shaw JE, Zimmet PZ et al. Breaks in sedentary time: beneficial associations with metabolic risk. Diabetes Care 2008; 31: 661–666.
25. Chastin S.F., Palarea-Albaladejo J., Dontje M.L., Skelton D.A. Combined effects of time spent in physical activity, sedentary behaviors and sleep on obesity and cardio-metabolic health markers: A novel compositional data analysis approach. PLoS ONE. 2015;10:10 doi: 10.1371/journal.pone.0139984.
26. Li TY, Rana JS, Manson JE, Willett WC, Stampfer MJ, Colditz GA, et al. Obesity as compared with physical activity in predicting risk of coronary heart disease in women. Circulation 2006; 113: 499–506.
27. Wilmot E.G., Edwardson C.L., Achana F.A., Davies M.J., Gorely T., Gray L.J., Khunti K., Yates T., Biddle S.J. Sedentary time in adults and the association with diabetes, cardiovascular disease and death: Systematic review and meta-analysis. Diabetologia. 2012;55:2895–2905. doi: 10.1007/s00125-012-2677-z.
28. Restaino RM, Walsh LK, Morishima T, Vranish JR, Martinez-Lemus LA, Fadel PJ, Padilla J. Endothelial dysfunction following prolonged sitting is mediated by a reduction in shear stress. Am J Physiol Heart Circ Physiol 310: H648–H653, 2016. doi:10.1152/ajpheart.00943.2015.
29. Thosar SS, Bielko SL, Mather KJ, Johnston JD, Wallace JP. Effect of prolonged sitting and breaks in sitting time on endothelial function. Med Sci Sports Exerc 47: 843–849, 2015. doi:10.1249/MSS.0000000000000479.
30. McLenachan JM, Williams JK, Fish RD, Ganz P, Selwyn AP. Loss of flow-mediated endothelium-dependent dilation occurs early in the development of atherosclerosis. Circulation 84: 1273–1278, 1991. doi:10.1161/01.CIR.84.3.1273.
31. Widlansky ME, Gokce N, Keaney JF Jr, Vita JA. The clinical implications of endothelial dysfunction. J Am Coll Cardiol 42: 1149–1160, 2003. doi:10.1016/S0735-1097(03)00994-X.
32. McDermott MM, Liu K, Ferrucci L, et al. Greater sedentary hours and slower walking speed outside the home predict faster declines in functioning and adverse calf muscle changes in peripheral arterial disease. J Am Coll Cardiol. 2011;57(23):2356-64.
33. Morishima T, Restaino RM, Walsh LK, Kanaley JA, Fadel PJ, Padilla J. Prolonged sitting-induced leg endothelial dysfunction is prevented by fidgeting. Am J Physiol Heart Circ Physiol 311: H177–H182, 2016. doi:10.1152/ajpheart.00297.2016.
34. Morishima T, Restaino RM, Walsh LK, Kanaley JA, Padilla J. Prior exercise and standing as strategies to circumvent sitting-induced leg endothelial dysfunction. Clin Sci (Lond) 131: 1045–1053, 2017. doi:10.1042/CS20170031.
35. Novakovic M, Jug B, Lenasi H. Clinical impact of exercise in patients with peripheral arterial disease. Vascular. 2017 Aug;25(4):412-422. doi: 10.1177/1708538116678752. Epub 2016 Nov 9.
36. Morris DR, Rodriguiez AJ, Moxon JV. Association of lower extremity performance with cardiovascular and all-cause mortality in patients with peripheral artery disease: A systematic review and meta-analysis. J Am Heart Assoc. 2014;3:e001105.

37. Nicolosi A, Glasser DB, Moreira ED, Villa M. Prevalence of erectile dysfunction and associated factors among men without concomitant disease: a population study. Int J Impot Res. 2003;15:253–257.
38. Bacon CG, Mittleman MA, Kawachi I, Giovannucci E, Glasser DB, Rimm EB. Sexual function in men older than 50 years of age: results from the health Professionals' follow-up study. Ann Intern Med. 2003;139:161–168.
39. Furukawa S, Sakai T, Niiya T, et al. Self-reported sitting time and prevalence of erectile dysfunction in Japanese patients with type 2 diabetes mellitus: The Dogo Study. J Diabetes Complications. 2017 Jan;31(1):53-57. doi: 10.1016/j.jdiacomp.2016.10.011. Epub 2016 Oct 18.
40. Padberg F. The physiology and hemodynamics of the normal venous circulation. In: Gloviczki P., Yao J., editors. Handbook of Venous Disorders. 2nd ed. Arnold Publisher; New York, NY, USA: 2001. pp. 25–35.
41. Lyndsay Orr Kathleen A. Klement Laura McCrossin Deirdre O'Sullivan Drombolis Pamela E. Houghton Sandi Spaulding Shauna Burke. A Systematic Review and Meta-analysis of Exercise Intervention for the Treatment of Calf Muscle Pump Impairment in Individuals with Chronic Venous Insufficiency. Ostomy Wound Manage. 2017;63(8):30-43. doi: 10.25270/owm.2017.08.3043.
42. Pocock E.S., Alsaigh T., Mazor R., Schmid-Schonbein G.W. Cellular and molecular basis of Venous insufficiency. Vasc. Cell. 2014;6:24. doi: 10.1186/s13221-014-0024-5.
43. Mansilha A, Sousa J. Pathophysiological Mechanisms of Chronic Venous Disease and Implications for Venoactive Drug Therapy. Int J Mol Sci. 2018;19(6):1669. Published 2018 Jun 5. doi:10.3390/ijms19061669.
44. Philbrick JT, Shumate R, Siadaty MS, Becker DM. Air travel and venous thromboembolism: a systematic review. J Gen Intern Med. 2007;22(1):107-14.
45. Suadicani P, Hannerz H, Bach E, Gyntelberg F. Jobs encompassing prolonged sitting in cramped positions and risk of venous thromboembolism: cohort study. JRSM Short Rep. 2012;3(2):8.
46. Aas M, Skretting A, Engeset A, Westgaard R, Nicolaysen G. Lymphatic drainage from subcutaneous tissue in the foot and leg in the sitting human. Acta Physiol Scand. 1985 Nov;125(3):505-11.
47. Madhavan, Cole JP, Pierce CS, McLeod KJ. Reversal of lower limb venous and lymphatic pooling by passive non-invasive calf muscle pump stimulation. Conf Proc IEEE Eng Med Biol Soc. 2006;1:2875-7.
48. Centers for Disease Control and Prevention Physical activity for everyone. 2011 http://wwwcdcgov/physicalactivity/everyone/glossary/indexhtml.
49. Larson-Meyer DE. A Systematic Review of the Energy Cost and Metabolic Intensity of Yoga. Med Sci Sports Exerc. 2016 Aug;48(8):1558-69.
50. Ray Long . The Key Muscles of Yoga: Scientific Keys, Volume I Paperback – November 1, 2009. BandhaYoga; 3 edition (November 1, 2009).
51. Watts AW, Rydell SA, Eisenberg ME, Laska MN, Neumark-Sztainer D. Yoga's potential for promoting healthy eating and physical activity behaviors among young adults: a mixed-methods study. Int J Behav Nutr Phys Act. 2018;15(1):42. Published 2018 May 2. doi:10.1186/s12966-018-0674-4.
52. Ross A, Friedmann E, Bevans M, Thomas S. National Survey of Yoga Practitioners: Mental and Physical Health Benefits. Complementary therapies in medicine. 2013;21(4):313-323. doi:10.1016/j.ctim.2013.04.001.
53. Tew GA, Howsam J, Hardy M, Bissell L. Adapted yoga to improve physical function and health-related quality of life in physically-inactive older adults: a randomised controlled pilot trial. BMC Geriatr. 2017;17(1):131. Published 2017 Jun 23. doi:10.1186/s12877-017-0520-6.

Sleep

1. Irwin MR. Why sleep is important for health: a psychoneuroimmunology perspective. Annu

Rev Psychol. 2014;66:143-72.
2. Miyazaki S, Liu CY, Hayashi Y. Sleep in vertebrate and invertebrate animals, and insights into the function and evolution of sleep. Neurosci Res. 2017 May;118:3-12. doi: 10.1016/j.neures.2017.04.017. Epub 2017 May 10.
3. Watson NF, Badr MS, Belenky G, et al. Recommended amount of sleep for a healthy adult: a joint consensus statement of the American Academy of Sleep Medicine and Sleep Research Society. Sleep. 2015;38:843–4.
4. Carskadon MA, Acebo C, Jenni OG. Regulation of adolescent sleep: implications for behavior. Ann N Y Acad Sci. 2004;1021:276–91.
5. Ohayon MM, Carskadon MA, Guilleminault C, Vitiello MV. Meta-analysis of quantitative sleep parameters from childhood to old age in healthy individuals: developing normative sleep values across the human lifespan. Sleep. 2004 Nov 1;27(7):1255–1273.
6. Irwin MR. Why sleep is important for health: a psychoneuroimmunology perspective. Annu Rev Psychol. 2014;66:143-72.
7. Nedeltcheva AV, Scheer FA. Metabolic effects of sleep disruption, links to obesity and diabetes. Curr Opin Endocrinol Diabetes Obes. 2014;21(4):293-8.
8. Institute of Medicine. Sleep disorders and sleep deprivation: An unmet public health problem. Washington, D.C.: National Academies Press; 2006.
9. Consensus Conference Panel, Watson NF, Badr MS, et al. Joint Consensus Statement of the American Academy of Sleep Medicine and Sleep Research Society on the Recommended Amount of Sleep for a Healthy Adult: Methodology and Discussion. Sleep. 2015;38(8):1161–1183. Published 2015 Aug 1. doi:10.5665/sleep.4886.
10. Spiegel K, Tasali E, Penev P, Van Cauter E. Brief communication: Sleep curtailment in healthy young men is associated with decreased leptin levels, elevated ghrelin levels, and increased hunger and appetite. Ann Intern Med. 2004;141:846–50.
11. Taheri S, et al. Short sleep duration is associated with reduced leptin, elevated ghrelin, and increased body mass index. PLoS medicine. 2004;1(3):e62.
12. Patel SR, et al. Association between reduced sleep and weight gain in women. American journal of epidemiology. 2006;164(10):947–54.
13. Knutson KL, Van Cauter E. Associations between sleep loss and increased risk of obesity and diabetes. Ann NY Acad Sci. 2008;1129:287–304.
14. Spaeth AM, Dinges DF, Goel N. Effects of experimental sleep restriction on weight gain, caloric intake, and meal timing in healthy adults. Sleep. 2013;36:981–90.
15. Nedeltcheva AV, et al. Sleep curtailment is accompanied by increased intake of calories from snacks. Am J Clin Nutr. 2009;89(1):126–33.
16. Markwald RR, et al. Impact of insufficient sleep on total daily energy expenditure, food intake, and weight gain. Proc Natl Acad Sci U S A. 2013;110(14):5695–700.
17. Donga E, et al. Partial sleep restriction decreases insulin sensitivity in type 1 diabetes. Diabetes care. 2010;33(7):1573–7.
18. Broussard JL, Ehrmann DA, Van Cauter E, Tasali E, Brady MJ. Impaired insulin signaling in human adipocytes after experimental sleep restriction: a randomized, crossover study. Ann Intern Med. 2012;157:549–57.
19. Spiegel K, Leproult R, Van Cauter E. Impact of sleep debt on metabolic and endocrine function. Lancet. 1999;354(9188):1435–9.
20. Cappuccio FP, D'Elia L, Strazzullo P, Miller MA. Quantity and quality of sleep and incidence of type 2 diabetes: a systematic review and meta-analysis. Diabetes Care. 2010;33:414–20.
21. Engeda J, et al. Association between duration and quality of sleep and the risk of pre-diabetes: evidence from NHANES. Diabet Med. 2013;30(6):676–80.
22. Moldofsky H, Lue FA, Davidson JR, Gorczynski R. Effects of sleep deprivation on human immune functions. FASEB J. 1989;3:1972–77.
23. Spiegel K, Sheridan JF, Van Cauter E. Effect of sleep deprivation on response to immunization. JAMA. 2002;288:1471–2.
24. Cohen S, Doyle WJ, Alper CM, Janicki-Deverts D, Turner RB. Sleep habits and susceptibility to the common cold. Arch Intern Med. 2009;169:62–7.
25. Ibarra-Coronado EG, Pantaleón-Martínez AM, Velazquéz-Moctezuma J, et al. The Bidirectional Relationship between Sleep and Immunity against Infections. J Immunol Res. 2015;2015:678164.
26. Jiao L, Duan Z, Sangi-Haghpeykar H, Hale L, White DL, El-Serag HB. Sleep duration and incidence of colorectal cancer in postmenopausal women. Br J Cancer. 2013;108:213–21.

27. 46. Kakizaki M, Kuriyama S, Sone T, et al. Sleep duration and the risk of breast cancer: the Ohsaki Cohort Study. Br J Cancer. 2008;99:1502–5.
28. Gomez-Gonzalez B, Dominguez-Salazar E, Hurtado-Alvarado G, et al. Role of sleep in the regulation of the immune system and the pituitary hormones. Ann N Y Acad Sci. 2012;1261:97–106.
29. Johnson EO, Roth T, Breslau N (2006) The association of insomnia with anxiety disorders and depression: Exploration of the direction of risk. J Psychiatr Res 40(8): 700–708. doi: 10.1016/j.jpsychires.2006.07.008.
30. Soldatos CR. Insomnia in relation to depression and anxiety: epidemiologic considerations. J Psychiatr Res. 2006 Dec;40(8):700-8. Epub 2006 Sep 15. J Psychosom Res. 1994;38 Suppl 1:3-8.
31. Cricco M, Simonsick EM, Foley DJ. The impact of insomnia on cognitive functioning in older adults. J Am Geriatr Soc. 2001 Sep;49(9):1185–1189.
32. Paiva T, Gaspar T, Matos MG. Sleep deprivation in adolescents: correlations with health complaints and health-related quality of life. Sleep Med. 2015 Apr;16(4):521-7. doi: 10.1016/j.sleep.2014.10.010. Epub 2015 Jan 20.
33. Johnson KD, Patel SR, Baur DM, et al. Association of sleep habits with accidents and near misses in United States transportation operators. J Occup Environ Med. 2014;56(5):510-5.
34. Grandner MA, et al. Mortality associated with short sleep duration: The evidence, the possible mechanisms, and the future. Sleep Med Rev. 2010;14(3):191–203.
35. Sivertsen B, Pallesen S, Glozier N, et al. Midlife insomnia and subsequent mortality: the Hordaland health study. BMC Public Health. 2014;14:720. Published 2014 Jul 15. doi:10.1186/1471-2458-14-720.
36. Aurora RN, Kim JS, Crainiceanu C, O'Hearn D, Punjabi NM. Habitual Sleep Duration and All-Cause Mortality in a General Community Sample. Sleep. 2016;39(11):1903–1909. Published 2016 Nov 1. doi:10.5665/sleep.6212.
37. Sabanayagam C, Shankar A. Sleep duration and cardiovascular disease: results from the National Health Interview Survey. Sleep. 2010;33(8):1037–42.
38. Tobaldini E, Pecis M, Montano N. Effects of acute and chronic sleep deprivation on cardiovascular regulation. Arch Ital Biol. 2014 Jun-Sep;152(2-3):103-10. doi: 10.12871/000298292014235.
39. Tobaldini E, Costantino G, Solbiati M, Cogliati C, Kara T, Nobili L, Montano N. Sleep, sleep deprivation, autonomic nervous system and cardiovascular diseases. Neurosci Biobehav Rev. 2017 Mar;74(Pt B):321-329. doi: 10.1016/j.neubiorev.2016.07.004. Epub 2016 Jul 7.
40. Wang Q, Xi B, Liu M, Zhang Y, Fu M. Short sleep duration is associated with hypertension risk among adults: a systematic review and meta-analysis. Hypertens Res. 2012;35:1012–8.
41. Gottlieb DJ, Redline S, Nieto FJ, et al. Association of usual sleep duration with hypertension: the Sleep Heart Health Study. Sleep. 2006;29:1009–14.
42. Guo XF, Zheng LQ, Wang J, et al. Epidemiological evidence for the link between sleep duration and high blood pressure: a systematic review and meta-analysis. Sleep Med. 2013; 14(4):324–32.
43. Anne-Laure Borel, Pierre-Yves Benhamou, Jean-Philippe Baguet, Isabelle Debaty, Patrick Levy, Jean-Louis Pépin, Jean-Michel Mallion. Short Sleep Duration Is Associated With a Blood Pressure Nondipping Pattern in Type 1 Diabetes. Diabetes Care Sep 2009, 32 (9) 1713-1715; DOI: 10.2337/dc09-0422.
44. Meier-Ewert HK, Ridker PM, Rifai N, Regan MM, Price NJ, et al. Effect of sleep loss on C-reactive protein, an inflammatory marker of cardiovascular risk. J Am Coll Cardiol. 2004;43:678–83.
45. Chennaoui M, et al. Effect of one night of sleep loss on changes in tumor necrosis factor alpha (TNF-alpha) levels in healthy men. Cytokine. 2011;56(2):318–24.
46. Spiegel K, Leproult R, Van Cauter E. Impact of sleep debt on metabolic and endocrine function. Lancet. 1999;354:1435–9.
47. Zhong X, Hilton HJ, Gates GJ, et al. Increased sympathetic and decreased parasympathetic cardiovascular modulation in normal humans with acute sleep deprivation. J Appl Physiol. 2005;98:2024–32.
48. Morgan E, Schumm LP, McClintock M, Waite L, Lauderdale DS. Sleep Characteristics and Daytime Cortisol Levels in Older Adults. Sleep. 2017;40(5):zsx043.
49. Libby P, Ridket PM, Maseri A. Inflammation and atherosclerosis. Circulation. 2002;105:1135–43.

50. Knutson KL, Spiegel K, Penev P, Van Cauter E: The metabolic consequences of sleep deprivation. Sleep medicine reviews, 2007; 11: 163-178.
51. Fernando Domínguez, et al. Association of Sleep Duration and Quality With Subclinical Atherosclerosis. Journal of the American College of Cardiology Jan 2019, 73 (2)134-144; DOI: 10.1016/j.jacc.2018.10.060.
52. Kowall B, Lehmann N, Mahabadi AA et al. Sleep characteristics and progression of coronary artery calcification: Results from the Heinz Nixdorf Recall cohort study. Atherosclerosis. 2018 Apr;271:45-52. doi: 10.1016/j.atherosclerosis.2018.02.013. Epub 2018 Feb 9.
53. Sands-Lincoln M, Loucks EB, Lu B, et al. Sleep duration, insomnia, and coronary heart disease among postmenopausal women in the Women's Health Initiative. J Womens Health. 2013; 22(6): 477–86.
54. Meisinger C , Heier M , Löwel H , Schneider A , Döring A. Sleep duration and sleep complaints and risk of myocardial infarction in middle-aged men and women from the general population: the MONICA/KORA Augsburg cohort study . Sleep. 2007;30:1121–7.
55. Amagai Y, Ishikawa S, Gotoh T, Kayaba K, Nakamura Y, Kajii E. Sleep duration and incidence of cardiovascular events in a Japanese population: the Jichi Medical School cohort study. J Epidemiol. 2010;20:106–10.
56. King CR, Knutson KL, Rathouz PJ, et al. Short sleep duration and incident coronary artery calcification. JAMA 2008;300(24):2859-2866.
57. Xiao Q, Keadle SK, Hollenbeck AR, Matthews CE. Sleep duration and total and cause-specific mortality in a large US cohort: interrelationships with physical activity, sedentary behavior, and body mass index. Am J Epidemiol. 2014;180(10):997-1006.
58. Ge BH, Guo XM. Short and long sleep durations are both associated with increased risk of stroke: a meta-analysis of observational studies. Int J Stroke. 2015; 10(2):177–84.
59. Chen JC, Brunner RL, Ren H, et al. Sleep duration and risk of ischemic stroke in postmenopausal women. Stroke. 2008; 39(12):3185–92.
60. Axelsson J, et al. Tolerance to shift work-how does it relate to sleep and wakefulness? International archives of occupational and environmental health. 2004;77(2):121–9.
61. Suwazono Y, et al. A longitudinal study on the effect of shift work on weight gain in male Japanese workers. Obesity. 2008;16(8):1887–93.
62. Morikawa Y, et al. Shift work and the risk of diabetes mellitus among Japanese male factory workers. Scandinavian journal of work, environment & health. 2005;31(3):179–83.
63. Tenkanen L, et al. Shift work, occupation and coronary heart disease over 6 years of follow-up in the Helsinki Heart Study. Scandinavian journal of work, environment & health. 1997;23(4):257–65.
64. Husnu T, Ersoz A, Bulent E et al. Obstructive sleep apnea syndrome and erectile dysfunction: does long term continuous positive airway pressure therapy improve erections? Afr Health Sci 2015; 15: 171–9.
65. McDermott MM, Guralnik JM, Ferrucci L, et al. Community walking speed, sedentary or lying down time, and mortality in peripheral artery disease. Vasc Med. 2016;21(2):120-9.
66. Szymański F, Puchalski B, Filipiak K. Obstructive sleep apnea, atrial fibrillation and erectile dysfunction: are they only coexisting conditions or a new clinical syndrome? The concept of the OSAFED syndrome. Pol Arch Med Wewn 2013; 123: 701–7.
67. Kohler T, Kim J, Feia K et al. Prevalence of androgen deficiency in men with erectile dysfunction. Urology 2008; 71: 693–7.
68. Lippi G, Mattiuzzi C, Franchini M. Sleep apnea and venous thromboembolism. A systematic review. Thromb Haemost. 2015 Nov;114(5):958-63. doi: 10.1160/TH15-03-0188. Epub 2015 May 21.
69. Sahajpal P, Ralte R. Impact of induced yogic relaxation training (IYRT) on stress-level, self-concept and quality of sleep among minority group individuals. J Indian Psychol 2000; 18: 66–73.
70. Ross A, Friedmann E, Bevans M, Thomas S. National survey of yoga practitioners: mental and physical health benefits. Complement Ther Med. 2013;21(4):313-23.
71. Khalsa SB. Treatment of chronic insomnia with yoga: a preliminary study with sleep-wake diaries. Appl Psychophysiol Biofeedback. 2004 Dec;29(4):269-78.
72. Fang R, Li X. A regular yoga intervention for staff nurse sleep quality and work stress: a randomised controlled trial. J Clin Nurs. 2015 Dec;24(23-24):3374-9. doi: 10.1111/jocn.12983. Epub 2015 Oct 19.
73. Rshikesan PB, Subramanya P, Nidhi R. Yoga practice to improve sleep quality and body

composition parameters of obese male - a randomized controlled trial. J Complement Integr Med. 2018 Oct 20;15(4). pii: /j/jcim.2018.15.issue-4/jcim-2016-0077/jcim-2016-0077.xml. doi: 10.1515/jcim-2016-0077.
74. Halpern J, Cohen M, Kennedy G, Reece J, Cahan C, Baharav A. Yoga for improving sleep quality and quality of life for older adults. Altern Ther Health Med. 2014 May-Jun;20(3):37-46.
75. Afonso RF, Hachul H, Kozasa EH, et al. Yoga decreases insomnia in postmenopausal women: a randomized clinical trial. Menopause. 2012;19(2):186–193.
76. Mansikkamaki K, Raitanen J, Nygard CH, et al. Sleep quality and aerobic training among menopausal women--a randomized controlled trial. Maturitas. 2012;72(4):339–345.
77. Ward L, Stebbings S, Athens J, Cherkin D, David Baxter G. Yoga for the management of pain and sleep in rheumatoid arthritis: a pilot randomized controlled trial. Musculoskeletal Care. 2018 Mar;16(1):39-47. doi: 10.1002/msc.1201. Epub 2017 Jun 16.
78. Ebrahimi M, Guilan-Nejad TN, Pordanjani AF. Effect of yoga and aerobics exercise on sleep quality in women with Type 2 diabetes: a randomized controlled trial. Sleep Sci. 2017;10(2):68-72.
79. McCall M. Yoga intervention may improve health-related quality of life (HRQL), fatigue, depression, anxiety and sleep in patients with breast cancer. Evid Based Nurs. 2018 Jan;21(1):9. doi: 10.1136/eb-2017-102673. Epub 2017 Nov 25.

Smoking/Tobacco Use

1. Phillips E, Wang TW, Husten CG, et al. Tobacco Product Use Among Adults — United States, 2015. MMWR Morb Mortal Wkly Rep 2017;66:1209–1215. DOI: http://dx.doi.org/10.15585/mmwr.mm6644a2.
2. Health U. D. O., Services H. Office on Smoking and Health. Vol. 3. Atlanta, GA: National Center for Chronic Disease Prevention and Health Promotion; 2012. Preventing tobacco use among youth and young adults: A report of the Surgeon General.
3. https://www.cdc.gov/tobacco/data_statistics/fact_sheets/secondhand_smoke/health_effects/index.htm.
4. Sleiman M, Gundel LA, Pankow JF, Jacob P, III, Singer BC, Destaillats H. Formation of carcinogens indoors by surface-mediated reactions of nicotine with nitrous acid, leading to potential thirdhand smoke hazards. Proc Natl Acad Sci USA. 2010b;107:6576–6581.
5. Matt G. E., Quintana P. J. E., Destaillats H., et al. Thirdhand tobacco smoke: Emerging evidence and arguments for a multidisciplinary research agenda. Environmental Health Perspectives. 2011;119(9):1218–1226. doi: 10.1289/ehp.1103500.
6. General S. The health consequences of smoking—50 years of progress: a report of the surgeon general - https://www.surgeongeneral.gov/library/reports/50-years-of-progress/index.html.
7. Liu Y, Pleasants RA, Croft JB, et al. Smoking duration, respiratory symptoms, and COPD in adults aged ≥45 years with a smoking history. Int J Chron Obstruct Pulmon Dis. 2015;10:1409–1416. Published 2015 Jul 21. doi:10.2147/COPD.S82259.
8. Lee PN, Forey BA, Coombs KJ. Systematic review with meta-analysis of the epidemiological evidence in the 1900s relating smoking to lung cancer. BMC Cancer 2012;12:385 10.1186/1471-2407-12-385.
9. Alberg AJ, Shopland DR, Cummings KM. The 2014 Surgeon General's report: commemorating the 50th Anniversary of the 1964 Report of the Advisory Committee to the US Surgeon General and updating the evidence on the health consequences of cigarette smoking. Am J Epidemiol. 2014;179(4):403–412.
10. White WB, Cain LR, Benjamin EJ, et al. High-Intensity Cigarette Smoking Is Associated With Incident Diabetes Mellitus In Black Adults: The Jackson Heart Study. J Am Heart Assoc. 2018;7(2):e007413. Published 2018 Jan 12. doi:10.1161/JAHA.117.007413.
11. U.S. Department of Health and Human Services . Oral Health in America: A Report of Surgeon General. Rockville, MD: U.S. Department of Health and Human Services, National Institute of Dental and Craniofacial Research, National Institutes of Health; 2000.

12. Sugiyama D, Nishimura K, Tamaki K, et al. Impact of smoking as a risk factor for developing rheumatoid arthritis: a meta-analysis of observational studies. Ann Rheum Dis. 2010;69(1):70–81.
13. Ye J, He J, Wang C, Wu H, Shi X, Zhang H, et al. Smoking and risk of age-related cataract: a meta-analysis. Investigative ophthalmology & visual science. 2012;53(7):3885–95. 10.1167/iovs.12-9820.
14. Harlev A, Agarwal A, Gunes SO, Shetty A, du Plessis SS. Smoking and Male Infertility: An Evidence-Based Review. World J Mens Health. 2015;33(3):143–160. doi:10.5534/wjmh.2015.33.3.143.
15. Waylen AL, Metwally M, Jones GL, Wilkinson AJ, Ledger WL. Effects of cigarette smoking upon clinical outcomes of assisted reproduction: A meta-analysis. Hum Reprod Update. 2009;15:31–44.
16. Department of Health and Human Services (US). Atlanta: HHS, Centers for Disease Control and Prevention, National Center for Chronic Disease Prevention and Health Promotion, Office on Smoking and Health (US); 2004. The health consequences of smoking: a report of the Surgeon General.
17. Department of Health and Human Services (US). Atlanta: HHS, Centers for Disease Control and Prevention, National Center for Chronic Disease Prevention and Health Promotion, Office on Smoking and Health (US); 2010. A report of the Surgeon General: how tobacco smoke causes disease: the biology and behavioral basis for smoking-attributable disease, 2010.
18. Dietz PM, England LJ, Shapiro-Mendoza CK, Tong VT, Farr SL, Callaghan WM. Infant morbidity and mortality attributable to prenatal smoking in the U.S. Am J Prev Med. 2010;39:45–52.
19. Gellert C, Schöttker B, Brenner H. Smoking and all-cause mortality in older people: systematic review and meta-analysis. Arch Intern Med. 2012;172(11):837–844. doi: 10.1001/archinternmed.2012.1397.
20. Taghizadeh N, Vonk JM, Boezen HM. Lifetime Smoking History and Cause-Specific Mortality in a Cohort Study with 43 Years of Follow-Up. PLoS One. 2016;11(4):e0153310. Published 2016 Apr 7. doi:10.1371/journal.pone.0153310.
21. Pan A, Wang Y, Talaei M, Hu FB. Relation of Smoking with Total Mortality and Cardiovascular Events Among Patients with Diabetes: A Meta-Analysis and Systematic Review. Circulation. 2015;132(19):1795-1804.
22. GBD 2013 Risk Factors Collaborators. Global, regional, and national comparative risk assessment of 79 behavioural, environmental and occupational, and metabolic risks or clusters of risks in 188 countries, 1990–2013: a systematic analysis for the Global Burden of Disease Study 2013. Lancet. 2015;386:2287–2323.
23. Ambrose JA, Barua RS. The pathophysiology of cigarette smoking and cardiovascular disease: an update. J Am Coll Cardiol 43: 1731–1737, 2004.
24. White WB. Smoking-related morbidity and mortality in the cardiovascular setting. Prev Cardiol 10, Suppl 2: 1–4, 2007.
25. Erhardt L. Cigarette smoking: an undertreated risk factor for cardiovascular disease. Atherosclerosis. 2009;205:23–32. doi: 10.1016/j.atherosclerosis.2009.01.007.
26. Howard G, Wagenknecht LE, Burke GL, Diez-Roux A, Evans GW, McGovern P, Nieto FJ, Tell GS. Cigarette smoking and progression of atherosclerosis: the Atherosclerosis Risk in Communities (ARIC) study. JAMA 279: 119–124, 1998.
27. Kianoush S, Yakoob MY, Al-Rifai M, et al. Associations of Cigarette Smoking With Subclinical Inflammation and Atherosclerosis: ELSA-Brasil (The Brazilian Longitudinal Study of Adult Health). J Am Heart Assoc. 2017;6(6):e005088. Published 2017 Jun 24. doi:10.1161/JAHA.116.005088.
28. Khalili P, Nilsson PM, Nilsson JA, Berglund G. Smoking as a modifier of the systolic blood pressure-induced risk of cardiovascular events and mortality: a population-based prospective study of middle-aged men. J Hypertens 20: 1759–1764, 2002.

29. Bowman T.S., Gaziano J.M., Buring J.E., Sesso H.D. A prospective study of cigarette smoking and risk of incident hypertension in women. J. Amer. Coll. Cardiol. 2007;50:2085–2092. doi: 10.1016/j.jacc.2007.08.017.
30. Halperin R.O., Gaziano J.M., Sesso H.D. Smoking and the risk of incident hypertension in middle-aged and older men. Amer. J. Hypertens. 2008;21:148–152. doi: 10.1038/ajh.2007.36.
31. Dochi M., Sakata K., Oishi M., Tanaka K., Kobayashi E., Suwazono Y. Smoking as an independent risk factor for hypertension: A 14-year longitudinal study in male Japanese workers. Tohoku J. Exp. Med. 2009;217:37–43. doi: 10.1620/tjem.217.37.
32. Linneberg A, Jacobsen RK, Skaaby T, et al. Effect of Smoking on Blood Pressure and Resting Heart Rate: A Mendelian Randomization Meta-Analysis in the CARTA Consortium. Circ Cardiovasc Genet. 2015;8(6):832–841. doi:10.1161/CIRCGENETICS.115.001225.
33. Bjartveit K, Tverdal A. Health consequences of smoking 1-4 cigarettes per day. Tob Control 2005;14:315-20. 10.1136/tc.2005.011932; A Report of the Surgeon General . How tobacco smoke causes disease: the biology and behavioral basis for smoking-attributable disease. 2010.
34. US Department of Health and Human Services. How Tobacco Smoke Causes Disease: The Biology and Behavioral Basis for Smoking-Attributable Disease: A Report of the Surgeon General. Atlanta, GA: US Department of Health and Human Services, Centers for Disease Control and Prevention, National Center for Chronic Disease Prevention and Health Promotion, Office on Smoking and Health; 2010.
35. Tungsubutra W, Tresukosol D, Buddhari W, Boonsom W, Sanguanwang S, Srichaiveth B. Acute coronary syndrome in young adults: The Thai ACS registry. JMed Assoc Thailand. 2007;90(1):81–90.
36. Teo KK, Ounpuu S, Hawken Set al. INTERHEART Study Investigators Tobacco use and risk of myocardial infarction in 52 countries in the INTERHEART study: a case-control study. Lancet 368: 647–658, 2006.
37. Canto JG, Kiefe CI, Rogers WJ, Peterson ED, Frederick PD, French WJ, Gibson CM, Pollack CV, Jr, Ornato JP, Zalenski RJ, Penney J, Tiefenbrunn AJ, Greenland P, NRMI Investigators Number of coronary heart disease risk factors and mortality in patients with first myocardial infarction. JAMA. 2011;306:2120–2127. doi: 10.1001/jama.2011.1654.
38. Tonstad S, Andrew Johnston J. Cardiovascular risks associated with smoking: a review for clinicians. Eur J Cardiovasc Prev Rehabil. 2006;13:507–514. doi: 10.1097/01.hjr.0000214609.06738.62.
39. Inoue-Choi M, Liao LM, Reyes-Guzman C, Hartge P, Caporaso N, Freedman ND. Association of Long-term, Low-Intensity Smoking With All-Cause and Cause-Specific Mortality in the National Institutes of Health-AARP Diet and Health Study. JAMA Intern Med 2017;177:87-95. 10.1001/jamainternmed.2016.7511.
40. Huxley RR, Woodward M. Cigarette smoking as a risk factor for coronary heart disease in women compared with men: a systematic review and meta-analysis of prospective cohort studies. Lancet. 2011;378:1297–1305. doi: 10.1016/S0140-6736(11)60781-2.
41. Inoue-Choi M, Liao LM, Reyes-Guzman C, Hartge P, Caporaso N, Freedman ND. Association of Long-term, Low-Intensity Smoking With All-Cause and Cause-Specific Mortality in the National Institutes of Health-AARP Diet and Health Study. JAMA Intern Med 2017;177:87-95. 10.1001/jamainternmed.2016.7511.
42. https://www.cdc.gov/tobacco/data_statistics/fact_sheets/health_effects/tobacco_related_mortality/index.htm.
43. Nakamura K, Barzi F, Lam TH, Huxley R, Feigin VL, Ueshima H, Woo J, Gu D, Ohkubo T, Lawes CM, Suh I, Woodward M Asia Pacific Cohort Studies Collaboration. Cigarette smoking, systolic blood pressure, and cardiovascular diseases in the Asia-Pacific region. Stroke. 2008;39:1694–1702. doi: 10.1161/STROKEAHA.107.496752.
44. Ischaemic stroke and combined oral contraceptives: results of an international, multicentre, case-control study. WHO Collaborative Study of Cardiovascular Disease and Steroid Hormone Contraception. Lancet. 1996;348:498–505.

45. Haemorrhagic stroke, overall stroke risk, and combined oral contraceptives: results of an international, multicentre, case-control study. WHO Collaborative Study of Cardiovascular Disease and Steroid Hormone Contraception. Lancet. 1996;348:505–510.
46. Ezzati M, Henley SJ, Thun MJ, Lopez AD. Role of smoking in global and regional cardiovascular mortality. Circulation 112: 489–497, 2005.
47. Meschia JF et al. American Heart Association Stroke Council; Council on Cardiovascular and Stroke Nursing; Council on Clinical Cardiology; Council on Functional Genomics and Translational Biology; Council on Hypertension. Guidelines for the primary prevention of stroke: a statement for healthcare professionals from the American Heart Association/American Stroke Association. Stroke. 2014;45:3754–3832.
48. Shah RS, Cole JW. Smoking and stroke: the more you smoke the more you stroke. Expert Rev Cardiovasc Ther. 2010;8:917–932. doi: 10.1586/erc.10.56.
49. Lofroth G. Environmental tobacco smoke: overview of chemical composition and Genotoxic components. Mutat Res 1989;222:73–80.
50. U.S. Department of Health and Human Services. The Health Consequences of Involuntary Exposure to Tobacco Smoke: A Report of the Surgeon General. U.S. Department of Health and Human Services, Centers for Disease Control and Prevention, National Center for Chronic Disease Prevention and Health Promotion, Office on Smoking and Health, 2006.
51. Oberg M., Jaakkola M. S., Woodward A., Peruga A., Prüss-Ustün A. 2011 Worldwide burden of disease from exposure to second-hand smoke: A retrospective analysis of data from 192 countries. Lancet, 377, 139–146.
52. Prof Bo Xi, Yajun Liang, Prof Yunxia Liu, Yinkun Yan, Min Zhao, Chuanwei Ma, MS et al. Tobacco use and second-hand smoke exposure in young adolescents aged 12–15 years: data from 68 low-income and middle-income countries. Lancet. 4, 11, PE795-E805, Nov 01, 2016.
53. U.S. Department of Health and Human Services. The Health Consequences of Smoking—50 Years of Progress: A Report of the Surgeon General. Atlanta: U.S. Department of Health and Human Services, Centers for Disease Control and Prevention, National Center for Chronic Disease Prevention and Health Promotion, Office on Smoking and Health, 2014.
54. Law MR, Morris JK, Wald NJ. Environmental tobacco smoke exposure and ischaemic heart disease: An evaluation of the evidence. BMJ. 1997;315:973–80.
55. He J, Vupputuri S, Allen K, Prerost MR, Hughes J, Whelton PK. Passive smoking and the risk of coronary heart disease – a meta-analysis of epidemiologic studies. N Engl J Med. 1999;340:920–6.
56. Angela M. Malek, Angela M. Malek, Mary Cushman, Daniel T. Lackland, George Howard, Leslie A. McClure, Secondhand Smoke Exposure and Stroke. AJPM. December 2015Volume 49, Issue 6, Pages e89–e97.
57. U.S. Department of Health and Human Services. The Health Consequences of Smoking—50 Years of Progress: A Report of the Surgeon General. Atlanta: U.S. Department of Health and Human Services, Centers for Disease Control and Prevention, National Center for Chronic Disease Prevention and Health Promotion, Office on Smoking and Health, 2014.
58. Lv X, Sun J, Bi Y, Xu M, Lu J, Zhao L, Xu Y. Risk of all-cause mortality and cardiovascular disease associated with secondhand smoke exposure: a systematic review and meta-analysis. Int J Cardiol. 2015;199:106–115. doi: 10.1016/j.ijcard.2015.07.011.
59. Acuff, L.; Fristoe, K.; Hamblen, J.; Smith, M.; Chen, J. Third-Hand Smoke: Old Smoke, New Concerns. J. Community Health 2016, 41, 680–687.
60. Matt, G.E.; Quintana, P.J.; Destaillats, H.; Gundel, L.A.; Sleiman, M.; Singer, B.C.; Jacob, P., III; Benowitz, N.; Winickoff, J.P.; Rehan, V.; et al. Thirdhand tobacco smoke: Emerging evidence and arguments for a multidisciplinary research agenda. Environ. Health Perspect. 2011, 119, 1218–1226.
61. Martins-Green, M.; Adhami, N.; Frankos, M.; Valdez, M.; Goodwin, B.; Lyubovitsky, J.; Dhall, S.; Garcia, M.; Egiebor, I.; Martinez, B. Cigarette smoke toxins deposited on surfaces: Implications for human health. PLoS ONE 2014, 9, e86391.
62. Moon SY, Kim TW, Kim YJ, Kim Y, Kim SY, Kang D. Public Facility Utility and Third-Hand Smoking Exposure without First and Second-Hand Smoking According to Urinary Cotinine

Level. Int J Environ Res Public Health. 2019 Mar 8;16(5). pii: E855. doi: 10.3390/ijerph16050855.
63. Jacob, P., 3rd; Benowitz, N.L.; Destaillats, H.; Gundel, L.; Hang, B.; Martins-Green, M.; Matt, G.E.; Quintana, P.J.; Samet, J.M.; Schick, S.F.; et al. Thirdhand Smoke: New Evidence, Challenges, and Future Directions. Chem. Res. Toxicol. 2017, 30, 270–294.
64. Chang CM, Corey CG, Rostron BL, Apelberg BJ. Systematic review of cigar smoking and all cause and smoking related mortality. BMC Public Health. 2015;15:390. doi: 10.1186/s12889-015-1617-5.
65. Thun MJ, Carter BD, Feskanich D, Freedman ND, Prentice R, Lopez AD, Hartge P, Gapstur SM. 50-Year trends in smoking-related mortality in the United States. N Engl J Med. 2013;368:351–364. doi: 10.1056/NEJMsa1211127.
66. Mackay D. F., Irfan M. O., Haw S., Pell J. P. (2010). Meta-analysis of the effect of comprehensive smoke-free legislation on acute coronary events. Heart, 96, 1525–1530.
67. Ockene IS, Miller NH. Cigarette smoking, cardiovascular disease, and stroke: a statement for healthcare professionals from the American Heart Association. American Heart Association Task Force on Risk Reduction. Circulation 96: 3243–3247, 1997.
68. Salonen JT. Stopping smoking and long-term mortality after acute myocardial infarction. Br Heart J. 1980;43:463-469.
69. Jha P, Ramasundarahettige C, Landsman V, Rostron B, Thun M, Anderson RN, McAfee T, Peto R. 21st-century hazards of smoking and benefits of cessation in the United States. N Engl J Med. 2013;368:341–350. doi: 10.1056/NEJMsa1211128.
70. Wennmalm A, Benthin G, Granstrom EF, Persson L, Petersson AS, Winell S. Relation between tobacco use and urinary excretion of thromboxane A2 and prostacyclin metabolites in young men. Circulation. 1991;83:1698–1704.
71. Benowitz NL. Cigarette smoking and cardiovascular disease: Pathophysiology and implications for treatment. Prog Cardiovasc Dis. 2003;46:91–111.
72. Winniford MD, Wheelan KR, Kremers MS, Ugolini V, van den Berg E, Niggemann EH, Jansen DE, Hillis LD. Smoking-induced coronary vasoconstriction in patients with atherosclerotic coronary artery disease: evidence for adrenergically mediated alterations in coronary artery tone. Circulation. 1986;73:662–667.
73. Krupski WC, Olive GC, Weber CA, Rapp JH. Comparative effects of hypertension and nicotine on injury-induced myointimal thickening. Surgery. 1987;102:409–415.
74. Folts JD, Bonebrake FC. The effects of cigarette smoke and nicotine on platelet thrombus formation in stenosed dog coronary arteries: inhibition with phentolamine. Circulation. 1982;65:465–469.
75. Aicher A, Heeschen C, Mohaupt M, Cooke JP, Zeiher AM, Dimmeler S. Nicotine strongly activates dendritic cell-mediated adaptive immunity: Potential role for progression of atherosclerotic lesions. Circulation. 2003;107:604–611.
76. Hellerstein MK, Benowitz NL, Neese RA, Schwartz JM, Hoh R, Jacob P, Hsieh J, Faix D. Effects of cigarette smoking and its cessation on lipid metabolism and energy expenditure in heavy smokers. J Clin Invest. 1994;93:265–272.
77. Roya S. Moheimani, May Bhetraratana, Fen Yin, Kacey M. Peters, Jeffrey Gornbein, Jesus A. Araujo, Holly R. Middlekauff. Increased Cardiac Sympathetic Activity and Oxidative Stress in Habitual Electronic Cigarette Users" Implications for Cardiovascular Risk. JAMA Cardiol. Published online February 1, 2017.
78. Nardos Temesgen, Ivan Pena, Tahir Tayeb, Talal Alzahrani. A cross sectional study reveals an association between electronic cigarette use and myocardial infarction. Poster, GW Annual Research Days 2017.
79. Maziak W, Ben Taleb Z, Bahelah R, et al. The global epidemiology of waterpipe smoking. Tob Control 2015;24:i3–12.
80. Akl EA, Gunukula SK, Aleem S, et al. The prevalence of waterpipe tobacco smoking among the general and specific populations: a systematic review. BMC Public Health 2011;11:244.
81. El-Zaatari ZM, Chami HA, Zaatari GS. Health effects associated with waterpipe smoking. Tob Control. 2015;24 Suppl 1(Suppl 1):i31-i43.

82. Waziry R, Jawad M, Ballout R and Akl E. The effects of waterpipe tobacco smoking on health outcomes: an updated systematic review and meta-analysis. International Journal of Epidemiology. 2017.
83. Kim KH, Kabir E and Jahan SA. Waterpipe tobacco smoking and its human health impacts. J Hazard Mater. 2016;317:229-236.
84. Maziak W. The waterpipe: an emerging global risk for cancer. Cancer Epidemiol. 2013;37:1-4.
85. Al-Numair K, Barber-Heidal K, Al-Assaf A and El-Desoky G. Water-pipe (shisha) smoking influences total antioxidant capacity and oxidative stress of healthy Saudi males. J Food Agri Environ 2007;5:17–22.
86. Selim GM, Elia RZ, El Bohey AS and El Meniawy KA. Effect of shisha vs. cigarette smoking on endothelial function by brachial artery duplex ultrasonography: an observational study. Anadolu Kardiyol Derg. 2013;13:759-65.
87. Azar RR, Frangieh AH, Mroué J, Bassila L, Kasty M, Hage G, Kadri Z. Acute effects of waterpipe smoking on blood pressure and heart rate: a real-life trial. Inhal Toxicol. 2016;28:339–342. doi: 10.3109/08958378.2016.1171934.
88. Yatsuya H, Folsom AR ARIC Investigators. Risk of incident cardiovascular disease among users of smokeless tobacco in the Atherosclerosis Risk in Communities (ARIC) study. Am J Epidemiol. 2010;172:600–605. doi: 10.1093/aje/kwq191.
89. Al Suwaidi J, Zubaid M, El-Menyar AA, Singh R, Asaad N, Sulaiman K, Al Mahmeed W, Al-Shereiqi S, Akbar M and Al Binali HA. Prevalence and outcome of cigarette and waterpipe smoking among patients with acute coronary syndrome in six Middle-Eastern countries. Eur J Prev Cardiol. 2012;19:118-25.
90. Islami F, Pourshams A, Vedanthan R, Poustchi H, Kamangar F, Golozar A, Etemadi A, Khademi H, Freedman ND, Merat S, Garg V, Fuster V, Wakefield J, Dawsey SM, Pharoah P, Brennan P, Abnet CC, Malekzadeh R and Boffetta P. Smoking water-pipe, chewing nass and prevalence of heart disease: a cross-sectional analysis of baseline data from the Golestan Cohort Study, Iran. Heart. 2013;99:272-8.
91. Sibai AM, Tohme RA, Almedawar MM, Itani T, Yassine SI, Nohra EA and Isma'eel HA. Lifetime cumulative exposure to waterpipe smoking is associated with coronary artery disease. Atherosclerosis. 2014;234:454-60.
92. Wu F, Chen Y, Parvez F, Segers S, Argos M, Islam T, Ahmed A, Rakibuz-Zaman M, Hasan R, Sarwar G and Ahsan H. A prospective study of tobacco smoking and mortality in Bangladesh. PLoS One. 2013;8:e58516.
93. Christen AG, Swanson BZ, Glover ED, Henderson AH. Smokeless tobacco: the folklore and social history of snuffing, sneezing, dipping and chewing. J Am Dent Assoc. 1982;105:821–829.
94. World Health Organization. Tobacco: Deadly in Any Form or Disguise. Geneva, Switzerland: World Health Organization; 2006. Accessed February 4, 2010.
95. World Health Organization. WHO Report on the Global Tobacco Epidemic, 2008. The MPOWER Package. Geneva, Switzerland: World Health Organization; 2008.
96. Substance Abuse and Mental Health Services Administration (SAMHSA). Results from the 2008 National Survey on Drug Use and Health: National Findings. Rockville, MD: SAMHSA, Office of Applied Studies; 2009. NSDUH Series H-36, HHS Publication No. SMA 09-4434.
97. Nelson DE, Mowery P, Tomar S, Marcus S, Giovino G, Zhao L. Trends in smokeless tobacco use among adults and adolescents in the United States. Am J Public Health. 2006;96:897–905.
98. Centers for Disease Control and Prevention. Smokeless tobacco facts: smokeless tobacco use in the United States. Available at: http://www.cdc.gov/tobacco/data_statistics/fact_sheets/smokeless/smokeless_facts/index.htm#use. Accessed August 30, 2010.
99. Norberg M, Stenlund H, Lindahl B, Boman K, Weinehall L. Contribution of Swedish moist snuff to the metabolic syndrome: a wolf in sheep's clothing? Scand J Public Health. 2006;34:576–583.

100. Persson PG, Carlsson S, Svanstrom L, Ostenson CG, Ependic S, Grill V. Cigarette smoking, orka mosit snuff use and glucose intolerance. J Intern Med. 2000;248:103–110.
101. Murray CJ, Abraham J, Ali MK, et al. The state of US Health, 1990–2010: burden of diseases, injuries, and risk factors. JAMA. 2013;310:591–608. doi: 10.1001/jama.2013.13805.
102. Hatsukami DK, Severson HH. Oral spit tobacco: addiction, prevention and treatment. Nicotine Tob Res.1999;1:21–44.
103. Mariann R. Piano et al. Impact of Smokeless Tobacco Products on Cardiovascular Disease: Implications for Policy, Prevention, and Treatment. A Policy Statement From the American Heart Association. Circulation, October 12, 2010, Vol 122, Issue 15.
104. Lee PN. Circulatory disease and smokeless tobacco in western populations: a review of the evidence. Int J Epidemiol. 2007;36:789–804.
105. Benowitz NL, Porchet H, Sheiner L, Jacob P. Nicotine absorption and cardiovascular effects with smokeless tobacco use: comparison with cigarettes and nicotine gum. Clin Pharmacol Ther. 1988;44:23–28.
106. Wennmalm A, Benthin G, Granstrom EF, Persson L, Petersson AS, Winell S. Relation between tobacco use and urinary excretion of thromboxane A2 and prostacyclin metabolites in young men. Circulation. 1991;83:1698–1704.
107. Lee PN. Circulatory disease and smokeless tobacco in western populations: a review of the evidence. Int J Epidemiol. 2007;36:789–804.
108. Boffetta P, Straif K. Use of smokeless tobacco and risk of myocardial infarction and stroke: systematic review with meta-analysis. BMJ. 2009;339:b3060.
109. Fowkes FG, Housley E, Riemersma RA, Macintyre CC, Cawood EH, Prescott RJ, Ruckley CV. Smoking, lipids, glucose intolerance and blood pressure as risk factors for peripheral atherosclerosis compared with ischemic heart disease in the Edinburgh Artery Study. Am J Epidemiol. 1992;135(4):331–340.
110. Patru S, Marcu IR, Matei D, Bighea AC. The Influence of Physical Exercise on Smoking Patients with Peripheral Arterial Disease. Curr Health Sci J. 2018;44(1):34–38.
111. Hirsch, A.T., Treat-Jacobsen, D., Lando, H.A., and Hatsukami, D.K. The role of tobacco cessation, antiplatelet and lipid-lowering therapies in the treatment of peripheral arterial disease. Vasc Med. 1997; 2: 243–251.
112. Newman, A.B., Siscovick, D.S., Manolio, T.A., Polak, J., Fried, L.P., Borhani, N.O. et al. Ankle-arm index as a marker of atherosclerosis in the Cardiovascular Health Study. Circulation. 1993; 88: 837–845.
113. Ricci, M.A., Fleishman, C., and Gerstein, N. The effects of cigarette smoking and smoking cessation aids on transcutaneous oxygen levels. J Vasc Med Biol. 1993; 4: 256–259.
114. Yataco, A.R. and Gardner, A.W. Acute reduction in ankle/brachial index following smoking in chronic smokers with peripheral arterial occlusive disease. Angiology. 1999; 50: 355–360.
115. Gardner, A.W. The effect of cigarette smoking on exercise capacity in patients with intermittent claudication. Vasc Med. 1996; 1: 181–186.
116. Gardner, A.W., Sieminski, D.J., and Killewich, L.A. The effect of cigarette smoking on free-living daily physical activity in older claudication patients. Angiology. 1997; 48: 947–955doi:10.12865/CHSJ.44.01.06.
117. Clark D, Cain LR, Blaha MJ, et al. Cigarette Smoking and Subclinical Peripheral Arterial Disease in Blacks of the Jackson Heart Study. J Am Heart Assoc. 2019;8(3):e010674. doi:10.1161/JAHA.118.010674.
118. Boc V, Božic Mijovski M, Pohar Perme M, Blinc A. Diabetes and smoking are more important for prognosis of patients with peripheral arterial disease than some genetic polymorphisms. Vasa. 2018 Dec 11:1-7. doi: 10.1024/0301-1526/a000766.
119. Ghalayini IFA-GM, Al-Azab R, Bani-Hani I, Matani YS, Barham AE, Harfeil MN, Haddad Y. Erectile dysfunction in a Mediterranean country: results of an epidemiological survey of a representative sample of men. Int J Impot Res. 2010;22:196–203.
120. Wu C, Zhang H, Gao Y, Tan A, Yang X, Lu Z, Zhang Y, Liao M, Wang M, Mo Z. The association of smoking and erectile dysfunction: results from the Fangchenggang Area Male Health and Examination Survey (FAMHES) J Androl. 2012;33:59–65.

121. Kovac JR, Labbate C, Ramasamy R, Tang D, Lipshultz LI. Effects of cigarette smoking on erectile dysfunction. Andrologia. 2014;47(10):1087–1092. doi:10.1111/and.12393.
122. Celermajer DS, Sorensen KE, Georgakopoulos D, Bull C, Thomas O, Robinson J, Deanfield JE. Cigarette smoking is associated with dose-related and potentially reversible impairment of endothelium-dependent dilation in healthy young adults. Circulation. 1993;88:2149–2155.
123. Butler R, Morris AD, Struthers AD. Cigarette smoking in men and vascular responsiveness. Br J Clin Pharmacol. 2001;52:145–149.
124. Peluffo G, Calcerrada P, Piacenza L, Pizzano N, Radi R. Superoxide-mediated inactivation of nitric oxide and peroxynitrite formation by tobacco smoke in vascular endothelium: studies in cultured cells and smokers. Am J Physiol Heart Circ Physiol. 2009;296:H1781–1792.
125. Guo X, Oldham MJ, Kleinman MT, Phalen RF, Kassab GS. Effect of cigarette smoking on nitric oxide, structural, and mechanical properties of mouse arteries. Am J Physiol Heart Circ Physiol. 2006;291:H2354–2361.
126. Holst AG, Jensen G, Prescott E (2010) Risk factors for venous thromboembolism: results from the Copenhagen City Heart Study. Circulation 121: 1896–1903.
127. Severinsen MT, Kristensen SR, Johnsen SP, Dethlefsen C, Tjonneland A, et al. (2009) Smoking and venous thromboembolism: a Danish follow-up study. J Thromb Haemost 7: 1297–1303.
128. Cheng YJ, Liu ZH, Yao FJ, et al. Current and former smoking and risk for venous thromboembolism: a systematic review and meta-analysis. PLoS Med. 2013;10(9):e1001515. doi:10.1371/journal.pmed.1001515.
129. Yarnell JW, Sweetnam PM, Rumley A, Lowe GD (2001) Lifestyle factors and coagulation activation markers: the Caerphilly Study. Blood Coagul Fibrinolysis 12: 721–728.
130. Yukizawa Y, Inaba Y, Watanabe S, Yajima S, Kobayashi N, et al. (2012) Association between venous thromboembolism and plasma levels of both soluble fibrin and plasminogen-activator inhibitor 1 in 170 patients undergoing total hip arthroplasty. Acta Orthop 83: 14–21.
131. Gary T, Hafner F, Froehlich H, Stojakovic T, Scharnagl H, et al. (2010) High factor VIII activity, high plasminogen activator inhibitor 1 antigen levels and low factor XII activity contribute to a thrombophilic tendency in elderly venous thromboembolism patients. Acta Haematol 124: 214–217.
132. Willi C, Bodenmann P, Ghali WA, Faris PD, Cornuz J (2007) Active smoking and the risk of type 2 diabetes: a systematic review and meta-analysis. JAMA 298: 2654–2664.
133. Yeh JM, Hur C, Schrag D, Kuntz KM, Ezzati M, et al. (2013) Contribution of H. pylori and smoking trends to US incidence of intestinal-type noncardia gastric adenocarcinoma: a microsimulation model. PLoS Med 10: e1001451 doi:10.1371/journal.pmed.1001451.
134. Khaw KT, Friesen MD, Riboli E, Luben R, Wareham N (2012) Plasma phospholipid fatty acid concentration and incident coronary heart disease in men and women: the EPIC-Norfolk prospective study. PLoS Med 9: e1001255.
135. Grumelli S, Corry DB, Song LZ, Song L, Green L, et al. (2004) An immune basis for lung parenchymal destruction in chronic obstructive pulmonary disease and emphysema. PLoS Med 1: e8.
136. Ross A, Friedmann E, Bevans M, Thomas S. National survey of yoga practitioners: mental and physical health benefits. Complement Ther Med. 2013;21(4):313-23.
137. McIver S, O'Halloran P, McGartland M. The impact of Hatha yoga on smoking behavior. Altern Ther Health Med 2004;10:22–23.
138. Kochupillai V, Kumar P, Singh D, et al. Effect of rhythmic breathing (Sudarshan Kriya and Pranayam) on immune functions and tobacco addiction. Ann N Y Acad Sci 2005;1056:242–252.
139. Elibero A, Janse Van Rensburg K, & Drobes DJ (2011). Acute effects of aerobic exercise and hatha yoga on craving to smoke. Nicotine & Tobacco Research, 13(11), 1140–1148.
140. Bock BC, Fava JL, Gaskins R, et al. Yoga as a complementary treatment for smoking cessation in women. J Womens Health 2012;21:240–248.

141. Bock BC, Fava JL, Gaskins R, et al. Yoga as a complementary treatment for smoking cessation in women. J Womens Health (Larchmt) 2012;21(2):240–248.
142. L Carim Todd, S Mitchell, B Oken. Does yoga improve smoking cessation outcomes? A systematic review of the literature. BMC Complement Altern Med. 2012; 12(Suppl 1): P389. Published online 2012 Jun 12.
143. Shahab L, Sarkar BK, West R. The acute effects of yogic breathing exercises on craving and withdrawal symptoms in abstaining smokers. Psychopharmacology (Berl). 2013 Feb;225(4):875-82.
144. Chia-Liang Dai, and Manoj Sharma. Between Inhale and Exhale: Yoga as an Intervention in Smoking Cessation. Journal of Evidence-Based Complementary & Alternative Medicine 2014, Vol. 19(2) 144-149.
145. Rosen RK, Thind H, Jennings E, Guthrie KM, Williams DM, Bock BC. "Smoking Does Not Go With Yoga:" A Qualitative Study of Women's Phenomenological Perceptions During Yoga and Smoking Cessation. Int J Yoga Therap. 2016;26(1):33-41.
146. Klinsophon T, Thaveeratitham P, Sitthipornvorakul E, Janwantanakul P. Effect of exercise type on smoking cessation: a meta-analysis of randomized controlled trials. BMC Research Notes. 2017;10:442. doi:10.1186/s13104-017-2762-y.

Social Isolation/Loneliness

1. Baumeister RF, Leary MR. The need to belong: desire for interpersonal attachments as a fundamental human motivation. Psychol Bull. 1995;117(3):497. doi: 10.1037/0033-2909.117.3.497.
2. Weiss RS. Reflections on the present state of loneliness research. Journal of Social Behavior and Personality. 1987;2(2):1–16.
3. Beutel ME, Klein EM, Brähler E, et al. Loneliness in the general population: prevalence, determinants and relations to mental health. BMC Psychiatry. 2017;17(1):97. Published 2017 Mar 20. doi:10.1186/s12888-017-1262-x.
4. Theeke LA: Predictors of loneliness in US adults over age sixty-five. Arch Psychiatr Nurs 2009; 23: 387–396.
5. Wilson C, Moulton B: Loneliness among older adults: a national survey of adults 45+ Prepared by Knowledge Networks and Insight Policy Research. Washington, DC, AARP, 2010.
6. Perissinotto CM, Stojacic Cenzer I, Covinsky KE: Loneliness in older persons: a predictor of functional decline and death. Arch Intern Med 2012; 172: 1078–1084.
7. Heinrich L, Gullone E. The clinical significance of loneliness: A literature review. Clin Psychol Rev. 2006;26:695–718. doi: 10.1016/j.cpr.2006.04.002.
8. Luanaigh CO, Lawlor BA. Loneliness and the health of older people. Int J Geriatr Psychiatry. 2008 Dec;23(12):1213-21. doi: 10.1002/gps.2054.
9. Friedler B, Crapser J, McCullough L. One is the deadliest number: the detrimental effects of social isolation on cerebrovascular diseases and cognition. Acta Neuropathol. 2015;129(4):493–509. doi: 10.1007/s00401-014-1377-9.
10. Courtin E, Knapp M. Social isolation, loneliness and health in old age: a scoping review. Health Soc Care Community. 2017 May;25(3):799-812. doi: 10.1111/hsc.12311. Epub 2015 Dec 28.
11. Leigh-Hunt N, Bagguley D, Bash K, Turner V, Turnbull S, Valtorta N, Caan W. An overview of systematic reviews on the public health consequences of social isolation and loneliness. Public Health. 2017 Nov;152:157-171. doi: 10.1016/j.puhe.2017.07.035. Epub 2017 Sep 12.
12. Greaves CJ, Farbus L. Effects of creative and social activity on the health and well-being of socially isolated older people: outcomes from a multi-method observational study. J R Soc Promot Health. 2006 May;126(3):134-42.
13. Cacioppo JT, Hughes ME, Waite LJ, Hawkley LC, Thisted RA. Loneliness as a specific risk factor for depressive symptoms: cross-sectional and longitudinal analyses. Psychol Aging. 2006;21(1):140–51.
14. Cacioppo JT, Hawkley LC, Thisted RA. Perceived social isolation makes me sad: 5-year cross-lagged analyses of loneliness and depressive symptomatology in the Chicago Health, Aging, and Social Relations Study. Psychol Aging. 2010;25:453–463.

15. Stickley A, Koyanagi A. Loneliness, common mental disorders and suicidal behavior: Findings from a general population survey. J Affect Disord. 2016 Jun;197:81-7. doi: 10.1016/j.jad.2016.02.054. Epub 2016 Mar 2.
16. Shankar A, Hamer M, McMunn A, Steptoe A. Social isolation and loneliness: relationships with cognitive function during 4 years of follow-up in the English Longitudinal Study of Ageing. Psychosom Med. 2013;75:161–170.
17. Donovan NJ, Wu Q, Rentz DM, Sperling RA, Marshall GA, Glymour MM. Loneliness, depression and cognitive function in older U.S. adults. Int J Geriatr Psychiatry. 2016;32(5):564-573.
18. Wilson RS, Krueger KR, Arnold SE, et al. Loneliness and risk of Alzheimer disease. Arch Gen Psychiatry. 2007;64:234–240.
19. Perissinotto CM, Stijacic Cenzer I, Covinsky KE. Loneliness in older persons: a predictor of functional decline and death. Arch Intern Med. 2012;172(14):1078-83.
20. Theeke LA, Goins RT, Moore J, Campbell H. Loneliness, depression, social support, and quality of life in older chronically ill Appalachians. Journal of Psychology. 2012;146(1–2):155–171.
21. Holt-Lunstad J, Smith TB, Baker M, Harris T, Stephenson D: Loneliness and social isolation as risk factors for mortality: a meta-analytic review. Perspect Psychol Sci 2015; 10: 227–237.
22. Penninx BW, van Tilburg T, Kriegsman DM, Deeg DJ, Boeke AJ, van Eijk JT. Effects of social support and personal coping resources on mortality in older age: The Longitudinal Aging Study Amsterdam. American Journal of Epidemiology. 1997;146(6):510–519.
23. Holwerda TJ, van Tilburg TG, Deeg DJ, Schutter N, Van R, Dekker J, Stek ML, Beekman AT, Schoevers RA. Impact of loneliness and depression on mortality: results from the Longitudinal Ageing Study Amsterdam. Br J Psychiatry. 2016 Aug;209(2):127-34. doi: 10.1192/bjp.bp.115.168005. Epub 2016 Apr 21.
24. Valtorta NK, Kanaan M, Gilbody S, Ronzi S, Hanratty B. Loneliness and social isolation as risk factors for coronary heart disease and stroke: systematic review and meta-analysis of longitudinal observational studies. Heart. 2016;102(13):1009-1016.
25. Hawkley LC, Burleson MH, Berntson GG, Cacioppo JT. Loneliness in everyday life: Cardiovascular activity, psychosocial context, and health behaviors. Journal of Personality and Social Psychology. 2003;85:105–120.
26. Hawkley LC, Masi CM, Berry JD, Cacioppo JT. Loneliness is a unique predictor of age-related differences in systolic blood pressure. Psychology and Aging. 2006;21(1):152–164.
27. Hawkley LC, Thisted RA, Masi CM, Cacioppo JT. Loneliness predicts increased blood pressure: Five-year cross-lagged analyses in middle-aged and older adults. Psychology and Aging. 2010;25(1):132–141.
28. Richard A, Rohrmann S, Vandeleur CL, Schmid M, Barth J, Eichholzer M. Loneliness is adversely associated with physical and mental health and lifestyle factors: Results from a Swiss national survey. PLoS One. 2017;12(7):e0181442. Published 2017 Jul 17. doi:10.1371/journal.pone.0181442.
29. Hawkley LC, Thisted RA, Cacioppo JT. Loneliness predicts reduced physical activity: cross-sectional & longitudinal analyses. Health Psychol. 2009;28(3):354–63. doi: 10.1037/a0014400 ; PubMed Central PMCID: PMC2791498.
30. Hawkley LC, Preacher KJ, Cacioppo JT. Loneliness impairs daytime functioning but not sleep duration. Health Psychology. 2010;29(2):124–129.
31. Petitte T, Mallow J, Barnes E, Petrone A, Barr T, Theeke L. A Systematic Review of Loneliness and Common Chronic Physical Conditions in Adults. Open Psychol J. 2015;8(Suppl 2):113–132. doi:10.2174/1874350101508010113.
32. Lauder W, Mummery K, Jones M, Caperchione C. A comparison of health behaviours in lonely and non-lonely populations. Psychology Health & Medicine. 2006;11:233–245.
33. Whisman MA. Loneliness and the metabolic syndrome in a population-based sample of middle-aged and older adults. Health Psychol. 2010;29:4.
34. Yanguas J, Pinazo-Henandis S, Tarazona-Santabalbina FJ. The complexity of loneliness. Acta Biomed. 2018 Jun 7;89(2):302-314. doi: 10.23750/abm.v89i2.7404.
35. Cole SW, Hawkley LC, Arevalo JM, Sung CY, Rose RM, Cacioppo JT. Social regulation of gene expression in human leukocytes. Genome Biology. 2007;8(9): R189.181–R189.113. PMCID: PMC2375027.
36. Danese A, Moffitt TE, Harrington H, Milne BJ, Polanczyk G, Pariante CM, et al. Adverse childhood experiences and adult risk factors for age-related disease: depression,

37. Ranjit N, Diez-Roux AV, Shea S, Cushman M, Seeman T, Jackson SA, et al. Psychosocial factors and inflammation in the multi-ethnic study of atherosclerosis. Arch Intern Med. 2007;167(2):174–81.
38. Richard A, Rohrmann S, Vandeleur CL, Schmid M, Barth J, Eichholzer M. Loneliness is adversely associated with physical and mental health and lifestyle factors: Results from a Swiss national survey. PLoS One. 2017;12(7):e0181442. Published 2017 Jul 17. doi:10.1371/journal.pone.0181442.
39. Akerlind I, Hornquist JO. Loneliness and alcohol abuse: a review of evidences of an interplay. Soc Sci Med. 1992;34(4):405–14.
40. Grippo AJ, Lamb DG, Carter CS, Porges SW. Social isolation disrupts autonomic regulation of the heart and influences negative affective behaviors. Biol Psychiatry. 2007;62(10):1162-70.
41. Cacioppo JT, Hawkley LC, Thisted RA. Perceived social isolation makes me sad: 5-year cross-lagged analyses of loneliness and depressive symptomatology in the chicago health, aging, and social relations study. Psychol Aging. 2010;25:453–63.
42. Bekhet AK, Zauszniewski JA. Mental health of elders in retirement communities: Is loneliness a key factor? Arch Psychiatr Nurs. 2012;26:214–24.
43. Petitte T, Mallow J, Barnes E, Petrone A, Barr T, Theeke L. A Systematic Review of Loneliness and Common Chronic Physical Conditions in Adults. Open Psychol J. 2015;8(Suppl 2):113–132. doi:10.2174/1874350101508010113.
44. Thurston RC, Kubzansky LD. Women, loneliness, and incident coronary heart disease. Psychosom Med. 2009;71:836–42.
45. Hegeman A, Schutter N, Comijs H, Holwerda T, Dekker J, Stek M, van der Mast R. Loneliness and cardiovascular disease and the role of late-life depression. Int J Geriatr Psychiatry. 2018 Jan;33(1):e65-e72. doi: 10.1002/gps.4716. Epub 2017 Apr 18.
46. Lofvenmark C, Mattiasson AC, Billing E, Edner M. Perceived loneliness and social support in patients with chronic heart failure. Eur J Cardiovasc Nurs. 2009;8:251–8.
47. Valtorta NK, Kanaan M, Gilbody S, Ronzi S, Hanratty B. Loneliness and social isolation as risk factors for coronary heart disease and stroke: systematic review and meta-analysis of longitudinal observational studies. Heart. 2016;102(13):1009-1016.
48. Cox AM, McKevitt C, Rudd AG, Wolfe CD. Socioeconomic status and stroke. Lancet Neurol. 2006;5:181–8.
49. Cacioppo JT, Hughes ME, Waite LJ, Hawkley LC, Thisted RA. Loneliness as a specific risk factor for depressive symptoms: Cross-sectional and longitudinal analyses. Psychol Aging. 2006;21:140–51.
50. B. Boden-Albala, E. Litwak, M.S.V. Elkind, T. Rundek, R. L. Sacco. Social isolation and outcomes post stroke. Neurology Jun 2005, 64 (11) 1888-1892; DOI:10.1212/01.WNL.0000163510.79351.AF.
51. Penninx BW, van Tilburg T, Kriegsman DM, Deeg DJ, Boeke AJ, van Eijk JT. Effects of social support and personal coping resources on mortality in older age: The Longitudinal Aging Study Amsterdam. American Journal of Epidemiology. 1997;146(6):510–519.
52. Wattanakit K, Williams JE, Schreiner PJ, Hirsch AT, Folsom AR. Association of anger proneness, depression and low social support with peripheral arterial disease: the Atherosclerosis Risk in Communities Study. Vasc Med. 2005 Aug;10(3):199-206.
53. Holt-Lunstad J, Smith TB, Layton JB. Social relationships and mortality risk: A meta-analytic review. PLoS Medicine. 2010;7:2–19.
54. Shor E, Roelfs DJ, Yogev T. The strength of family ties: A meta-analysis and meta-regression of self-reported social support and mortality. Social Networks. 2013;35:626–638.
55. Hill TD, Uchino BN, Eckhardt JL, Angel JL. Perceived Social Support Trajectories and the All-Cause Mortality Risk of Older Mexican American Women and Men. Research on aging. 2016;38(3):374-398. doi:10.1177/0164027515620239.
56. Masi CM, Chen HY, Hawkley LC, Cacioppo JT. A meta-analysis of interventions to reduce loneliness. Pers Soc Psychol Rev. 2010;15(3):219-66.
57. Bucher HC. Social support and prognosis following first myocardial infarction. J Gen Int Med. 1994;9:409–417.
58. Ross A, Bevans M, Friedmann E, Williams L, Thomas S. "I Am a Nice Person When I Do Yoga!!!": A Qualitative Analysis of How Yoga Affects Relationships. Journal of holistic

nursing : official journal of the American Holistic Nurses' Association. 2014;32(2):67-77. doi:10.1177/0898010113508466.
59. Kinser PA, Bourguignon C, Taylor AG, Steeves R. "A Feeling of Connectedness": Perspectives on a Gentle Yoga Intervention for Women with Major Depression. Issues in mental health nursing. 2013;34(6):402-411. doi:10.3109/01612840.2012.762959.
60. Ross A, Friedmann E, Bevans M, Thomas S. National Survey of Yoga Practitioners: Mental and Physical Health Benefits. Complementary therapies in medicine. 2013;21(4):313-323. doi:10.1016/j.ctim.2013.04.001.
61. Creswell JD, Irwin MR, Burklund LJ, Lieberman MD, Arevalo JM, Ma J, et al. Mindfulness-based stress reduction training reduces loneliness and pro-inflammatory gene expression in older adults: a small randomized controlled trial. Brain Behav Immun (2012) 26(7):1095–10110.1016/j.bbi.2012.07.006.

Spirituality

1. Fetzer Institute, National Institute on Aging Working Group (1999) Multidimensional measurement of religiousness/spirituality for use in health research Kalamazoo, MI: Fetzer Institute. 96 p.
2. de Jager Meezenbroek EC, Garssen B, van den Berg M, van Dierendonck D, Visser A, et al. (2012) Measuring spirituality as a universal human experience: A review of spirituality questionnaires. J Relig Health 51: 336–354. doi: 10.1007/s10943-010-9376-1.
3. Weaver AJ, Pargament KI, Flannelly KJ, Oppenheimer JE. Trends in the scientific study of religion, spirituality, and health: 1965–2000. Journal of Religion and Health. 2006;45:208–214. doi: 10.1007/s10943-006-9011-3.
4. McCaffrey A. M., Eisenberg D. M., Legedza A. T. R., Davis R. B., Phillips R. S. Prayer for health concerns: results of a national survey on prevalence and patterns of use. Archives of Internal Medicine. 2004;164(8):858–862. doi: 10.1001/archinte.164.8.858.
5. Yates J. S., Mustian K. M., Morrow G. R., et al. Prevalence of complementary and alternative medicine use in cancer patients during treatment. Supportive Care in Cancer. 2005;13(10):806–811. doi: 10.1007/s00520-004-0770-7.
6. Roberts L, Ahmed I, Hall S, Davison A. Intercessory prayer for the alleviation of ill health. Cochrane Database Syst Rev. 2009 Apr 15;(2):CD000368. doi: 10.1002/14651858.CD000368.pub3.
7. Jors K, Büssing A, Hvidt NC, Baumann K. Personal Prayer in Patients Dealing with Chronic Illness: A Review of the Research Literature. Evidence-based Complementary and Alternative Medicine : eCAM. 2015;2015:927973. doi:10.1155/2015/927973.
8. Ginting H, Näring G, Kwakkenbos L, Becker ES. Spirituality and Negative Emotions in Individuals With Coronary Heart Disease. J Cardiovasc Nurs. 2015 Nov-Dec;30(6):537-45. doi: 10.1097/JCN.0000000000000201.
9. Stefanek M, McDonald PG, Hess SA. Religion, spirituality and cancer: Current status and methodological challenges. Psycho-Oncology. 2005;14:450–463. doi: 10.1002/pon.861.
10. Sawatzky R, Ratner PA, Chiu L. A meta-analysis of the relationship between spirituality and quality of life. Social Indicators Research. 2005;72:153–188. doi: 10.1007/s11205-004-5577-x.
11. Hemmati R, Bidel Z, Nazarzadeh M et al. Religion, Spirituality and Risk of Coronary Heart Disease: A Matched Case-Control Study and Meta-Analysis. J Relig Health. 2018 Oct 22. doi: 10.1007/s10943-018-0722-z.
12. Najafi Ghezeljeh T, Emami A. Strategies for recreating normal life: Iranian coronary heart disease patients' perspectives on coping strategies. Journal of Clinical Nursing. 2014;23:2151–2160. doi: 10.1111/jocn.12428.
13. Abu HO, Ulbricht C, Ding E, et al. Association of religiosity and spirituality with quality of life in patients with cardiovascular disease: a systematic review. Qual Life Res. 2018;27(11):2777–2797. doi:10.1007/s11136-018-1906-4.
14. Monk-Turner E, Turner C. Does yoga shape body, mind and spiritual health and happiness: Differences between yoga practitioners and college students. Int J Yoga. 2010;3(2):48-54.
15. Park CL, Riley KE, Bedesin E, Stewart VM. Why practice yoga? Practitioners' motivations for adopting and maintaining yoga practice. J Health Psychol. 2016 Jun;21(6):887-96. doi: 10.1177/1359105314541314. Epub 2014 Jul 16.

16. Genovese JEC, Fondran KM. The Psychology of Yoga Practitioners: A Cluster Analysis. Int J Yoga Therap. 2017 Nov;27(1):51-58. doi: 10.17761/1531-2054-27.1.51.
17. Varambally S, Gangadhar BN. Yoga: a spiritual practice with therapeutic value in psychiatry. Asian J Psychiatr. 2012 Jun;5(2):186-9. doi: 10.1016/j.ajp.2012.05.003. Epub 2012 May 18.
18. Ando M, Morita T, Akechi T, Ito S, Tanaka M, Ifuku Y, Nakayama T. The efficacy of mindfulness-based meditation therapy on anxiety, depression, and spirituality in Japanese patients with cancer. J Palliat Med. 2009 Dec;12(12):1091-4. doi: 10.1089/jpm.2009.0143.
19. Nakau M, Imanishi J, Imanishi J, Watanabe S, Imanishi A, Baba T, Hirai K, Ito T, Chiba W, Morimoto Y. Spiritual care of cancer patients by integrated medicine in urban green space: a pilot study. Explore (NY). 2013 Mar-Apr;9(2):87-90. doi: 10.1016/j.explore.2012.12.002.

Stroke

1. Go AS, Mozaffarian D, Roger VL, Benjamin EJ, et al. American Heart Association Statistics Committee and Stroke Statistics Subcommittee Heart disease and stroke statistics–2014 update: a report from the American Heart Association. Circulation. 2014;129:e28–e292.
2. Mackay J, Mensah GA: The Atlas of Heart Disease and Stroke. Geneva: World Health Organization, 2002.; Chong JY, Sacco RL: Epidemiology of stroke in young adults: race/ethnic differences. J Thromb Thrombolysis, 2005, 20: 77–83., WHO 2015.
3. Heron M. Deaths: leading causes for 2007. Natl Vital Stat Rep. 2011;59:1–95.
4. Go AS, Mozaffarian D, Roger VL, et al. American Heart Association Statistics Committee and Stroke Statistics Subcommittee: heart disease and stroke statistics—2013 update: a report from the American Heart Association. Circulation, 2013, 127: 6–245.
5. Silva SM, Corrêa FI, Faria CDC de M, Buchalla CM, Silva PF da C, Corrêa JCF. Evaluation of post-stroke functionality based on the International Classification of Functioning, Disability, and Health: a proposal for use of assessment tools. Journal of Physical Therapy Science. 2015;27(6):1665-1670. doi:10.1589/jpts.27.1665.
6. Murray CJ, Vos T, Lozano R, et al. Disability-adjusted life years (DALYs) for 291 diseases and injuries in 21 regions, 1990–2010: a systematic analysis for the Global Burden of Disease Study 2010. Lancet, 2012, 380: 2197–2223.
7. Samsa GP, Matchar DB, Goldstein L, Bonito A, Duncan PW, Lipscomb J, Enarson C, Witter D, Venus P, Paul JE, Weinberger M. Utilities for major stroke: results from a survey of preferences among persons at increased risk for stroke. Am Heart J. 1998;136(pt 1):703–713.
8. Saposnik G and C. J. Estol, "Translational research: from observational studies to health policy: how a cohort study can help improve outcomes after stroke," Stroke, vol. 42, no. 12, pp. 3336–3337, 2011.
9. Meschia JF, Bushnell C, Boden-Albala B, et al. Guidelines for the primary prevention of stroke: a statement for healthcare professionals from the American Heart Association/American Stroke Association. Stroke. 2014;45(12):3754–3832. doi:10.1161/STR.0000000000000046.
10. Kannel WB, Benjamin EJ. Status of the epidemiology of atrial fibrillation. Med Clin North Am. 2008;92:17–40. ix.
11. Banerjee C, Moon YP, Paik MC, Rundek T, Mora-McLaughlin C, Vieira JR, Sacco RL, Elkind MS. Duration of diabetes and risk of ischemic stroke: the Northern Manhattan Study. Stroke. 2012;43:1212–1217.
12. He FJ, Nowson CA, MacGregor GA. Fruit and vegetable consumption and stroke: meta-analysis of cohort studies. Lancet. 2006;367:320–326.
13. Iso H, Jacobs DR, Jr, Wentworth D, Neaton JD, Cohen JD. Serum cholesterol levels and six-year mortality from stroke in 350,977 men screened for the multiple risk factor intervention trial. N Engl J Med. 1989;320:904–910.
14. Chobanian AV, Bakris GL, Black HR, et al. National Heart, Lung, and Blood Institute Joint National Committee on Prevention, Detection, Evaluation, and Treatment of High Blood Pressure; National High Blood Pressure Education Program Coordinating Committee The Seventh Report of the Joint National Committee on Prevention,

Detection, Evaluation, and Treatment of High Blood Pressure: the JNC 7 report. JAMA. 2003;289:2560–2572.
15. Suk SH, Sacco RL, Boden-Albala B, Cheun JF, Pittman JG, Elkind MS, Paik MC, Northern Manhattan Stroke Study Abdominal obesity and risk of ischemic stroke: the Northern Manhattan Stroke Study. Stroke. 2003;34:1586–1592.
16. Wendel-Vos GC, Schuit AJ, Feskens EJ, Boshuizen HC, Verschuren WM, Saris WH, Kromhout D. Physical activity and stroke: a meta-analysis of observational data. Int J Epidemiol. 2004;33:787–798.
17. Rodriguez BL, D'Agostino R, Abbott RD, Kagan A, Burchfiel CM, Yano K, Ross GW, Silbershatz H, Higgins MW, Popper J, Wolf PA, Curb JD. Risk of hospitalized stroke in men enrolled in the Honolulu Heart Program and the Framingham Study: A comparison of incidence and risk factor effects. Stroke. 2002;33:230–236.
18. Dhanunjaya Lakkireddy, DonitaAtkins, JayasreePillarisett, et al. Effect of Yoga on Arrhythmia Burden, Anxiety, Depression, and Quality of Life in Paroxysmal Atrial Fibrillation: The YOGA My Heart Study. Journal of the American College of Cardiology. Volume 61, Issue 11, 19 March 2013, Pages 1177-1182.
19. Cui J, Yan J, Yan L, Pan L, Le J, Guo Y. Effects of yoga in adults with type 2 diabetes mellitus: A meta-analysis. Journal of Diabetes Investigation. 2017;8(2):201-209. doi:10.1111/jdi.12548.
20. Tyagi A, Cohen M. Yoga and hypertension: a systematic review. Altern Ther Health Med. 2014 Mar-Apr;20(2):32-59.
21. Cramer H, Sibbritt D, Park CL, Adams J, Lauche R. Is the practice of yoga or meditation associated with a healthy lifestyle? Results of a national cross-sectional survey of 28,695 Australian women. J Psychosom Res. 2017 Oct;101:104-109. doi: 10.1016/j.jpsychores.2017.07.013. Epub 2017 Jul 27.
22. Tew GA, Howsam J, Hardy M, Bissell L. Adapted yoga to improve physical function and health-related quality of life in physically-inactive older adults: a randomised controlled pilot trial. BMC Geriatr. 2017;17(1):131. Published 2017 Jun 23. doi:10.1186/s12877-017-0520-6.
23. Youkhana S, Dean CM, Wolff M, Sherrington C, Tiedemann A. Yoga-based exercise improves balance and mobility in people aged 60 and over: a systematic review and meta-analysis. Age Ageing. 2016 Jan;45(1):21-9. doi: 10.1093/ageing/afv175. Epub 2015 Dec 25.
24. Innes KE, Selfe TK. Yoga for Adults with Type 2 Diabetes: A Systematic Review of Controlled Trials. Journal of Diabetes Research. 2016;2016:6979370. doi:10.1155/2016/6979370.
25. Rshikesan PB, Subramanya P, Nidhi R. Yoga Practice for Reducing the Male Obesity and Weight Related Psychological Difficulties-A Randomized Controlled Trial. J Clin Diagn Res. 2016;10(11):OC22-OC28.
26. Rosen RK, Thind H, Jennings E, Guthrie KM, Williams DM, Bock BC. "Smoking Does Not Go With Yoga:" A Qualitative Study of Women's Phenomenological Perceptions During Yoga and Smoking Cessation. Int J Yoga Therap. 2016;26(1):33–41. doi:10.17761/1531-2054-26.1.33.
27. Lawrence M, Celestino Junior FT, Matozinho HH, Govan L, Booth J, Beecher J. Yoga for stroke rehabilitation. Cochrane Database Syst Rev. 2017 Dec 8;12:CD011483. doi: 10.1002/14651858.CD011483.pub2.
28. Thayabaranathan T, Andrew NE, Immink MA, Hillier S, Stevens P, Stolwyk R, Kilkenny M, Cadilhac DA. Determining the potential benefits of yoga in chronic stroke care: a systematic review and meta-analysis. Top Stroke Rehabil. 2017 May;24(4):279-287. doi: 10.1080/10749357.2016.1277481. Epub 2017 Jan 19.
29. Harris A, Austin M, Blake TM, Bird ML. Perceived benefits and barriers to yoga participation after stroke: A focus group approach. Complement Ther Clin Pract. 2019 Feb;34:153-156. doi: 10.1016/j.ctcp.2018.11.015. Epub 2018 Nov 30.

Stroke Rehabilitation

1. Mackay J, Mensah GA: The Atlas of Heart Disease and Stroke. Geneva: World Health Organization, 2002.; Chong JY, Sacco RL: Epidemiology of stroke in young adults: race/ethnic differences. J Thromb Thrombolysis, 2005, 20: 77–83., WHO 2015.

2. Go AS, Mozaffarian D, Roger VL, et al. American Heart Association Statistics Committee and Stroke Statistics Subcommittee: heart disease and stroke statistics—2013 update: a report from the American Heart Association. Circulation, 2013, 127: 6–245.
3. Silva SM, Corrêa FI, Faria CDC de M, Buchalla CM, Silva PF da C, Corrêa JCF. Evaluation of post-stroke functionality based on the International Classification of Functioning, Disability, and Health: a proposal for use of assessment tools. Journal of Physical Therapy Science. 2015;27(6):1665-1670. doi:10.1589/jpts.27.1665.
4. Murray CJ, Vos T, Lozano R, et al. Disability-adjusted life years (DALYs) for 291 diseases and injuries in 21 regions, 1990–2010: a systematic analysis for the Global Burden of Disease Study 2010. Lancet, 2012, 380: 2197–2223.
5. Saposnik G and C. J. Estol, "Translational research: from observational studies to health policy: how a cohort study can help improve outcomes after stroke," Stroke, vol. 42, no. 12, pp. 3336–3337, 2011.
6. Langhorne P., Bernhardt J., Kwakkel G. (2011). Stroke rehabilitation. Lancet 377, 1693–1702. 10.1016/S0140-6736(11)60325-5.
7. Roth EJ. Heart disease in patients with stroke. Part II: Impact and implications for rehabilitation. Archives of physical medicine and rehabilitation. 1994;75(1):94–94.
8. Liu M, Tsuji T, Tsujiuchi K, Chino N. Comorbidities in stroke patients as assessed with a newly developed comorbidity scale. Am J Phys Med Rehabil. 1999;78:416–24.
9. Gaete JM1, Bogousslavsky J. Post-stroke depression. Expert Rev Neurother. 2008 Jan;8(1):75-92.
10. Carolee J. Winstein, Joel Stein, Ross Arena, et al. Guidelines for Adult Stroke Rehabilitation and Recovery. A Guideline for Healthcare Professionals from the American Heart Association/American Stroke Association. Stroke. 2016;47:e98-e169.
11. Brewer L, Horgan F, Hickey A, Williams D. Stroke rehabilitation: recent advances and future therapies. QJM. 2013;106(1):11–25.
12. Sun F, Wang J, Wen X. Acupuncture in stroke rehabilitation: Literature retrieval based on international databases. Neural Regeneration Research. 2012;7(15):1192-1199. doi:10.3969/j.issn.1673-5374.2012.15.011.
13. Bastille JV, Gill-Body KM. A yoga-based exercise program for people with chronic poststroke hemiparesis. Phys Ther. 2004;84:33–48.
14. Zettergren KK, Lubeski JM, Viverito JM. Effects of a yoga program on postural control, mobility, and gait speed in community-living older adults: a pilot study. J Geriatr Phys Ther. 2011 Apr-Jun;34(2):88-94.
15. Garrett R, Immink MA, Hillier S. Becoming connected: The lived experience of yoga participation after stroke. Disabil Rehabil. 2011:1–12.
16. Bastille JV, Gill-Body KM. A yoga-based exercise program for people with chronic poststroke hemiparesis. Phys Ther. 2004; 84:33–48.
17. Bastille JV, Gill-Body KM. A yoga-based exercise program for people with chronic poststroke hemiparesis. Phys Ther. 2004;84:33–48.
18. Schmid A. A, Marieke Van Puymbroeck, Peter A. Altenburger et al. Poststroke Balance Improves with Yoga. A Pilot Study. Stroke. 2012; 43: 2402-2407.
19. Schmid AA, Miller KK, Van Puymbroeck M, DeBaun-Sprague E. Yoga leads to multiple physical improvements after stroke, a pilot study. Complement Ther Med. 2014 Dec;22(6):994-1000. doi: 10.1016/j.ctim.2014.09.005. Epub 2014 Oct 7.
20. Immink MA, Hillier S, Petkov J. Randomized controlled trial of yoga for chronic poststroke hemiparesis: motor function, mental health, and quality of life outcomes. Top Stroke Rehabil. 2014 May-Jun;21(3):256-71. doi: 10.1310/tsr2103-256.
21. Asimina Lazaridou, Phaethon Philbrook, and Aria A. Tzika. Yoga and Mindfulness as Therapeutic Interventions for Stroke Rehabilitation: A Systematic Review. Evidence-Based Complementary and Alternative Medicine. Volume 2013.
22. Thayabaranathan T, Andrew NE1, Immink MA et al. Determining the potential benefits of yoga in chronic stroke care: a systematic review and meta-analysis. Top Stroke Rehabil. 2017 May;24(4):279-287. doi: 10.1080/10749357.2016.1277481. Epub 2017 Jan 19.

23. Lawrence M, Celestino Junior FT, Matozinho HH, Govan L, Booth J, Beecher J. Yoga for stroke rehabilitation. Cochrane Database Syst Rev. 2017 Dec 8;12:CD011483. doi: 10.1002/14651858.CD011483.pub2.

Vascular Dementia

1. Jellinger K.A., Attems J. Is there pure vascular dementia in old age? J. Neurol. Sci. 2010;299(1–2):150–154.
2. Gorelick PB, Scuteri A, Black SE, Decarli C, Greenberg SM, Iadecola C, Launer LJ, Laurent S, Lopez OL, Nyenhuis D, Petersen RC, et al. Vascular contributions to cognitive impairment and dementia: a statement for healthcare professionals from the american heart association/american stroke association. Stroke. 2011;42:2672–2713.
3. Lambert C, Zeestraten E, Williams O, et al. Identifying preclinical vascular dementia in symptomatic small vessel disease using MRI. Neuroimage Clin. 2018;19:925-938. Published 2018 Jun 20. doi:10.1016/j.nicl.2018.06.023.
4. Lopez O. L., Kuller L. H., Becker J. T., Jagust W. J., DeKosky S. T., Fitzpatrick A., et al. (2005). Classification of vascular dementia in the Cardiovascular Health Study Cognition Study. Neurology 64, 1539–1547 10.1212/01.WNL.0000159860.19413.C4.
5. Grinberg L. T., Thal D. R. (2010). Vascular pathology in the aged human brain. Acta Neuropathol. 119, 277–290 10.1007/s00401-010-0652-7.
6. Jellinger KA. Pathology and pathogenesis of vascular cognitive impairment-a critical update. Front Aging Neurosci. 2013;5:17. Published 2013 Apr 10. doi:10.3389/fnagi.2013.00017.
7. De Leeuw F.E., De Groot J.C., Achten E., Oudkerk M., Ramos L.M.P., Heijboer R., Hofman A., Jolles J., Van Gijn J., Breteler M.M.B. Prevalence of cerebral white matter lesions in elderly people: a population based magnetic resonance imaging study, The Rotterdam Scan Study. J. Neurol. Neurosurg. Psychiatry. 2001;70(1):9–14.
8. Pantoni L. Cerebral small vessel disease: from pathogenesis and clinical characteristics to therapeutic challenges. Lancet Neurol. 2010;9(7):689–701.
9. Gouw A.A., Seewann A., van der Flier W.M., Barkhof F., Rozemuller A.M., Scheltens P., Geurts J.J. Heterogeneity of small vessel disease: a systematic review of MRI and histopathology correlations. J. Neurol. Neurosurg. Psychiatry. 2011;82(2):126–135.
10. Chang-Quan H, Hui W, Chao-Min W, et al. The association of antihypertensive medication use with risk of cognitive decline and dementia: a meta-analysis of longitudinal studies. Int J Clin Pract 2011; 65: 1295–1305.
11. Rouch L, Cestac P, Hanon O, et al. Antihypertensive drugs, prevention of cognitive decline and dementia: a systematic review of observational studies, randomized controlled trials and meta-analyses, with discussion of potential mechanisms. CNS Drugs 2015; 29: 113–130.
12. Ninomiya T. Diabetes mellitus and dementia. Curr Diab Rep 2014; 14: 487.
13. Attems J., Jellinger K., Thal D. R., Van Nostrand W. (2011). Review: sporadic cerebral amyloid angiopathy. Neuropathol. Appl. Neurobiol. 37, 75–93 10.1111/j.1365-2990.2010.01137.x.
14. Ballard C, Neill D, O'Brien J, McKeith IG, Ince P, Perry R. Anxiety, depression and psychosis in vascular dementia: prevalence and associations. J Affect Disord. 2000;59:97–106.
15. Gorelick PB, Scuteri A, Black SE, Decarli C, Greenberg SM, Iadecola C, Launer LJ, Laurent S, Lopez OL, Nyenhuis D, Petersen RC, et al. Vascular contributions to cognitive impairment and dementia: a statement for healthcare professionals from the american heart association/american stroke association. Stroke. 2011;42:2672–2713.
16. Richard E, Reitz C, Honig LH, et al. Late-life depression, mild cognitive impairment, and dementia. JAMA Neurol 2013; 70: 374–382.
17. Mourao RJ, Mansur G, Malloy-Diniz LF, et al. Depressive symptoms increase the risk of progression to dementia in subjects with mild cognitive impairment: systematic review and meta-analysis. Int J Geriatr Psychiatry 2016; 31: 905–911.
18. Tyagi A, Cohen M. Yoga and hypertension: a systematic review. Altern Ther Health Med. 2014 Mar-Apr;20(2):32-59.
19. Cui J, Yan J, Yan L, Pan L, Le J, Guo Y. Effects of yoga in adults with type 2 diabetes mellitus: A meta-analysis. Journal of Diabetes Investigation. 2017;8(2):201-209.

doi:10.1111/jdi.12548.
20. Cramer H, Lauche R, Langhorst J, Dobos G. Yoga for depression: a systematic review and meta-analysis. Depress Anxiety. 2013 Nov;30(11):1068-83. doi: 10.1002/da.22166. Epub 2013 Aug 6.

Vascular Elasticity

1. Lee H, Oh B. Aging and arterial stiffness. Circ J. 2010;74(11):2257–2262.
2. Lyle AN, Raaz U. Killing Me Unsoftly: Causes and Mechanisms of Arterial Stiffness. Arterioscler Thromb Vasc Biol. 2017;37(2):e1-e11.
3. Prenner SB, Chirinos JA. Arterial stiffness in diabetes mellitus. Atherosclerosis. 2015 Feb;238(2):370-9. doi: 10.1016/j.atherosclerosis.2014.12.023. Epub 2014 Dec 20.
4. Li P, Wang L, Liu C. Overweightness, obesity and arterial stiffness in healthy subjects: a systematic review and meta-analysis of literature studies. Postgrad Med. 2017 Mar;129(2):224-230. doi: 10.1080/00325481.2017.1268903. Epub 2016 Dec 15.
5. Mozos I, Maidana JP, Stoian D, Stehlik M. Gender Differences of Arterial Stiffness and Arterial Age in Smokers. Int J Environ Res Public Health. 2017;14(6):565. Published 2017 May 26. doi:10.3390/ijerph14060565.
6. Tsai TC, Wu JS, Yang YC, Huang YH, Lu FH, Chang CJ. Long sleep duration associated with a higher risk of increased arterial stiffness in males. Sleep. 2014;37(8):1315–1320. Published 2014 Aug 1. doi:10.5665/sleep.3920.
7. Dao HH, Essalihi R, Bouvet C, Moreau P. Evolution and modulation of age related medial elastocalcinosis: impact on large artery stiffness and isolated systolic hypertension. Cardiovasc Res. 2005;66:307–317.
8. Franklin SS, Gustin Wt, Wong ND, Larson MG, Weber MA, Kannel WB, Levy D. Hemodynamic patterns of age-related changes in blood pressure. The Framingham Heart Study. Circulation. 1997;96:308–15.
9. Daniel H. O'Leary, M.D., Joseph F. Polak, M.D., M.P.H., Richard A. Kronmal, Ph.D., Teri A. Manolio, M.D., M.H.S., Gregory L. Burke, M.D., M.S., and Sidney K. Wolfson, Jr., M.D. for the Cardiovascular Health Study Collaborative Research Group. Carotid-Artery Intima and Media Thickness as a Risk Factor for Myocardial Infarction and Stroke in Older Adults. N Engl J Med 1999; 340:14-22. DOI: 10.1056/NEJM199901073400103.
10. Laurent S, Cockcroft J, Van BL, et al. Expert consensus document on arterial stiffness: methodological issues and clinical applications. European Heart Journal. 2006;27(21):2588–2605.
11. van Popele NM, Grobbee DE, Bots ML, et al. Association between arterial stiffness and atherosclerosis: the Rotterdam Study. Stroke. 2001;32:454–60.
12. O'Rourke MF, Hashimoto J. Mechanical factors in arterial aging: a clinical perspective. J Am Coll Cardiol. 2007;50:1–13.
13. Mattace-Raso FU, van der Cammen TJ, Hofman A, van Popele NM, Bos ML, Schalekamp MA, Asmar R, Reneman RS, Hoeks AP, Breteler MM, Witteman JC. Arterial stiffness and risk of coronary heart disease and stroke: the Rotterdam Study. Circulation. 2006;113:657–663.
14. Chen YT, Vaccarino V, Williams CS, Butler J, Berkman LF, Krumholz HM. Risk factors for heart failure in the elderly: a prospective community-based study. Am J Med. 1999;106:605–612.
15. Laurent S, Katsahian S, Fassot C, Tropeano AI, Gautier I, Laloux B, Boutouyrie P. Aortic stiffness is an independent predictor of fatal stroke in essential hypertension. Stroke. 2003;34:1203–1206.
16. Kim J, Cha MJ, Lee DH, et al. The association between cerebral atherosclerosis and arterial stiffness in acute ischemic stroke. Atherosclerosis. 2011;219:887–91.
17. Safar M, Levy B, Struijker-Boudier H. Current perspectives on arterial stiffness and pulse pressure in hypertension and cardiovascular diseases. Circulation. 2003;107:2864–9.
18. Sutton-Tyrrell K, Najjar SS, Boudreau RM, Venkitachalam L, Kupelian V, Simonsick EM, Havlik R, Lakatta EG, Spurgeon H, Kritchevsky S, Pahor M, Bauer D, Newman A. Elevated aortic pulse wave velocity, a marker of arterial stiffness, predicts cardiovascular events in well-functioning older adults. Circulation. 2005;111:3384–3390.
19. Mattace-Raso FU, van der Cammen TJ, Hofman A, van Popele NM, Bos ML, Schalekamp MA, Asmar R, Reneman RS, Hoeks AP, Breteler MM, Witteman JC. Arterial stiffness and

risk of coronary heart disease and stroke: the Rotterdam Study. Circulation. 2006;113:657–663.
20. G.F. Mitchell, S.J. Hwang, R.S. Vasan, et al.Arterial stiffness and cardiovascular events: The Framingham Heart Study.Circulation, 121 (2010), pp. 505-511.
21. Ben-Shlomo Y, Spears M, Boustred C, et al. Aortic pulse wave velocity improves cardiovascular event prediction: an individual participant meta-analysis of prospective observational data from 17,635 subjects. J Am Coll Cardiol. 2013;63:636–646. doi: 10.1016/j.jacc.2013.09.063.
22. Vlachopoulos C, Aznaouridis K, Stefanadis C. Prediction of cardiovascular events and all-cause mortality with arterial stiffness: a systematic review and meta-analysis. J Am Coll Cardiol. 2010;55(13):1318–1327.
23. Chen Y, Shen F, Liu J, Yang GY. Arterial stiffness and stroke: de-stiffening strategy, a therapeutic target for stroke. Stroke Vasc Neurol. 2017;2(2):65-72. Published 2017 Mar 17. doi:10.1136/svn-2016-000045.
24. Gunsoo HanYounghwa LeeWisug KoByungjun Cho. Effect of Exercise Therapy on Elasticity of the Blood Vessels. June 2012. Journal of Physical Therapy Science 24(5):401-403. doi: 10.1589/jpts.24.401.
25. Patil S.G., Aithala M.R., Das K.K. Effect of yoga on arterial stiffness in elderly with increased pulse pressure: a randomized controlled study. Complement Ther Med. 2015;23(4):562–569.
26. Metri KG, Pradhan B, Singh A, Nagendra HR. Effect of 1-Week Yoga-Based Residential Program on Cardiovascular Variables of Hypertensive Patients: A Comparative Study. Int J Yoga. 2018;11(2):170=174.
27. Hunter SD, Dhindsa MS, Cunningham E, Tarumi T, Alkatan M, Nualnim N, Tanaka H. The effect of Bikram yoga on arterial stiffness in young and older adults. J Altern Complement Med. 2013 Dec;19(12):930-4. doi: 10.1089/acm.2012.0709. Epub 2013 Jun 5.

Vascular Inflammation

1. Khansari N, Shakiba Y, Mahmoudi M. Chronic inflammation and oxidative stress as a major cause of age-related diseases and cancer. Recent Pat Inflamm Allergy Drug Discov. 2009 Jan;3(1):73-80.
2. Janice K, Glaser K, Belury MA. Omega-3 supplementation lowers inflammation in healthy middle aged and older adults. Brain Behav Immun. 2013;6:988–95.
3. Cox AJ, West NP, Cripps AW. Obesity, inflammation, and the gut microbiota. Lancet Diabetes Endocrinol. 2015 Mar;3(3):207-15. doi: 10.1016/S2213-8587(14)70134-2. Epub 2014 Jul 22.
4. Koene RJ, Prizment AE, Blaes A, Konety SH. Shared Risk Factors in Cardiovascular Disease and Cancer. Circulation. 2016;133: 1104–1114. doi: 10.1161/CIRCULATIONAHA.115.020406.
5. Berk M, Williams LJ, Jacka FN, et al. So depression is an inflammatory disease, but where does the inflammation come from?. BMC Med. 2013;11:200. Published 2013 Sep 12. doi:10.1186/1741-7015-11-200.
6. Felger JC. Imaging the Role of Inflammation in Mood and Anxiety-related Disorders. Curr Neuropharmacol. 2018;16(5):533-558.
7. Rapaport MH, McAllister CG, Pickar D, Nelson DL, Paul SM. Elevated levels of soluble interleukin 2 receptors in schizophrenia. Arch Gen Psychiatry. 1989;46(3):291–2.
8. Shadfar S, Hwang CJ, Lim MS, Choi DY, Hong JT. Involvement of inflammation in Alzheimer's disease pathogenesis and therapeutic potential of anti-inflammatory agents. Arch Pharm Res. 2015;38(12):2106–2119. doi: 10.1007/s12272-015-0648-x.
9. Deon D, Ahmed S, Tai K, Scaletta N, Herrero C, Lee IH, Krause A, Ivashkiv LB. Cross-talk between IL-1 and IL-6 signaling pathways in rheumatoid arthritis synovial fibroblasts. J Immunol. 2001;167:5395–5403.
10. Lia Ginaldi, Maria Cristina Di Benedetto, Massimo De Martinis. Osteoporosis, inflammation and ageing. Immunity & Ageing20052:14. https://doi.org/10.1186/1742-4933-2-14.
11. Page RC. The role of inflammatory mediators in the pathogenesis of periodontal disease. J Periodontal Res. 1991;26(3):230–42.
12. Pedicino D, Liuzzo G, Trotta F, Giglio AF, Giubilato S, Martini F, Zaccardi F, Scavone G, Previtero M, Massaro G, Cialdella P, Cardillo MT, Pitocco D, Ghirlanda G, Crea F. Adaptive

12. immunity, inflammation, and cardiovascular complications in type 1 and type 2 diabetes mellitus. J Diabetes Res. 2013;2013:184258. doi: 10.1155/2013/184258.
13. Donath MY. Targeting inflammation in the treatment of type 2 diabetes: time to start. Nat Rev Drug Discov. 2014;13(6):465–76.
14. Aggarwal BB, Shishodia S, Sandur SK, Pandey MK, Sethi G. Inflammation and cancer: How hot is the link? Biochem Pharmacol. 2006;72:1605–1621.
15. Colotta F, Allavena P, Sica A, Garlanda C, Mantovani A. Cancer-related inflammation, the seventh hallmark of cancer: links to genetic instability. Carcinogenesis. 2009;30(7):1073–1081. doi: 10.1093/carcin/bgp127.)
16. Harris TB, Ferrucci L, Tracy RP, Corti MC, Wacholder S, Ettinger WH Jr, Heimovitz H, Cohen HJ, Wallace R. Associations of elevated interleukin-6 and C-reactive protein levels with mortality in the elderly. Am J Med. 1999 May;106(5):506-12.
17. Krabbe KS, Pedersen M, Bruunsgaard H. Inflammatory mediators in the elderly. Exp Gerontol. 2004;39:687–699.
18. Ross R. Atherosclerosis – an inflammatory disease. N Engl J Med 1999; 340: 115–26.; Blake GJ, Ridker PM. Novel clinical markers of vascular wall inflammation. Circ Res 2001; 89: 763–71.
19. Shah SH, Newby LK. C-reactive protein: a novel marker of cardiovascular risk. Cardiol Rev. 2003;11(4):169–79.
20. Blake GJ, Ridker PM. Inflammatory bio-markers and cardiovascular risk prediction. J Intern Med. 2002;252(4):283–94.
21. Virdis A, Dell'agnello U, Taddei S. Impact of inflammation on vascular disease in hypertension. Maturitas. 2014;78(3):179–183.
22. Ridker PM, Rifai N, Stampfer MJ, Hennekens CH. Plasma concentration of interleukin-6 and the risk of future myocardial infarction among apparently healthy men. Circulation. 2000;101(15):1767–1772.
23. Popa C, Netea MG, van Riel PL, van der Meer JW, Stalenhoef AF. The role of TNF-alpha in chronic inflammatory conditions, intermediary metabolism, and cardiovascular risk. J Lipid Res. 2007 Apr;48(4):751-62. Epub 2007 Jan 2.
24. Ridker PM, Hennekens CH, Buring JE, Rifai N. C-reactive protein and other markers of inflammation in the prediction of cardiovascular disease in women. The New England Journal of Medicine. 2000;342(12):836–843.
25. Stone NJ, Robinson JG, Lichtenstein AH, et al. 2013 ACC/AHA guideline on the treatment of blood cholesterol to reduce atherosclerotic cardiovascular risk in adults: a report of the American College of Cardiology/American Heart Association Task Force on Practice Guidelines. J Am Coll Cardiol. 2014;63(25 Pt B):2889–2934.
26. Kuller LH, Tracy RP, Shaten J, Meilahn EN. Relation of C-reactive protein and coronary heart disease in the MRFIT nested case–control study. Multiple Risk Factor Intervention Trial. Am J Epidemiol 1996; 144: 537–47.
27. Koenig W, Sund M, Frohlich M et al. C-Reactive protein, a sensitive marker of inflammation, predicts future risk of coronary heart disease in initially healthy middle-aged men: results from the MONICA (Monitoring Trends and Determinants in Cardiovascular Disease) Augsburg Cohort Study, 1984–92. Circulation 1999; 99: 237–42.
28. Shah SH, Newby LK. C-reactive protein: a novel marker of cardiovascular risk. Cardiol Rev. 2003 Jul-Aug;11(4):169-79.
29. Ludewig B, Zinkernagel RM, Hengartner H. Arterial inflammation and atherosclerosis. Trends Cardiovasc Med. 2002;12(4):154–9.; Libby P (2002) Inflammation in atherosclerosis. Nature 420, 868–874.
30. Ridker P.M. Inflammatory biomarkers and risks of myocardial infarction, stroke, diabetes, and total mortality: implications for longevity. Nutr. Rev. 2007;65(12 Pt 2):S253–S259.
31. Welsh P, Murray HM, Ford I, Trompet S, de Craen AJ, Jukema JW et al., PROSPER Study Group (2011). Circulating interleukin-10 and risk of cardiovascular events: a prospective study in the elderly at risk. Arterioscler Thromb Vasc Biol 31: 2338–2344.
32. Danesh J, Kaptoge S, Mann AG, Sarwar N, Wood A, Angleman SB et al. (2008). Long-term interleukin-6 levels and subsequent risk of coronary heart disease: two new prospective studies and a systematic review. PLoS Med 5: e78.
33. Neumann F-J, Ott I, Gawaz M, Richardt G, Holzapfel H, Jochum M, et al. Cardiac release of cytokines and inflammatory responses in acute myocardial infarction. Circulation. 1995;92(4):748–55.

34. Frangogiannis NG, Smith CW, Entman ML. The inflammatory response in myocardial infarction. Cardiovascular research. 2002;53(1):31–47.
35. Del Zoppo G, Ginis I, Hallenbeck JM, Iadecola C, Wang X, Feuerstein GZ. Inflammation and stroke: putative role for cytokines, adhesion molecules and iNOS in brain response to ischemia. Brain Pathol. 2000;10(1):95–112.
36. Chamorro Á Role of inflammation in stroke and atherothrombosis. Cerebrovasc Dis. 2004;17(Suppl. 3):1–5.
37. Muir KW, Tyrrell P, Sattar N, Warburton E. Inflammation and ischaemic stroke. Curr Opin Neurol. 2007 Jun;20(3):334-42.
38. Tzoulaki I, Murray GD, Lee AJ, Rumley A, Lowe GD, Fowkes FGR. Inflammatory, haemostatic, and rheological markers for incident peripheral arterial disease: Edinburgh Artery Study. Eur Heart J. 2007;28(3):354–62.
39. Ridker PM, Stampfer MJ, Rifai N. Novel risk factors for systemic atherosclerosis: a comparison of C-reactive protein, fibrinogen, homocysteine, lipoprotein (a), and standard cholesterol screening as predictors of peripheral arterial disease. JAMA. 2001;285(19):2481–5.
40. Kaptoge S, Di Angelantonio E, Lowe G, et al. C-reactive protein concentration and risk of coronary heart disease, stroke, and mortality: an individual participant meta-analysis. Lancet. 2010;375(9709):132–140.
41. Conen D, Ridker PM, Everett BM, et al. A multimarker approach to assess the influence of inflammation on the incidence of atrial fibrillation in women. Eur Heart J. 2010;31(14):1730-6.
42. Ridker PM, Stampfer MJ, Rifai N. Novel risk factors for systemic atherosclerosis: a comparison of C-reactive protein, fibrinogen, homocysteine, lipoprotein(a), and standard cholesterol screening as predictors of peripheral arterial disease. JAMA. 2001 May 16;285(19):2481-5.
43. Lindahl B, Toss H, Siegbahn A, Venge P, Wallentin L. Markers of myocardial damage and inflammation in relation to long-term mortality in unstable coronary artery disease. FRISC Study Group. Fragmin during Instability in Coronary Artery Disease. N Engl J Med. 2000 Oct 19;343(16):1139-47.
44. Thea Morris, Melanie Stables, Adrian Hobbs, Patricia de Souza, Paul Colville-Nash, Tim Warner, Justine Newson, Geoffrey Bellingan, Derek W. Gilroy. Effects of Low-Dose Aspirin on Acute Inflammatory Responses in Humans. The Journal of Immunology August 1, 2009, 183 (3) 2089-2096; DOI: 10.4049/jimmunol.0900477.
45. Kennon S, Price CP, Mills PG, Ranjadayalan K, Cooper J, Clarke H, Timmis AD. The effect of aspirin on C-reactive protein as a marker of risk in unstable angina. J Am Coll Cardiol. 2001 Apr;37(5):1266-70.
46. Patrono, C., G. Ciabattoni, E. Pinca, F. Pugliese, G. Castrucci, A. De Salvo, M. A. Satta, B. A. Peskar. 1980. Low dose aspirin and inhibition of thromboxane B2 production in healthy subjects. Thromb. Res. 17: 317-327.
47. Blake GJ, Ridker PM. Are statins anti-inflammatory? Curr Cont Trials Cardiovasc Medical 2000; 1: 161–5.89.
48. Ridker PM, Rifai N, Lowenthal SP. Rapid reduction C-reactive protein with cerivastatin among 785 patients with primary hypercholesterolemia. Circulation 2001; 103: 1191–3.
49. Babelova A, Sedding DG, Brandes RP (2013). Anti-atherosclerotic mechanisms of statin therapy. Curr Opin Pharmacol 13: 260–264. ;Sirtori CR (2014). The pharmacology of statins. Pharmacol Res 88: 3–11.
50. Knoops K.T., de Groot L.C., Kromhout D., Perrin A.E., Moreiras-Varela O., Menotti A., van Staveren W.A. Mediterranean diet, lifestyle factors, and 10-year mortality in elderly European men and women: The HALE project. JAMA. 2004;292:1433–1439. doi: 10.1001/jama.292.12.1433.
51. Estruch R., Martinez-Gonzalez M.A., Corella D., Salas-Salvado J., Ruiz-Gutierrez V., Covas M.I., Fiol M., Gomez-Gracia E., Lopez-Sabater M.C., Vinyoles E., et al. Effects of a Mediterranean-style diet on cardiovascular risk factors: A randomized trial. Ann. Intern. Med. 2006;145:1–11. doi: 10.7326/0003-4819-145-1-200607040-00004.
52. Lavie CJ, Arena R, Swift DL, et al. Exercise and the cardiovascular system: clinical science and cardiovascular outcomes. Circ Res. 2015;117(2):207-19.
53. Tsoupras A, Lordan R, Zabetakis I. Inflammation, not Cholesterol, Is a Cause of Chronic Disease. Nutrients. 2018;10(5):604. Published 2018 May 12.

54. Woods JA, Wilund KR, Martin SA, Kistler BM. Exercise, inflammation and aging. Aging Dis. 2011;3(1):130-40.doi:10.3390/nu10050604.
55. Vijayaraghava A, Doreswamy V, Narasipur OS, Kunnavil R, Srinivasamurthy N. Effect of Yoga Practice on Levels of Inflammatory Markers After Moderate and Strenuous Exercise. Journal of Clinical and Diagnostic Research : JCDR. 2015;9(6):CC08-CC12. doi:10.7860/JCDR/2015/12851.6021.
56. Kim S, Ju S. Elderly-customized hatha yoga effects on the vascular inflammation factors of elderly women. Journal of Physical Therapy Science. 2017;29(10):1708-1711. doi:10.1589/jpts.29.1708.
57. Kiecolt-Glaser JK, Christian L, Preston H, et al. Stress, inflammation, and yoga practice. Psychosom Med. 2010;72(2):113-21.
58. Vijayaraghava A, Doreswamy V, Narasipur OS, Kunnavil R, Srinivasamurthy N. Effect of Yoga Practice on Levels of Inflammatory Markers After Moderate and Strenuous Exercise. Journal of Clinical and Diagnostic Research : JCDR. 2015;9(6):CC08-CC12. doi:10.7860/JCDR/2015/12851.6021.
59. Pullen PR, Nagamia SH, Mehta PK, Thompson WR, Benardot D, Hammoud R, Parrott JM, Sola S, Khan BV. Effects of yoga on inflammation and exercise capacity in patients with chronic heart failure. J Card Fail. 2008;14:407–413.
60. Kiecolt-Glaser et al., 2010). Kiecolt-Glaser J. K., Christian L., Preston H., Houts C. R., Malarkey W. B., Emery C. F., et al. . (2010). Stress, inflammation, and yoga practice. Psychosom. Med. 72, 113–121. 10.1097/PSY.0b013e3181cb9377.
61. Kiecolt-Glaser J.K., Christian L.M., Andridge R., Hwang B.S., Malarkey W.B., Belury M.A., Emery C.F., Glaser R. Adiponectin, leptin, and yoga practice. Physiol. Behav. 2012;107:809–813. doi: 10.1016/j.physbeh.2012.01.016.
62. Sarvottam K., Magan D., Yadav R.K., Mehta N., Mahapatra S.C. Adiponectin, interleukin-6, and cardiovascular disease risk factors are modified by a short-term yoga-based lifestyle intervention in overweight and obese men. J. Altern. Complement. Med. 2013;19:397–402. doi: 10.1089/acm.2012.0086.
63. Yadav R.K., Magan D., Mehta N., Sharma R., Mahapatra S.C. Efficacy of a short-term yoga-based lifestyle intervention in reducing stress and inflammation: Preliminary results. J. Altern. Complement. Med. 2012;18:662–667. doi: 10.1089/acm.2011.0265.
64. Barbaresko J., Koch M., Schulze M.B., Nöthlings U. Dietary pattern analysis and biomarkers of low-grade inflammation: A systematic literature review. Nutr. Rev. 2013;71:511–527. doi: 10.1111/nure.12035.
65. Piccand E., Vollenweider P., Guessous I., Marques-Vidal P. Association between dietary intake and inflammatory markers: Results from the CoLaus study. Public Health Nutr. 2018;18:1–8.
66. Badimon L., Chagas P., Chiva-Blanch G. Diet and Cardiovascular Disease: Effects of Foods and Nutrients in Classical and Emerging Cardiovascular Risk Factors. Curr. Med. Chem. 2017 doi: 10.2174/0929867324666170428103206.
67. Ross A, Friedmann E, Bevans M, Thomas S. National survey of yoga practitioners: mental and physical health benefits. Complement Ther Med. 2013;21(4):313-23.

Venous Diseases

1. Beebe-Dimmer JL, Pfeifer JR, Engle JS, Schottenfeld D. The epidemiology of chronic venous insufficiency and varicose veins. Ann Epidemiol. 2005;15(3):175–84. doi: 10.1016/j.annepidem.2004.05.015.
2. Fowkes FG, Evans CJ, Lee AJ. Prevalence and risk factors of chronic venous insufficiency. Angiology. 2001;52 Suppl 1:S5–15. ; Robertson L, Evans C, Fowkes FG. Epidemiology of chronic venous disease. Phlebology.2008;23(3):103–11. doi: 10.1258/phleb.2007.007061.
3. Eberhardt RT, Raffetto JD. Chronic venous insufficiency. Circulation. 2005;111(18):2398–409. doi: 10.1161/01.CIR.0000164199.72440.08.
4. Lal BK. Venous ulcers of the lower extremity: definition, epidemiology, and economic and social burdens. Semin Vasc Surg. 2015;28(1):3–5.
5. Donnell TF, Passman MA, Marston WA, et al. Management of venous leg ulcers: clinical practice guidelines of the Society for Vascular Surgery® and the American Venous Forum. J Vasc Surg. 2014;60(2):3S–59S.)
6. Bergan J, Pascarella L. Venous anatomy, physiology, and pathophysiology. In: Bergan JJ,

editor. The vein book. New York: Elsevier; 2007. pp. 39–45.
7. J.F., Gillot C. Anatomy of the foot venous pump: Physiology and influence on chronic venous disease. Phlebology. 2012;27:219–230. doi: 10.1258/phleb.2012.012b01.
8. Ludbrook J. The musculo-venous pumps of the human lower limb. Am. Heart J.1966;71:635–641. doi: 10.1016/0002-8703(66)90313-9.
9. Meissner MH. Lower extremity venous anatomy. Semin Intervent Radiol. 2005;22:147–156.
10. Meissner MH, Moneta G, Burnand K, Gloviczki P, Lohr JM, Lurie F, Mattos MA, McLafferty RB, Mozes G, Rutherford RB, et al. The hemodynamics and diagnosis of venous disease. J Vasc Surg. 2007;46(Suppl):4S–24S. doi: 10.1016/j.jvs.2007.09.043.
11. Bergan J, Pascarella L. Venous anatomy, physiology, and pathophysiology. In: Bergan JJ, editor. The vein book. New York: Elsevier; 2007. pp. 39–45.
12. Bundens WP. The chronically swollen leg: finding the cause: theory and practice Venous Ulcers. New York: Elsevier; 2007. pp. 67–74.).
13. Scott TE, LaMorte WW, Gorin DR, Menzoian JO. Risk factors for chronic venous insufficiency: A dual case-control study. J Vasc Surg. 1995; 22:622–8.
14. Jawien A. The influence of environmental factors in chronic venous insufficiency. Angiology.2003;54 (Suppl 1):S19–31.)
15. Bergan J, Pascarella L. Venous anatomy, physiology, and pathophysiology. In: Bergan JJ, editor. The vein book. New York: Elsevier; 2007. pp. 39–45.
16. Beebe-Dimmer JL, Pfeifer JR, Engle JS, Schottenfeld D. The epidemiology of chronic venous insufficiency and varicose veins. Ann Epidemiol. 2005;15(3):175–84. doi: 10.1016/j.annepidem.2004.05.015.
17. Lopez AP, Phillips TJ. Venous Ulcers. Wounds. 1998;10:149–57.
18. Shaydakov ME, Comerota AJ, Lurie F. Primary venous insufficiency increases risk of deep vein thrombosis. J Vasc Surg Venous Lymphat Disord. 2016 Apr;4(2):161-6. doi: 10.1016/j.jvsv.2015.09.008. Epub 2015 Nov 6.
19. Becker F, Fourgeau P, Carpentier PH, Ouchène A. Quantification of early cutaneous manifestations of chronic venous insufficiency by automated analysis of photographic images: Feasibility and technical considerations. Phlebology. 2018 Jun;33(5):309-314. doi: 10.1177/0268355517703840. Epub 2017 Apr 12.
20. Callam M.J. Epidemiology of varicose veins. Br. J. Surg. 1994;81:167–173. doi: 10.1002/bjs.1800810204.
21. Evans CJ, Fowkes FG, Ruckley CV, Lee AJ. Prevalence of varicose veins and chronic venous insufficiency in men and women in the general population: Edinburgh Vein Study. J Epidemiol Community Health. 1999;53(3):149–153.
22. Partsch H. Varicose veins and chronic venous insufficiency. Vasa 2009 Nov;38(4):293-301.
23. Evans CJ, Fowkes FG, Ruckley CV, Lee AJ. Prevalence of varicose veins and chronic venous insufficiency in men and women in the general population: Edinburgh Vein Study. J Epidemiol Community Health. 1999;53(3):149–153.
24. Ren S, Liu P, Zou N, Tan X. Better outcomes of varicose veins with EVLT alone than in combination with Trivex by GRA. J Grey Syst. 2008;20(3):195–204.
25. Liu P, Ren S, Yang Y, Liu J, Ye Z, Lin F. Intravenous catheter-guided laser ablation: a novel alternative for branch varicose veins. Int Surg. 2011;96(4):331–336.
26. Ren S, Liu P. Initial clinical experiences in treating 27 cases of varicose veins with EVLT plus TRIVEX. J US China Med Sci. 2005;2(1):4–8.
27. Maurins U, Hoffmann BH, Lösch C, et al. Distribution and prevalence of reflux in the superficial and deep venous system in the general population—results from the Bonn Vein Study, Germany. J Vasc Surg. 2008; 48: 680–687.
28. Gloviczki P, Comerota AJ, Dalsing MC, et al; for the Society for Vascular Surgery; American Venous Forum. The care of patients with varicose veins and associated chronic venous diseases: clinical practice guidelines of the Society for Vascular Surgery and the American Venous Forum. J Vasc Surg. 2011; 53 (5 suppl): 2S–48S.
29. Vasquez MA, Munschauer CE. Venous Clinical Severity Score and quality-of-life assessment tools: application to vein practice. Phlebology. 2008;23(6):259–275.
30. Gloviczki P, Comerota AJ, Dalsing MC, et al; for the Society for Vascular Surgery; American Venous Forum. The care of patients with varicose veins and associated chronic venous diseases: clinical practice guidelines of the Society for Vascular Surgery and the American Venous Forum. J Vasc Surg. 2011; 53 (5 suppl): 2S–48S.
31. Gloviczki P et al. Society for Vascular Surgery; American Venous Forum. The care of patients

with varicose veins and associated chronic venous diseases: clinical practice guidelines of the Society for Vascular Surgery and the American Venous Forum. J Vasc Surg. 2011 May;53(5 Suppl):2S-48S. doi: 10.1016/j.jvs.2011.01.079.
32. Biemans AA, Kockaert M, Akkersdijk GP, van den Bos RR, de Maeseneer MG, Cuypers P, et al. Comparing endovenous laser ablation, foam sclerotherapy, and conventional surgery for great saphenous varicose veins. J Vasc Surg. 2013;58(3):727–734.e1.
33. Tellings SS, Ceulen RP, Sommer A. Surgery and endovenous techniques for the treatment of small saphenous varicose veins: a review of the literature. Phlebology. 2011;26(5):179–184.
34. Bush RG. Hammond K.Treatment of incompetent vein of Giacomini (thigh extension branch) Ann Vasc Surg. 2007;21(2):245–248.
35. Rasmussen LH, Lawaetz M, Bjoern L, Vennits B, Blemings A, Eklof B. Randomized clinical trial comparing endovenous laser ablation, radiofrequency ablation, foam sclerotherapy and surgical stripping for great saphenous varicose veins. Br J Surg. 2011;98(8):1079–1087.
36. Attaran RR. Latest Innovations in the Treatment of Venous Disease. J Clin Med. 2018;7(4):77. Published 2018 Apr 11. doi:10.3390/jcm7040077.
37. Rathbun S. The surgeon general's call to action to prevent deep vein thrombosis and pulmonary embolism. Circulation. 2009;119:e480–e482.
38. Cushman M. Epidemiology and risk factors for venous thrombosis. Semin Hematol. 2007;44:62–69. ; , Rathbun S. The surgeon general's call to action to prevent deep vein thrombosis and pulmonary embolism. Circulation. 2009;119:e480–e482.
39. Barker RC, Marval P. Venous thromboembolism: risks and prevention. Contin Educ Anaesth Crit Care Pain. 2011;11:18–23.
40. Silverstein MD, Heit JA, Mohr DN, Petterson TM, O'Fallon WM, Melton LJ. Trends in the incidence of deep vein thrombosis and pulmonary embolism. Arch Intern Med. 1998;158:585.
41. Tagalakis V, Patenaude V, Kahn SR, Suissa S. Incidence of and mortality from venous thromboembolism in a real-world population: the Q-VTE Study Cohort. Am J Med. 2013;126:832.e13–e21.
42. Heit JA, Ashrani A, Crusan DJ, McBane RD, Petterson TM, Bailey KR. Reasons for the persistent incidence of venous thromboembolism. Thromb Haemost. 2017;117:390–400
43. Delluc A, Tromeur C, Le Ven F, et al. Current incidence of venous thromboembolism and comparison with 1998: a community-based study in Western France. Thromb Haemost. 2016;116:967–74.
44. Kahn SR. The post-thrombotic syndrome: the forgotten morbidity of deep venous thrombosis. J Thromb Thrombolysis. 2006;21(1):41–48.
45. Centers for Disease Control and Prevention. Venous thromboembolism (blood clots). Atlanta: CDC, 2015. Available at www.cdc.gov/ncbddd/dvt/data.html.
46. Roberts LN, Patel RK, Donaldson N, et al. Post-thrombotic syndrome is an independent determinant of health-related quality of life following both first proximal and distal deep vein thrombosis . Haematologica. 2014;99(3):e41–e43.
47. Doherty S. Pulmonary embolism An update. Aust Fam Phys 2017 Nov; 46(11):816-820.
48. Wells P, Anderson D. The diagnosis and treatment of venous thromboembolism. Hematology. 2013;2013:457–463.
49. Centers for Disease Control and Prevention. Venous thromboembolism (blood clots). Atlanta: CDC, 2015. Available at www.cdc.gov/ncbddd/dvt/data.html.
50. Heart Disease and Stroke Statistics—2018 Update: A Report From the American Heart Association. Circulation 2018;Jan 31:[Epub ahead of print]. From: https://www.acc.org/latest-in-cardiology/ten-points-to-remember/2018/02/09/11/59/heart-disease-and-stroke-statistics-2018-update.
51. Wang KL, Chu PH, Lee CH, et al. Management of Venous Thromboembolisms: Part I. The Consensus for Deep Vein Thrombosis. Acta Cardiol Sin. 2016;32(1):1-22.
52. Hull R, Hirsh J, Sackett DL, et al. Clinical validity of a negative venogram in patients with clinically suspected venous thrombosis. Circulation. 1981;64(3):622–625.
53. Goodacre S, Sampson F, Thomas S, et al. Systematic review and meta-analysis of the diagnostic accuracy of ultrasonography for deep vein thrombosis. BMC Med Imaging. 2005;5:6.
54. Wells PS, Anderson DR, Rodger M, et al. Evaluation of D-dimer in the diagnosis of suspected deep-vein thrombosis. N Engl J Med. 2003;349(13):1227–1235.
55. Kanne JP, Lalani TA. Role of computed tomography and magnetic resonance imaging for

deep venous thrombosis and pulmonary embolism. Circulation. 2004;109(12 Suppl 1):I15–I21.
56. Agnelli G, Prandoni P, Santamaria MG, et al. Warfarin Optimal Duration Italian Trial Investigators. Three months versus one year of oral anticoagulant therapy for idiopathic deep venous thrombosis. N Engl J Med. 2001;345(3):165–169.
57. Goldhaber SZ. Prevention of recurrent idiopathic venous thromboembolism. Circulation. 2004;110(24 Suppl 1):IV20–IV24.
58. Prandoni P, Lensing AW, Prins MH, Frulla M, Marchiori A, Bernardi E. Below-knee elastic compression stockings to prevent the post-thrombotic syndrome: a randomized, controlled trial. Ann Intern Med. 2004;141:249–256.
59. Kim NH, Delcroix M, Jais X, et al. Chronic thromboembolic pulmonary hypertension. Eur Respir J. 2019;53(1):1801915. Published 2019 Jan 24. doi:10.1183/13993003.01915-2018.
60. Simonneau G, Torbicki A, Dorfmüller P, et al. The pathophysiology of chronic thromboembolic pulmonary hypertension. Eur Respir Rev 2017; 26: 160112.
61. Heart Disease and Stroke Statistics—2017 Update. A Report From the American Heart Association.https://www.ncbi.nlm.nih.gov/pmc/articles/PMC5408160/.
62. Prandoni P, Lensing A, Cogo A, Cuppini S, Villalta S, Carta M, et al. The long-term clinical course of acute deep venous thrombosis. Ann Intern Med. 1996;125:1–7.
63. Stain M, Schonauer V, Minar E, Bialonczyk C, Hirschl M, Weltermann A, et al. The post-thrombotic syndrome: risk factors and impact on the course of thrombotic disease. J Thromb Haemost. 2005;3:2671–2676.
64. Brandjes DP, Buller HR, Heijboer H, Huisman MV, de Rijk M, Jagt H, et al. Randomised trial of effect of compression stockings in patients with symptomatic proximal-vein thrombosis. Lancet. 1997;349:759–762.
65. Prandoni P, Lensing AW, Prins MH, Frulla M, Marchiori A, Bernardi E, et al. Below-knee elastic compression stockings to prevent the post-thrombotic syndrome: a randomized, controlled trial. Ann Intern Med. 2004;141:249–256.
66. Partsch H. Investigations on the pathogenesis of venous leg ulcers. Acta Chir Scand Suppl. 1988;544:25–29. ;11.
67. Junger M, Steins A, Hahn M, Hafner HM. Microcirculatory dysfunction in chronic venous insufficiency (CVI) Microcirculation. 2000;7(6 Pt 2):S3–S12.
68. Leu HJ. Morphology of chronic venous insufficiency—light and electron microscopic examinations. Vasa. 1991;20(4):330–342.
69. Thomas PR, Nash GB, Dormandy JA. White cell accumulation in dependent legs of patients with venous hypertension: a possible mechanism for trophic changes in the skin. Br Med J (Clin Res Ed) 1988;296(6638):1693–1695.
70. Mani R, White JE, Barrett DF, Weaver PW. Tissue oxygenation, venous ulcers and fibrin cuffs. J R Soc Med. 1989;82(6):345–346.
71. Nicolaides A.N., Hussein M.K., Szendro G., Christopoulos D., Vasdekis S., Clarke H. The relation of venous ulceration with ambulatory venous pressure measurements. J Vasc Surg. 1993;17(2):414–419.
72. Agale SV (2013) Chronic leg ulcers: epidemiology, aetiopathogenesis, and management. Ulcers. https://doi.org/10.1155/2013/413604.
73. Bryant RA. Acute and chronic wounds. 2nd ed. St. Louis, MO: Mosby, 2000.
74. Rice JB, Cummings AKG, Skornicki, Parsons N. Burden of venous leg ulcers in the United States. J Med Econ. 2014;17(5):347–356.
75. Graham ID, Harrison MB, Nelson EA, Lorimer K, Fisher A. Prevalence of lower-limb ulceration: a systematic review of prevalence studies. Adv Skin Wound Care. 2003;16:305–316. doi: 10.1097/00129334-200311000-00013.
76. Lal BK. Venous ulcers of the lower extremity: definition, epidemiology, and economic and social burdens. Semin Vasc Surg. 2015;28(1):3–5.
77. Scottish Intercollegiate Guidelines Network (2010) Guideline No. 120: Management of chronic venous leg ulcers. http://www.sign.ac.uk/guidelines/fulltext/120/.
78. Tew GA, Gumber A, McIntosh E, et al. Effects of supervised exercise training on lower-limb cutaneous microvascular reactivity in adults with venous ulcers. Eur J Appl Physiol. 2017;118(2):321-329.
79. Jünger M, Wollina U, Kohnen R, Rabe E. Efficacy and tolerability of an ulcer compression stocking for therapy of chronic venous ulcer compared with a below-knee compression bandage: results from a prospective, randomized, multicentre trial. Current Medical

Research & Opinion. 2004;20:1613–1623.
80. Cullum N, Nelson EA, Fletcher AW, Sheldon TA. In: The Cochrane Library. Issue 4. Oxford: Update Software; 2002. Compression for venous leg ulcers (Cochrane Review); Scottish Intercollegiate Guidelines Network (2010) Guideline No. 120: Management of chronic venous leg ulcers. http://www.sign.ac.uk/guidelines/fulltext/120/.
81. Eberhardt RT, Raffetto JD. Chronic venous insufficiency. Circulation. 2014;130:333–346. doi: 10.1161/CIRCULATIONAHA.113.006898.
82. Kahle B, Hermanns HJ, Gallenkemper G. Evidence-based treatment of chronic leg ulcers. Dtsch Arztebl Int. 2011;108(14):231-7.
83. Eberhardt RT, Raffetto JD. Chronic venous insufficiency. Circulation. 2005;111:2398–2409.); Bergan J. Molecular mechanisms in chronic venous insufficiency. Ann Vasc Surg. 2007;21(3):260–266.
84. Barron GS, Jacob SE, Kirsner RS. Dermatologic complications of chronic venous disease: medical management and beyond. Ann Vasc Surg. 2007;21:652–662.
85. Eberhardt RT, Raffetto JD. Chronic venous insufficiency. Circulation. 2005;111:2398–2409; DaSilva A, Navarro M, Batalheiro J. The importance of chronic venous insufficiency: various preliminary data on its medico-social consequences. Phlebologie. 1992;45:439–443.
86. Briggs M, Flemming K. Living with leg ulceration: a synthesis of qualitative research. J Adv Nurs 2007;59:319–328.
87. Dias TY, Costa IK, Melo MD, Torres SM, Maia EM, Torres Gde V. Quality of life assessment of patients with and without venous ulcer. Rev Lat Am Enfermagem. 2014;22(4):576-81.
88. Brown A. Does social support impact on venous ulcer healing or recurrence? Br J Community Nurs. 2008 Mar;13(3):S6, S8, S10.

Other Lifestyles

1. Menotti A, Puddu PE, Maiani G, Catasta G. Lifestyle behaviour and lifetime incidence of heart diseases. Int J Cardiol. 2015 Dec 15;201:293-9. doi: 10.1016/j.ijcard.2015.08.050. Epub 2015 Aug 4.
2. Victoria Miller, Andrew Mente, Mahshid Dehghan, Sumathy Rangarajan, Xiaohe Zhang, Sumathi Swaminathan, et al. PURE: diet and cardiovascular disease: The Lancet: August 29, 2017.
3. Su C. Y. Aromatherapy and health care. Science Development. 2012;469:26–31.
4. Ju M-S, Lee S, Bae I, Hur M-H, Seong K, Lee MS. Effects of Aroma Massage on Home Blood Pressure, Ambulatory Blood Pressure, and Sleep Quality in Middle-Aged Women with Hypertension. Evidence-based Complementary and Alternative Medicine: eCAM. 2013;2013:403251.
5. Kim I-H, Kim C, Seong K, Hur M-H, Lim HM, Lee MS. Essential Oil Inhalation on Blood Pressure and Salivary Cortisol Levels in Prehypertensive and Hypertensive Subjects. Evidence-based Complementary and Alternative Medicine : eCAM. 2012;2012:984203.
6. Shimada K., Fukuda S., Maeda K., et al. Aromatherapy alleviates endothelial dysfunction of medical staff after night-shift work: preliminary observations. Hypertension Research. 2011;34(2):264–267.
7. Yazdi Z., Sadeghniiat-Haghighi K., Javadi A. R. H. S., Rikhtegar G. Sleep quality and insomnia in nurses with different circadian chronotypes: morningness and eveningness orientation. Work. 2014;47(4):561–567.
8. Chang Y-Y, Lin C-L, Chang L-Y. The Effects of Aromatherapy Massage on Sleep Quality of Nurses on Monthly Rotating Night Shifts. Evidence-based Complementary and Alternative Medicine : eCAM. 2017;2017:3861273.
9. Mi-Yeon Cho, Eun Sil Min, Myung-Haeng Hur, and Myeong Soo Lee. Effects of Aromatherapy on the Anxiety, Vital Signs, and Sleep Quality of Percutaneous Coronary Intervention Patients in Intensive Care Units. Evidence-Based Complementary and Alternative Medicine, Volume 2013, Article ID 381381, 6 pages
10. Mirbastegan Na, Ganjloo Jb, Bakhshandeh Bavarsad Mc, Rakhshani MHd Effects of Aromatherapy on Anxiety and Vital Signs of Myocardial Infarction Patients in Intensive Care Units. IMJM Volume 15 Number 2, Dec 2016.
11. D'Aiuto F, Ready D, Tonetti MS. Periodontal disease and C-reactive protein-associated cardiovascular risk. J Periodont Res 2004;39:236-41.

12. Loos BG, Craandijk J, Hoek FJ, Wertheim-van Dillen PM, van der Velden U. Elevation of systemic markers related to cardiovascular diseases in the peripheral blood of periodontitis patients. J Periodontol 2000;71:1528-34.
13. de Oliveira Cesar, Watt Richard, Hamer Mark. Toothbrushing, inflammation, and risk of cardiovascular disease: results from Scottish Health Survey BMJ 2010; 340: c2451.
14. Peter Libby, Paul M. Ridker and Attilio Maseri. Inflammation and Atherosclerosis. Circulation. 2002;105:1135-1143.
15. Kuwabara M, Motoki Y, Ichiura K et al. Association between toothbrushing and risk factors for cardiovascular disease: a large-scale, cross-sectional Japanese study. BMJ Open. 2016 Jan 14;6(1): e009870.
16. Persson GR, Persson RE. Cardiovascular disease and periodontitis: an update on the associations and risk. J Clin Periodontol 2008;35:362-79.
17. DeStefano F, Anda RF, Kahn HS, Williamson DF, Russell CM. Dental disease and risk of coronary heart disease and mortality. BMJ 1993;306:688-91.
18. Beck J, Garcia R, Heiss G, Vokonas PS, Offenbacher S. Periodontal disease and cardiovascular disease. J Periodontol 1996;67:1123-37.
19. Ashe MC, Miller WC, Eng JJ, Noreau L. Older adults, chronic disease and leisure-time physical activity. Gerontology. 2008;55:64–72.
20. Parmer SM, Salisbury-Glennon J, Shannon D, Struempler B. School gardens: An experiential learning approach for a nutrition education program to increase fruit and vegetable knowledge, preference, and consumption among second-grade students. Journal of Nutrition Education and Behavior. 2009;41:212–217.
21. Davis JN, Ventura EE, Cook LT, Gyllenhammer LE, Gatto NM. LA Sprouts: A gardening, nutrition, and cooking intervention for Latino youth improves diet and reduces obesity. Journal of the American Dietetic Association. 2011;111:1224–1230.
22. E. Ekblom-Bak, B. Ekblom, M. Vikstrom, U. de Faire, M.-L. Hellenius. The importance of non-exercise physical activity for cardiovascular health and longevity. British Journal of Sports Medicine, 2013.
23. Hartig T, Mitchell R, de Vries S, Frumkin H. Nature and health. Annu Rev Public Health. 2014;35:207–228.
24. Shiue I. Gardening is beneficial for adult mental health: Scottish Health Survey, 2012-2013. Scand J Occup Ther. 2016 Jul;23(4):320-5. doi: 10.3109/11038128.2015.1085596. Epub 2015 Sep 16.
25. Clatworthy J, Hinds J, Camic PM. Gardening as a mental health intervention: a review. Ment Health Rev (Brighton) 2013;18(4):214–225.
26. Wakefield S, Yeudall F, Taron C, Reynolds J, Skinner A. Growing urban health: Community gardening in South-East Toronto. Health Promotion International. 2007;22:92–101.
27. Magnus K, Matroos A, Strackee J. Walking, cycling, or gardening, with or without seasonal interruption, in relation to acute coronary events. Am J Epidemiol. 1979 Dec;110(6):724-33.
28. Ho SH, Lin CJ, Kuo FL. The effects of gardening on quality of life in people with stroke. Work. 2016 Jun 27;54(3):557-67. doi: 10.3233/WOR-162338.
29. Twohig-Bennett C, Jones A. The health benefits of the great outdoors: A systematic review and meta-analysis of greenspace exposure and health outcomes. Environ Res. 2018 Oct;166:628-637. doi: 10.1016/j.envres.2018.06.030. Epub 2018 Jul 5.
30. Lêng CH, Wang J-D. Daily home gardening improved survival for older people with mobility limitations: an 11-year follow-up study in Taiwan. Clinical Interventions in Aging. 2016;11:947-959.
31. https://www.yogapedia.com/definition/5020/karma-yoga.
32. Saihara K, Hamasaki S, Ishida S, Kataoka T, et al. Enjoying hobbies is related to desirable cardiovascular effects. Heart Vessels. 2010 Mar;25(2):113-20.
33. Lu L, Argyle M. Leisure satisfaction and happiness as a function of leisure activity. Gaoxiong Yi Xue Ke Xue Za Zhi. 1994 Feb;10(2):89-96.
34. Po-Ju Chang, Linda Wray, and Yeqiang Lin. Social Relationships, Leisure Activity, and Health in Older Adults. Health Psychology. 2014, Vol. 33, No. 6, 516 –523.
35. Alves AJ, Viana JL, Cavalcante SL, et al. Physical activity in primary and secondary prevention of cardiovascular disease: Overview updated. World Journal of Cardiology. 2016;8(10):575-583.

36. Telles S, Sharma SK, Singh N, Balkrishna A. Characteristics of Yoga Practitioners, Motivators, and Yoga Techniques of Choice: A Cross-sectional Study. Front Public Health. 2017;5:184. Published 2017 Jul 27. doi:10.3389/fpubh.2017.00184.
37. United States Census Bureau. Families and Living Arrangements: America's Families and Living Arrangements: 2014: Adults. Table A1: Marital status of people 15 years and over, by age, sex, personal earnings, race, and Hispanic origin. 2014. https://www.census.gov/hhes/families/data/cps2014A.html.
38. Kiecolt-Glaser JK, Newton TL. Marriage and health: His and hers. Psychological Bulletin. 2001;127:472–503.
39. http://www.acc.org/about-acc/press-releases/2014/03/28/09/55/alviar-marital-status.
40. Ben-Shlomo, Smith, Shipley, & Marmot, 1993); Ben-Shlomo Y, Smith GD, Shipley M, Marmot MG. Magnitude and causes of mortality differences between married and unmarried men. Journal of Epidemiology and Community Health. 1993;47:200–205.
41. Cheung YB. Marital status and mortality in British women: A longitudinal study. International Journal of Epidemiology. 2000;29:93–99.
42. https://c.ymcdn.com/sites/iayt.site-ym.com/resource/resmgr/bibliographies-members/stats.pdf) accessed 1/31/19.
43. Kabat-Zinn, 2003; Kabat-Zinn J. (2003). Mindfulness-based interventions in context: past, present, and future. Clin. Psychol. Sci.Pract. 10, 144–156.
44. Gotink RA, Chu P, Busschbach JJ, Benson H, Fricchione GL, Hunink MG. Standardised mindfulness-based interventions in healthcare: an overview of systematic reviews and meta-analyses of RCTs. PLoS One. 2015;10(4):e0124344. doi: 10.1371/journal.pone.0124344.
45. Kabat-Zinn J. Full catastrophe living: How to cope with stress, pain and illness using mindfulness meditation. New York: NY: Bantam Dell; 1990.
46. Strauss C, Cavanagh K, Oliver A, Pettman D. Mindfulness-based interventions for people diagnosed with a current episode of an anxiety or depressive disorder: a meta-analysis of randomised controlled trials. PLoS One. 2014;9(4):e96110. Published 2014 Apr 24. doi:10.1371/journal.pone.0096110.
47. Boyd JE, Lanius RA, McKinnon MC. Mindfulness-based treatments for posttraumatic stress disorder: a review of the treatment literature and neurobiological evidence. J Psychiatry Neurosci. 2017;43(1):7–25. doi:10.1503/jpn.170021.
48. Indranill Basu Ray, Arthur R. Menezes, Pavan Malur, et al. Meditation and Coronary Heart Disease: A Review of the Current Clinical Evidence. Ochsner J. 2014 Winter; 14(4): 696–703.
49. William B. Malarkey, David Jarjoura, Maryanna Klatt, et al. Workplace based mindfulness practice and inflammation: A randomized trial. Brain Behav Immun. 2013 Jan; 27(1): 145–154.
50. Carlson LE, Speca M, Faris P, et al. One-year pre-post intervention follow-up of psychological, immune, endocrine and blood pressure outcomes of mindfulness-based stress reduction (MBSR) in breast and prostate cancer outpatients. Brain Behav Immun. 2007 Nov; 21(8):1038-49.
51. Hartmann M, Kopf S, Kircher C, et al. Sustained effects of a mindfulness-based stress-reduction intervention in type 2 diabetic patients: design and first results of a randomized controlled trial (the Heidelberger Diabetes and Stress-study). Diabetes Care. 2012 May; 35(5):945-7.
52. Paul-Labrador M, Polk D, Dwyer JH, et al. Effects of a randomized controlled trial of transcendental meditation on components of the metabolic syndrome in subjects with coronary heart disease. Arch Intern Med. 2006, 166(11):1218-24.
53. Zeidan F, Martucci KT, Kraft RA, McHaffie JG, Coghill RC. Neural correlates of mindfulness meditation-related anxiety relief. Social Cognitive and Affective Neuroscience. 2014;9(6):751-759.
54. Clara Strauss, Kate Cavanagh, Annie Oliver, et al. Mindfulness-Based Interventions for People Diagnosed with a Current Episode of an Anxiety or Depressive Disorder: A Meta-Analysis of Randomised Controlled Trials. PLoS One. 2014; 9(4): e96110.
55. Ridder HMO, Stige B, Qvale LG, Gold C. Individual music therapy for agitation in dementia: an exploratory randomized controlled trial. Aging Ment Health. 2013;17(6):67–678.
56. Bradt J, Dileo C, Shim M. Music interventions for preoperative anxiety. Cochrane

Database Syst Rev. 2013 Jun 6; (6):CD006908.
57. Yaman Aktaş Y, Karabulut N. Relief of Procedural Pain in Critically Ill Patients by Music Therapy: A Randomized Controlled Trial. Complement Med Res. 2019 Mar 20:1-9. doi: 10.1159/000495301.
58. Nilsson U. The Anxiety and Pain Reducing Effect of Music Intervention. A Systematic Review. AORN Journal. 2008;87:780–807. https://doi.org/10.1016/j.aorn.2007.09.013 PMid:18395022.
59. Iyendo TO. Exploring the effect of sound and music on health in hospital settings: A narrative review. Int J Nurs Stud. 2016 Nov;63:82-100. doi: 10.1016/j.ijnurstu.2016.08.008. Epub 2016 Aug 20.
60. Van der Heijden MJE, Oliai Araghi S, van Dijk M, Jeekel J, Hunink MGM. The Effects of Perioperative Music Interventions in Pediatric Surgery: A Systematic Review and Meta-Analysis of Randomized Controlled Trials. Laks J, ed. PLoS ONE. 2015;10(8): e0133608.
61. White JM. Effects of relaxing music on cardiac autonomic balance and anxiety after acute myocardial infarction. American Journal of Critical Care. 1999;8:220–230.
62. Bradt J, Dileo C, Potvin N. Music for stress and anxiety reduction in coronary heart disease patients. Cochrane Database Syst Rev. 2013 Dec 28;(12):CD006577.
63. Möckel M, Röcker L, Störk T, et al. Immediate physiological responses of healthy volunteers to different types of music: cardiovascular, hormonal and mental changes. Eur J Appl Physiol Occup Physiol. 1994; 68(6):451-9.
64. Mirbagher Ajorpaz N, Mohammadi A, Najaran H, Khazaei S. Effect of Music on Postoperative Pain in Patients Under Open Heart Surgery. Nursing and Midwifery Studies. 2014;3(3): e20213.
65. Alter DA, O'Sullivan M, Oh PI, et al. Synchronized personalized music audio-playlists to improve adherence to physical activity among patients participating in a structured exercise program: a proof-of-principle feasibility study. Sports Medicine - Open. 2015;1:23.
66. Teppo Sarkamo, Mari Tervaniemi, Sari Laitinen et al. Music listening enhances cognitive recovery and mood after middle cerebral artery stroke. Brain (2008), 131, 866 – 876.
67. Naresh Sen. Evaluation of heart rate variability and cardiac autonomic control on exposure to Indian music and slow music yoga asana before sleep at night. Poster Session 5: Cardiovascular rehabilitation. Monday 27 August,2018.
68. U.S. Pet Ownership & Demographics Sourcebook. 2012 https://www.avma.org/kb/resources/statistics/pages/market-research-statistics-us-pet-ownership-demographics-sourcebook.aspx.
69. Anderson WP, Reid CM, Jennings GL. Pet owners have lower levels of accepted risk factors for cardiovascular disease. Med J Aust. 1992 Sep 7;157(5):298-301.
70. Arhant-Sudhir K, Arhant-Sudhir R, Sudhir K. Pet ownership and cardiovascular risk reduction: supporting evidence, conflicting data and underlying mechanisms. Clin Exp Pharmacol Physiol. 2011 Nov;38(11):734-8.
71. Levine GN, Allen K, Braun LT, et al. Pet ownership and cardiovascular risk: a scientific statement from the American Heart Association. Circulation 2013;127:2353–63.
72. Oka K., Shibata A. Dog ownership and health-related physical activity among japanese adults. Journal of Physical Activity and Health. 2009;6(4):412–418.
73. Lentino C, Visek AJ, McDonnell K, DiPietro L. Dog walking is associated with a favorable risk profile independent of a moderate to high volume of physical activity. J Phys Act Health. 2012;9:414–20.
74. Katherine Jacobs Bao & George Schreer (2016) Pets and Happiness: Examining the Association between Pet Ownership and Wellbeing, Anthrozoös, 29:2, 283-296. DOI: 10.1080/08927936.2016.1152721.
75. Wright J. D., Kritz-Silverstein D., Morton D. J., Wingard D. L., Barrett-Connor E. Pet ownership and blood pressure in old age. Epidemiology. 2007;18(5):613–618. doi: 10.1097/EDE.0b013e3181271398.
76. Qureshi AI, Memon MA, Vazquez G, Suri MFK. Cat ownership and risk of fatal cardiovascular diseases. Results from the second national health and nutrition examination study mortality follow-up study. J Vasc Interv Neurol. 2009;2(1):132–5.
77. Xie ZY, Zhao D, Chen BR, et al. Association between pet ownership and coronary artery disease in a Chinese population. Medicine (Baltimore). 2017;96(13):e6466.
78. Friedmann E, Katcher AH, Lynch JL, Thomas SA. Animal companions and one-year

survival of patients after discharge from a coronary care unit. Public Health Rep. 1980;95(4):307–12.
79. Friedmann E, Thomas SA, H S, for the HAT Investigators Pets, depression and long-term survival in community living patients following myocardial infarction. Anthrozoös. 2011;24(3):273–85.
80. Lai H-K, Tsang H, Wong C-M. Meta-analysis of adverse health effects due to air pollution in Chinese populations. BMC Public Health. 2013; 13:360.
81. www.who.int.
82. Ito K, Mathes R, Ross Z, Nádas A, Thurston G, Matte T. Fine Particulate Matter Constituents Associated with Cardiovascular Hospitalizations and Mortality in New York City. Environmental Health Perspectives. 2011;119(4):467-473.
83. Pope CA 3rd, Dockery DW. Health effects of fine particulate air pollution: lines that connect. J Air Waste Manag Assoc. 2006; 56: 709–742.
84. Hoek G, Krishnan RM, Beelen R, et al. Long-term air pollution exposure and cardio-respiratory mortality: a review. Environmental Health. 2013;12:43.
85. Ljungman PL, Mittleman MA. Ambient Air Pollution and Stroke. Stroke; a journal of cerebral circulation. 2014;45(12):3734-3741.
86. Shah ASV, Lee KK, McAllister DA, et al. Short term exposure to air pollution and stroke: systematic review and meta-analysis. The BMJ. 2015;350:h1295.
87. Shah AS, Langrish JP, Nair H, et al. Global association of air pollution and heart failure: a systematic review and meta-analysis. Lancet. 2013;382(9897):1039-1048.
88. Wichmann J, Folke F, Torp-Pedersen C, et al. Out-of-Hospital Cardiac Arrests and Outdoor Air Pollution Exposure in Copenhagen, Denmark. ten Cate H, ed. PLoS ONE. 2013;8(1): e53684.
89. Hoek G, Krishnan RM, Beelen R, et al. Long-term air pollution exposure and cardio-respiratory mortality: a review. Environmental Health. 2013;12:43.
90. Guo Y, Li S, Tawatsupa B, Punnasiri K, Jaakkola JJK, Williams G. The association between air pollution and mortality in Thailand. Scientific Reports. 2014;4:5509.
91. Babisch W. Noise and health. Environ Health Perspect 2005;113(1):A14–5. 10.1289/ehp.113-a14.
92. Barbara Hoffmann, Susanne Moebus, Andreas Stang, et al. Residence close to high traffic and prevalence of coronary heart disease. Eur Heart J (2006) 27 (22): 2696-2702.
93. Babisch W. Transportation noise and cardiovascular risk: Updated review and synthesis of epidemiological studies indicate that the evidence has increased. Noise Health. 2006;8:1–29.
94. Angel Mario Dzhambov. Long¬term noise exposure and the risk for type 2 diabetes: A metaanalysis. Noise Health. 2015 Jan¬Feb; 17(74): 23–33.
95. Seidler A, Hegewald J, Seidler AL, et al. Association between aircraft, road and railway traffic noise and depression in a large case-control study based on secondary data. Environ Res. 2017 Jan;152:263-271. doi: 10.1016/j.envres.2016.10.017. Epub 2016 Nov 3.
96. Rylander R, Bjorkman M. Annoyance by aircraft noise around small airports. J Sound Vibrat 1997;205(4):533–7 10.1006/jsvi.1997.1022.
97. Münzel T, Daiber A, Steven S, et al. Effects of noise on vascular function, oxidative stress, and inflammation: mechanistic insight from studies in mice. Eur Heart J. 2017 Feb 17.
98. Eriksson C, Rosenlund M, Pershagen G, Hilding A, Ostenson CG, Bluhm G. Aircraft noise and incidence of hypertension. Epidemiology 2007;18(6):716–21. 10.1097/EDE.0b013e3181567e77.
99. Babisch WF, Beule B, Schust M, Kersten N, Ising H. Traffic noise and risk of myocardial infarction, Epidemiology, 2005, vol. 16 (pg. 33-40).
100. Seidler A, Wagner M, Schubert M, et al. Aircraft, road and railway traffic noise as risk factors for heart failure and hypertensive heart disease-A case-control study based on secondary data. Int J Hyg Environ Health. 2016 Nov;219(8):749-758.
101. Vandasova Z, Vencálek O, Puklová V. Specific and combined subjective responses to noise and their association with cardiovascular diseases. Noise Health. 2016 Nov-Dec;18(85):338-346.
102. Davies HW, Teschke K, Kennedy SM, et al. Occupational exposure to noise and mortality from acute myocardial infarction, Epidemiology, 2005, vol. 16: 25-32.
103. Booth FW, Roberts CK, Laye MJ. Lack of exercise is a major cause of chronic diseases. Compr Physiol. 2012;2(2):1143–1211. doi:10.1002/cphy.c110025.

104. Haskell, W. L., Lee, I-M., Pate, R. R., et al. (2007). Physical activity and public health: Updated recommendation for adults from the American College of Sports Medicine and the American Heart Association. Circulation, Volume 116, Issue 9, 2007, pages 1081-1093.
105. Teramoto M, Bungum TJ: Mortality and longevity of elite athletes. J Sci Med Sport 2010; 13: 410–6.
106. Blair SN, Goodyear NN, Gibbons LW, et al. Physical fitness and incidence of hypertension in healthy normotensive men and women. JAMA 1984;252:487-90.
107. Berg A, Halle M, Franz I, et al. Physical activity and lipoprotein metabolism: epidemiological evidence and clinical trials. Eur J Med Res 1997;2:259-64.
108. Tremblay A, Despres JP, Leblanc C, et al. Effect of intensity of physical activity on body fatness and fat distribution. Am J Clin Nutr 1990;51:153-7.
109. AbouAssi H, Slentz CA, Mikus CR, et al. The effects of aerobic, resistance, and combination training on insulin sensitivity and secretion in overweight adults from STRRIDE AT/RT: a randomized trial. J Appl Physiol (1985). 2015;118(12):1474–1482. doi:10.1152/japplphysiol.00509.2014.
110. Wallberg-Henriksson H, Rincon J, Zierath JR. Exercise in the management of non-insulin-dependent diabetes mellitus. Sports Med 1998;25:25-35.
111. Adamopoulos S, Parissis J, Kroupis C, et al. Physical training reduces peripheral markers of inflammation in patients with chronic heart failure. Eur Heart J 2001;22:791-7.
112. Warburton DE, Haykowsky MJ, Quinney HA, et al. Blood volume expansion and cardiorespiratory function: effects of training modality. Med Sci Sports Exerc 2004;36:991-1000.
113. Dunn AL, Trivedi MH, O'Neal HA. Physical activity dose–response effects on outcomes of depression and anxiety. [discussion 609-10]. Med Sci Sports Exerc 2001;33:S587-97.
114. Ray US, Pathak A, Tomer OS. Hatha yoga practices: Energy expenditure, respiratory changes and intensity of exercise. Evid Based Complement Alternat Med. 2011; 2011:241294.
115. Sovová E, Čajka V, Pastucha D, et al. Positive effect of yoga on cardiorespiratory fitness: A pilot study. Int J Yoga. 2015 Jul-Dec;8(2):134-8.
116. Tracy BL, Hart CE. Bikram yoga training and physical fitness in healthy young adults. J Strength Cond Res. 2013 Mar;27(3):822-30. doi: 10.1519/JSC.0b013e31825c340f.
117. Hart CE, Tracy BL. Yoga as steadiness training: effects on motor variability in young adults. J Strength Cond Res. 2008 Sep;22(5):1659-69. doi: 10.1519/JSC.0b013e31818200dd.
118. Amin DJ, Goodman M. The effects of selected asanas in Iyengar yoga on flexibility: pilot study. J Bodyw Mov Ther. 2014 Jul;18(3):399-404. doi: 10.1016/j.jbmt.2013.11.008. Epub 2013 Nov 8.
119. Polsgrove MJ, Eggleston BM, Lockyer RJ. Impact of 10-weeks of yoga practice on flexibility and balance of college athletes. Int J Yoga. 2016;9(1):27-34.
120. Donohue B, Miller A, Beisecker M, et al. Effects of brief yoga exercises and motivational preparatory interventions in distance runners: results of a controlled trial. Br J Sports Med. 2006;40(1):60-3; discussion 60-3.
121. Bera TK, Rajapurkar MV. Body composition, cardiovascular endurance and anaerobic power of yogic practitioner. Indian J Physiol Pharmacol. 1993;37:225–8.
122. Parikh HN, Patel HM, Pathak NR, Chandwani S. Effect of yoga practices on respiratory parameters in healthy young adults. Natl J Integr Res Med. 2014;3:37–41.
123. Yadav RK, Das S. Effect of yogic practice on pulmonary functions in young females. Indian J Physiol Pharmacol. 2001;45:493–6.
124. Pansare M S, Kulkarni A N, Pendse U B. Effect of yogic training on serum LDH levels. J Sports Med Phys Fitness 198929177–178.
125. Ives J C. Beyond mind-body exercise hype. Phys Sportmed 20002867–81, Kulmatycki L, Bukowska K. Differences in experiencing relaxation by sport coaches in relation to sport type and gender. Hum Mov. 2007;8(2):98–103.
126. Brunelle JF, Blais-Coutu S, Gouadec K, Bédard É, Fait P. Influences of a yoga intervention on the postural skills of the Italian short track speed skating team. Open Access J Sports Med. 2015;6:23-35. Published 2015 Feb 12. doi:10.2147/OAJSM.S68337.
127. Weisburger JH. Tea and health: a historical perspective. Cancer Lett. 1997;114(1–2):315–317.

128. Hayakawa S, Saito K, Miyoshi N, Ohishi T, Oishi Y, Miyoshi M, Nakamura Y. Anti-Cancer Effects of Green Tea by Either Anti- or Pro- Oxidative Mechanisms. Asian Pac J Cancer Prev. 2016;17(4):1649-54.
129. Noguchi-Shinohara M, Yuki S, Dohmoto C, et al. Consumption of green tea, but not black tea or coffee, is associated with reduced risk of cognitive decline. PLoS One. 2014;9(5):e96013. Published 2014 May 14. doi:10.1371/journal.pone.0096013.
130. Sun K, Wang L, Ma Q, et al. Association between tea consumption and osteoporosis: A meta-analysis. Medicine (Baltimore). 2017;96(49):e9034.
131. Balentine DA, Wiseman SA, Bouwens LC. The chemistry of tea flavonoids. Crit Rev Food Sci Nutr. 1997;37 (8):693–704.
132. Basu A, Lucas EA. Mechanisms and effects of green tea on cardiovascular health. Nutr Rev. 2007 Aug;65(8 Pt 1):361-75.
133. Greyling A, Ras RT, Zock PL, et al. The Effect of Black Tea on Blood Pressure: A Systematic Review with Meta-Analysis of Randomized Controlled Trials. Schillaci G, ed. PLoS ONE. 2014;9(7): e103247.
134. The InterAct Consortium. Tea Consumption and Incidence of Type 2 Diabetes in Europe: The EPIC-InterAct Case-Cohort Study. Herder C, ed. PLoS ONE. 2012;7(5): e36910.
135. Stensvold I, Tverdal A, Solvoll K, Foss OP. Tea consumption. relationship to cholesterol, blood pressure, and coronary and total mortality. Prev Med. 1992;21:546–53.
136. Wu CH, Lu FH, Chang TC, et al. Relationship among habitual tea consumption, percent body fat, and body fat distribution. Obesity. 2003;11(9):1088–1095.
137. Donnelly GF. The tea ceremony: connecting with self and others. Holist Nurs Pract. 2007 Sep-Oct;21(5):215.
138. Neyestani TR, Shariatzade N, Kalayi A, et al. Regular daily intake of black tea improves oxidative stress biomarkers and decreases serum C-reactive protein levels in type 2 diabetic patients. Ann Nutr Metab. 2010;57:40–9.
139. Steptoe A, Gibson EL, Vuononvirta R, Hamer M, Wardle J, Rycroft JA, et al. The effects of chronic tea intake on platelet activation and inflammation: a double-blind placebo controlled trial. Atherosclerosis. 2007;193:277–82.
140. Peters U, Poole C, Arab L. Does tea affect cardiovascular disease? a meta-analysis. Am J Epidemiol. 2001;154:495–503.
141. Bøhn SK, Ward NC, Hodgson JM, et al. Effects of tea and coffee on cardiovascular disease risk. Food Funct. 2012;3(6):575–91.; 12.
142. Wen W, Xiang Y-B, Zheng W, et al. The association of alcohol, tea, and other modifiable lifestyle factors with myocardial infarction and stroke in Chinese men. CVD prevention and control. 2008;3(3):133-140.
143. De Koning Gans JM, Uiterwaal CS, van der Schouw YT, Boer JM, Grobbee DE, Verschuren WM, et al. Tea and coffee consumption and cardiovascular morbidity and mortality. Arterioscler Thromb Vasc Biol. 2010;30:1665–71.
144. De Koning Gans JM, Uiterwaal CS, van der Schouw YT, Boer JM, Grobbee DE, Verschuren WM, et al. Tea and coffee consumption and cardiovascular morbidity and mortality. Arterioscler Thromb Vasc Biol. 2010;30:1665–71.
145. Mineharu Y, Koizumi A, Wada Y, et al. Coffee, green tea, black tea and Oolong tea consumption and risk of mortality from cardiovascular disease in Japanese men and women. J Epidemiol Community Health. 2011;65(3):230–240.
146. Diener E, Lucas RE, Oishi S. Subjective well-being: the science of happiness and life satisfaction. In: Snyder CR, Lopez SJ, editors. Handbook of Positive Psychology. New York: Oxford University Press; 2002.
147. Ryff CD, Singer BH, Dienberg Love G. Positive health: connecting well-being with biology. Philos Trans R Soc Lond B Biol Sci. 2004;359:1383–94.
148. Ulrich RS, Simons RF, Losito BD, Fiorito E, Miles MA, Zelson M. Stress recovery during exposure to natural and urban environments. J Environ Psychol. 1991;11:201–30.
149. Staats H, Gatersleben B, Hartig T. Change in mood as a function of environmental design: arousal and pleasure on a simulated forest hike. J Environ Psychol. 1997;17:283–300.
150. Cohen S, Doyle WJ, Skoner DP, Rabin BS, Gwaltney JM., Jr Social ties and susceptibility to the common cold. JAMA. 1997;277:1940–4.
151. Gump BB, Matthews KA. Are vacations good for your health? The 9-year mortality experience after the multiple risk factor intervention trial. Psychosom Med.

2000;62:608–12.
152. Tominaga K, Andow J, Koyama Y, Numao S, Kurokawa E, Ojima M, Nagai M. Family environment, hobbies and habits as psychosocial predictors of survival for surgically treated patients with breast cancer. Jpn J Clin Oncol. 1998;28:36–4122–24.
153. Epel ES, Puterman E, Lin J, et al. Meditation and vacation effects have an impact on disease-associated molecular phenotypes. Translational Psychiatry. 2016;6(8): e880.
154. Elaine D. Eaker, Joan Pinsky, William P. Castelli; Myocardial Infarction and Coronary Death among Women: Psychosocial Predictors from a 20-Year Follow-up of Women in the Framingham Study, American Journal of Epidemiology, Volume 135, Issue 8, 15 April 1992, Pages 854–864.
155. Multiple Risk Factor Intervention Trial Risk Factor Changes and Mortality Results. JAMA. 1982;248(12):1465–1477.
156. Gump BB, Matthews KA. Are vacations good for your health? The 9-year mortality experience after the multiple risk factor intervention trial. Psychosom Med. 2000 Sep-Oct;62(5):608-12.
157. Holick M. F., Chen T. C. Vitamin D deficiency: a worldwide problem with health consequences. The American Journal of Clinical Nutrition. 2008;87(4, supplement) :1080S–1086S.
158. Institute of Medicine, Food and Nutrition Board. Dietary Reference Intakes for Calcium and Vitamin D. Washington, DC: National Academy Press, 2010.
159. Holick MF. Vitamin D. In: Shils ME, Shike M, Ross AC, Caballero B, Cousins RJ, eds. Modern Nutrition in Health and Disease, 10th ed. Philadelphia: Lippincott Williams & Wilkins, 2006.
160. Norman AW, Henry HH. Vitamin D. In: Bowman BA, Russell RM, eds. Present Knowledge in Nutrition, 9th ed. Washington DC: ILSI Press, 2006.4.
161. Theodoratou E, Tzoulaki I, Zgaga L, Ioannidis JP. Vitamin D and multiple health outcomes. BMJ. 2014;348:g2035.
162. T. Pincikova, D. Paquin-Proulx, J. K. Sandberg, M. Flodström-Tullberg, L. Hjelte. Vitamin D treatment modulates immune activation in cystic fibrosis.Clin Exp Immunol. 2017 Sep; 189(3): 359–371. Published online 2017 May 24.
163. Holick MF. Vitamin D and sunlight: strategies for cancer prevention and other health benefits. Clin J Am Soc Nephrol. 2008;3(5):1548–1554.
164. Yamshchikov AV, Desai NS, Blumberg HM, Ziegler TR, Tangpricha V. Vitamin D for treatment and prevention of infectious diseases: a systematic review of randomized controlled trials. Endocr Pract. 2009;15(5):438–449. doi:10.4158/EP09101.ORR.
165. Doğan Bulut S, Bulut S, Görkem Atalan D, et al. The Relationship between Symptom Severity and Low Vitamin D Levels in Patients with Schizophrenia. PLoS One. 2016;11(10):e0165284. Published 2016 Oct 27. doi:10.1371/journal.pone.0165284.
166. Wacker M, Holick MF. Sunlight and Vitamin D: A global perspective for health. Dermato-endocrinology. 2013;5(1):51-108.
167. Melamed ML, Michos ED, Post W, Astor B. 25-hydroxyvitamin D levels and the risk of mortality in the general population. Arch Intern Med. 2008;168:1629–1637.
168. Kienreich K., Tomaschitz A., Verheyen N., et al. Vitamin D and cardiovascular disease. Nutrients. 2013;5(8):3005–3021.
169. Earthman C.P., Beckman L.M., Masodkar K., Sibley S.D. The link between obesity and low 25-hydroxyvitamin D concentrations: Considerations and implications. Int. J. Obes. (Lond.) 2012;36:387–396.
170. Jorde R., Grimnes G. Vitamin D and metabolic health with special reference to the effect of vitamin D on serum lipids. Prog. Lipid Res. 2011;50:303–312.
171. Forouhi NG, Ye Z, Rickard AP, et al. Circulating 25-hydroxyvitamin D concentration and the risk of type 2 diabetes: results from the European Prospective Investigation into Cancer (EPIC)-Norfolk cohort and updated meta-analysis of prospective studies. Diabetologia. 2012;55(8):2173–2182.
172. Witham M.D., Nadir M.A., Struthers A.D. Effect of vitamin D on blood pressure: A systematic review and meta-analysis. J. Hypertens. 2009;27:1948–1954.
173. Wang TJ, Pencina MJ, Booth SL, et al. Vitamin D deficiency and risk of cardiovascular disease. Circulation. 2008;117(4):503–511.
174. Bae S, Singh SS, Yu H, Lee JY, Cho BR, Kang PM. Vitamin D signaling pathway plays an important role in the development of heart failure after myocardial infarction. J Appl

Physiol (1985) 2013;114(8):979–87.
175. Chowdhury R., Stevens S., Ward H., Chowdhury S., Sajjad A., Franco O.H. Circulating vitamin D, calcium and risk of cerebrovascular disease: A systematic review and meta-analysis. Eur. J. Epidemiol. 2012;27:581–591.
176. Melamed ML, Munter P, Michos ED, Uribarri J, Weber C, Sharma J, Raggi P. Serum 25-hydroxyvitamin D levels and the prevalence of peripheral arterial disease. Atheroscler Thromb VascBiol. 2008;28:1179–1185.
177. Pilz S, Marz W, Wellnitz B, Seelhorst U, Fahrleitner-Pammer A, Dimai HP, Boehm BO, Dobnig H. Association of vitamin D deficiency with heart failure and sudden cardiac death in a large cross-sectional study of patients referred for coronary angiography. J Clin Endocrinol Metab. 2008;93:3927–3935.
178. Zittermann A., Prokop S. The role of vitamin D for cardiovascular disease and overall mortality. Advances in Experimental Medicine and Biology. 2014;810:106–119.
179. Ford JA, MacLennan GS, Avenell A, Bolland M, Grey A, Witham M; RECORD Trial Group. Cardiovascular disease and vitamin D supplementation: trial analysis, systematic review, and meta-analysis. Am J Clin Nutr. 2014 Sep;100(3):746-55. doi: 10.3945/ajcn.113.082602. Epub 2014 Jul 23.
180. Schnatz PF, Manson JE. Vitamin D and cardiovascular disease: an appraisal of the evidence. Clin Chem. 2013;60(4):600-9.
181. https://ods.od.nih.gov/factsheets/VitaminD-HealthProfessional/
182. Chandola T, Brunner E, Marmot M. Chronic stress at work and the metabolic syndrome: Prospective study. BMJ. 2006;332(7540):521–525. doi: 10.1136/bmj.38693.435301.80.
183. Maslach C., Jackson S.E., Leiter M.P. Maslach Burnout Inventory. 2nd ed. Consulting Psychologists Press; Palo Alto, CA, USA: 1986.
184. Konze AK, Rivkin W, Schmidt KH. Is Job Control a Double-Edged Sword? A Cross-Lagged Panel Study on the Interplay of Quantitative Workload, Emotional Dissonance, and Job Control on Emotional Exhaustion. Int J Environ Res Public Health. 2017;14(12):1608. Published 2017 Dec 20. doi:10.3390/ijerph14121608.
185. Frone MR, Tidwell MO. The meaning and measurement of work fatigue: Development and evaluation of the Three-Dimensional Work Fatigue Inventory (3D-WFI). J Occup Health Psychol. 2015;20(3):273-288.
186. Maruyama S, Morimoto K. Effects of long workhours on life-style, stress and quality of life among intermediate Japanese managers. Scand J Work Environ Health 1996;22(5):353-359.
187. Yoo DH, Kang M, Paek D, Min B, Cho S. Effect of Long Working Hours on Self reported Hypertension among Middle-aged and Older Wage Workers. Annals of Occupational and Environmental Medicine. 2014;26:25.
188. Kawakami N, Araki S, Takatsuka N, Shimizu H, Ishibashi H. Overtime, psychosocial working conditions, and occurrence of non- insulin dependent diabetes mellitus in Japanese men. Journal of Epidemiology and Community Health. 1999;53(6):359-363.
189. Kobayashi T, Suzuki E, Takao S, Doi H. Long working hours and metabolic syndrome among Japanese men: a cross-sectional study. BMC Public Health. 2012;12:395.
190. Virtanen M, Stansfeld SA, Fuhrer R, Ferrie JE, Kivimäki M. Overtime work as a predictor of major depressive episode: A 5-year follow-up of the Whitehall II study. PloS One. 2012;7: e30719.
191. Kang MY, Park H, Seo JC, et al. Long working hours and cardiovascular disease: a meta-analysis of epidemiologic studies. J Occup Environ Med. 2012 May;54(5):532-7.
192. Virtanen M, Ferrie JE, Singh-Manoux A, et al. Overtime work and incident coronary heart disease: The Whitehall II prospective cohort study. Eur Heart J. 2010;31:1737–1744.
193. Ke DS. Overwork, stroke, and karoshi-death from overwork. Acta Neurol Taiwan. 2012 Jun;21(2):54-9.
194. Conway SH, Pompeii LA, Roberts RE, Follis JL, Gimeno D. Dose-Response Relation Between Work Hours and Cardiovascular Disease Risk: Findings From the Panel Study of Income Dynamics. J Occup Environ Med. 2016 Mar;58(3):221-6. doi: 10.1097/JOM.0000000000000654.
195. Rosengren A, Hawken S, Ounpuu S, Sliwa K, Zubaid M, Almahmeed W, Blackett K, Sitti-amorn C, Sato H, Yuself S. Association of psychosocial risk factors with risk of acute myocardial infarction in 11,119 cases and 13,648 controls from 52 countries (the

INTERHEART study): case-control study. The Lancet. 2004;364:953–962. doi: 10.1016/S0140-6736(04)17019-0.
196. Kivimäki M, Virtanen M, Elovainio M, Kouvonen A, Vaananen A, Vahtera J. Work stress in the etiology of coronary heart disease - a meta-analysis. Scand J Work Environ Health. 2006;32(6):431–442. doi: 10.5271/sjweh.1049.
197. Kivimäki M, Kawachi I. Work Stress as a Risk Factor for Cardiovascular Disease. Curr Cardiol Rep. 2015;17(9):630.
198. Ke DS. Overwork, stroke, and karoshi-death from overwork. Acta Neurol Taiwan. 2012 Jun;21(2):54-9.
199. Wolever RQ, Bobinet KJ, McCabe K, Mackenzie ER, Fekete E, Kusnick CA, Baime M. Effective and viable mind-body stress reduction in the workplace: a randomized controlled trial. J Occup Health Psychol. 2012 Apr;17(2):246-258. doi: 10.1037/a0027278. Epub 2012 Feb 20.
200. Fang R, Li X. A regular yoga intervention for staff nurse sleep quality and work stress: a randomised controlled trial. J Clin Nurs. 2015 Dec;24(23-24):3374-9. doi: 10.1111/jocn.12983. Epub 2015 Oct 19.
201. Alexander GK, Rollins K, Walker D, Wong L, Pennings J. Yoga for Self-Care and Burnout Prevention Among Nurses. Workplace Health Saf. 2015 Oct;63(10):462-70; quiz 471. doi: 10.1177/2165079915596102.
202. de Bruin EI, Formsma AR, Frijstein G, Bögels SM. Mindful2Work: Effects of Combined Physical Exercise, Yoga, and Mindfulness Meditations for Stress Relieve in Employees. A Proof of Concept Study. Mindfulness (N Y). 2016;8(1):204-217.
203. Granath J, Ingvarsson S, von TU, Lundberg U. Stress management: a randomized study of cognitive behavioural therapy and yoga. Cogn Behav Ther. 2006;35(1):3–10. http://dx.doi.org/10.1080/16506070500401292.
204. Edmondson D, Richardson S, Falzon L, et al. Posttraumatic stress disorder prevalence and risk of recurrence in acute coronary syndrome patients: a meta-analytic review. PLoS ONE. 2012;7:e38915.
205. Roest AM, Martens EJ, de Jonge P, Denollet J. Anxiety and risk of incident coronary heart disease: a meta-analysis. J Am Coll Cardiol. 2010;56(1): 38-46.
206. Posadzki P, Kuzdzal A, Lee MS, Ernst E. Yoga for heart rate variability: A systematic review and meta-analysis of randomized clinical trials. Appl Psychophysiol Biofeedback. 2015;40:239–49.
207. Singh VP, Khandelwal B, Sherpa NT. Psycho-neuro-endocrine-immune mechanisms of action of yoga in type II diabetes. Anc Sci Life. 2015;35(1):12-7.

Yoga program for the heart and circulatory system

1. Iyengar BKS. Light on Yoga—The Classic Guide to Yoga by the World's Foremost Authority. New Delhi, India: HarperCollins; 2004.
2. Adam Burke, Chun Nok Lam, Barbara Stussman and Hui Yang. Meditation Prevalence and patterns of use of mantra, mindfulness and spiritual meditation among adults in the United States. BMC Complementary and Alternative MedicineBMC series – open, inclusive and trusted201717:316. https://doi.org/10.1186/s12906-017-1827-8.

Yoga Nidra

1. Satyananda SS. Yoga nidra. 6 th ed. India: Yoga publication Trust; 2009.
2. Parker S, Bharati SV, Fernandez M. Defining yoga-nidra: traditional accounts, physiological research, and future directions. Int J Yoga Therap. 2013;23(1):11-6.
3. Markil N, Whitehurst M, Jacobs PL, Zoeller RF. Yoga Nidra relaxation increases heart rate variability and is unaffected by a prior bout of Hatha yoga. Altern Complement Med. 2012 Oct;18(10):953-8. doi: 10.1089/acm.2011.0331. Epub 2012 Aug 6.
4. Lou HC, Kjaer TW, Friberg L, Wildschiodtz G, Holm S, Nowak M. A 15O-H2O PET study of meditation and the resting state of normal consciousness. Hum Brain Mapp. 1999;7(2):98-105.
5. Mandlik, V., Jain, P., and Jain, K. (2002). Effect of Yoga Nidra on EEG (Electro - Encephalo - Graph). Yoga Vidya Dham. Available at www.yogapoint.com

6. livealifeyoulove.com.

Yoga and Safety

1. Ross A, Friedmann E, Bevans M, Thomas S. National Survey of Yoga Practitioners: Mental and Physical Health Benefits. Complementary therapies in medicine. 2013;21(4):313-323. doi:10.1016/j.ctim.2013.04.001.
2. https://nccih.nih.gov/research/statistics/2007/camsurvey_fs1.htm - accessed 2/23/18.
3. https://nccih.nih.gov/health/yoga - accessed 2/13/18.
4. Agarwal SK. Evidence Based Therapeutic Effects of Yoga. 2017.Available at: https://www.amazon.com/Evidence-Based-Therapeutic-EffectsYoga/dp/1983936367/ref=sr_1_3?s=books&ie=UTF8&qid=1517713441 &sr=1-3&keywords=agarwal+shashi+k.
5. Dangerfield A (2009) Yoga wars. BBC news magazine. 23 January 2009. Available: http://news.bbc.co.uk/1/hi/7844691.stm. Accessed 20 February 2013.
6. Penman S, Cohen M, Stevens P, Jackson S. Yoga in Australia: Results of a national survey. International Journal of Yoga. 2012;5(2):92-101. doi:10.4103/0973-6131.98217.
7. Cramer H, Krucoff C, Dobos G (2013) Adverse Events Associated with Yoga: A Systematic Review of Published Case Reports and Case Series. PLoS ONE 8(10): e75515. https://doi.org/10.1371/journal.pone.0075515
8. Swain TA, McGwin G. Yoga-Related Injuries in the United States From 2001 to 2014. Orthopaedic Journal of Sports Medicine. 2016;4(11):2325967116671703. doi:10.1177/2325967116671703.
9. Fishman LM, Saltonstall E, Genis S. Yoga therapy in practice; understanding and preventing yoga injuries. Int J Yoga Ther. 2009;19:123–128.
10. Cowen VS. Functional fitness improvements after a worksite-based yoga initiative. J Bodyw Mov Ther. 2010;14(1):50–4. doi: 10.1016/j.jbmt.2009.02.006.
11. Takeno M, Shimizu Y, Nakamura S. A case of femoral shaft fracture occurring during stretching exercise. J Clinical Sports Med. 1986;3(1):75–8.
12. Patel SC, Parker DA. Isolated rupture of the lateral collateral ligament during yoga practice: a case report. J Orthop Surg (Hong Kong) 2008;16(3):378–80.
13. Shah NJ, Shah UN. Central retinal vein occlusion following Sirsasana (headstand posture) Indian J Ophthalmol. 2009;57(1):69–70. doi: 10.4103/0301-4738.44496.
14. Johnson DB, Tierney MJ, Sadighi PJ. Kapalabhati pranayama: breath of fire or cause of pneumothorax? A case report. Chest. 2004;125(5):1951–2.
15. Holton MK, Barry AE. Do side-effects/injuries from yoga practice result in discontinued use? Results of a national survey. Int J Yoga. 2014;7:152–154.
16. Matsushita T, Oka T. A large-scale survey of adverse events experienced in yoga classes. Biopsychosoc Med. 2015;9:9. Published 2015 Mar 18. doi:10.1186/s13030-015-0037-1.
17. Mace C, Eggleston B. Self-Reported Benefits and Adverse Outcomes of Hot Yoga Participation. Int J Yoga Therap. 2016 Jan;26(1):49-53.
18. Saoji AA, Raghavendra BR, Manjunath NK. Effects of yogic breath regulation: A narrative review of scientific evidence. J Ayurveda Integr Med. 2018 Jan 30. pii: S0975-9476(17)30322-4. doi: 10.1016/j.jaim.2017.07.008.
19. Johnson DB, Tierney MJ, Sadighi PJ. Kapalabhati pranayama: breath of fire or cause of pneumothorax? A case report. Chest. 2004 May;125(5):1951-2.
20. Cebolla A, Demarzo M, Martins P, Soler J, Garcia-Campayo J. Unwanted effects: Is there a negative side of meditation? A multicentre survey. PLoS One. 2017;12(9):e0183137. Published 2017 Sep 5. doi:10.1371/journal.pone.0183137.
21. Cramer H, Ward L, Saper R, Fishbein D, Dobos G, Lauche R. The Safety of Yoga: A Systematic Review and Meta-Analysis of Randomized Controlled Trials. Am J Epidemiol. 2015. August;182: 281–293. doi: 10.1093/aje/kwv071.
22. Walsh R., Rochs L. Precipitation of acute psychotic episodes by intensive meditation in individuals with a history of schizophrenia. American Journal of Psychiatry. 1979. August;136: 1085–1086. doi: 10.1176/ajp.136.8.1085.
23. French AP, Schmid AC, Ingalls E. Transcendental meditation, altered reality testing, and behavioral change: a case report. J Nerv Ment Dis. 1975. July;161: 55–58.
24. Lustyk MKB, Chawla N, Nolan RS, Marlatt GA. Mindfulness meditation research: issues of participant screening, safety procedures, and researcher training. Adv Mind Body

Med. 2009;24: 20–30.
25. Kuijpers HJ., van der Heijden FMMA, Tuinier S, Verhoeven WMA. Meditation-Induced Psychosis. Psychopathology. 2007. September;40: 461–464. doi: 10.1159/000108125.
26. Lustyk MKB, Chawla N, Nolan RS, Marlatt GA. Mindfulness meditation research: issues of participant screening, safety procedures, and researcher training. Adv Mind Body Med. 2009;24: 20–30.
27. Banks K, Newman E, Saleem J. An Overview of the Research on Mindfulness-Based Interventions for Treating Symptoms of Posttraumatic Stress Disorder: A Systematic Review. J Clin Psychol. 2015. October;71: 935–963. doi: 10.1002/jclp.22200.
28. Jaseja H. Meditation potentially capable of increasing susceptibility to epilepsy—a follow-up hypothesis. Med Hypotheses. 2006;66: 925–928. doi: 10.1016/j.mehy.2005.11.043.

Yoga *Nidra* with Positive Affirmations

1. Suzanne N. Haber. Neuroanatomy of Reward: A View from the Ventral Striatum. Neurobiology of Sensation and Reward.Gottfried JA, editor. Boca Raton (FL): CRC Press/Taylor & Francis; 2011.
2. Dfarhud D, Malmir M, Khanahmadi M. "Happiness & Health: The Biological Factors-Systematic Review Article." Iranian Journal of Public Health 43.11 (2014): 1468–1477.

Yoga *Nidra* with Happy Visualization

1. Folkman S, Moskowitz JT. Positive affect and the other side of coping. American Psychologist. 2000;55:647–654.
2. Baur V, Hanggi J, Langer N, Jancke L (2013): Resting-state functional and structural connectivity within an insula-amygdala route specifically index state and trait anxiety. Biol Psychiatry 73:85–92.
3. Clewett D, Bachman S, Mather M (2014): Age-related reduced prefrontal-amygdala structural connectivity is associated with lower trait anxiety. Neuropsychology 28:631–642.
4. Tugade MM, Fredrickson BL. Resilient individuals use positive emotions to bounce back from negative emotional experiences. J Pers Soc Psychol. 2004;86:320–333.
5. Adcock RA, Thangavel A, Whitfield-Gabrieli S, Knutson B, Gabrieli JDE. Reward-motivated learning: mesolimbic activation precedes memory formation. Neuron. 2006;50:507–517.
6. Balleine BW, Delgado MR, Hikosaka O. The role of the dorsal striatum in reward and decision-making. J Neurosci. 2007;27:8161–8165.
7. Tugade MM, Fredrickson BL. Resilient individuals use positive emotions to bounce back from negative emotional experiences. J Pers Soc Psychol. 2004;86:320–333.
8. Ranganathan VK, Siemionow V, Liu JZ, Sahgal V, Yue GH. From mental power to muscle power--gaining strength by using the mind. Neuropsychologia. 2004;42(7):944-56.
9. Kramer M. The dream experience. A systematic exploration. New York: Brunner-Routledge; 2007. 243 ; Hartmann E, Brezler T. A Systematic Change in Dreams after 9/11/01. Sleep. 2008;31(2):213-218.
10. Weinstein N, Campbell R, Vansteenkiste M. Linking psychological need experiences to daily and recurring dreams. Motivation and Emotion. 2018;42(1):50-63. doi:10.1007/s11031-017-9656-0.

Yoga Nidra with Gratitude Recital

1. Wong Y. J., Owen J., Gabana N. T., Brown J. W., McInnis S., Toth P., et al. (2016). Does gratitude writing improve the mental health of psychotherapy clients? Evidence from a randomized controlled trial. Psychother. Res. 10.1080/10503307.2016.1169332.
2. Redwine L. S., Henry B. L., Pung M. A., Wilson K., Chinh K., Knight B., et al. (2016). Pilot randomized study of a gratitude journaling intervention on heart rate variability and inflammatory biomarkers in patients with stage B heart failure. Psychosom. Med. 78 667–676. 10.1097/PSY.0000000000000316.
3. Karns CM, Moore WE, Mayr U. The Cultivation of Pure Altruism via Gratitude: A

Functional MRI Study of Change with Gratitude Practice. Frontiers in Human Neuroscience. 2017;11:599. doi:10.3389/fnhum.2017.00599.

Health Benefits of Yoga

1. Agarwal SK. Health benefits of yoga. (Book) CreateSpace. 2018
2. Butzer B, van Over M, Noggle Taylor JJ, Khalsa SB. Yoga May Mitigate Decreases in High School Grades. Evid Based Complement Alternat Med. 2015;2015:259814. doi: 10.1155/2015/259814. Epub 2015 Aug 10.
3. Larson-Meyer DE. A Systematic Review of the Energy Cost and Metabolic Intensity of Yoga. Med Sci Sports Exerc. 2016 Aug;48(8):1558-69. doi: 10.1249/MSS.0000000000000922.
4. Witkiewitz K, Bowen S. Depression, craving, and substance use following a randomized trial of mindfulness-based relapse prevention. J Consult Clin Psychol. 2010;78(3):362–74.
5. Kumar SB, Yadav R, Yadav RK, Tolahunase M, Dada R. Telomerase activity and cellular aging might be positively modified by a yoga-based lifestyle intervention. J Altern Complement Med. 2015 Jun;21(6):370-2. doi: 10.1089/acm.2014.0298. Epub 2015 May 12.
6. Reddy S, Dick AM, Gerber MR, Mitchell K. The Effect of a Yoga Intervention on Alcohol and Drug Abuse Risk in Veteran and Civilian Women with Posttraumatic Stress Disorder. Journal of Alternative and Complementary Medicine. 2014;20(10):750-756. doi:10.1089/acm.2014.0014.
7. Deshpande S, Nagendra HR, Raghuram N. A randomized control trial of the effect of yoga on verbal aggressiveness in normal healthy volunteers. International Journal of Yoga. 2008;1(2):76-82. doi:10.4103/0973-6131.41034.
8. Gordon L, McGrowder DA, Pena YT, Cabrera E, Lawrence-Wright MB. Effect of yoga exercise therapy on oxidative stress indicators with end-stage renal disease on hemodialysis. Int J Yoga. 2013 Jan;6(1):31-8. doi: 10.4103/0973-6131.105944.
9. Michalsen A, Grossman P, Acil A, Langhorst J, Ludtke R, Esch T, et al. Rapid stress reduction and anxiolysis among distressed women because of a three-month intensive yoga program. Med Sci Monit (2005) 11(12):CR555–61.
10. Cheung C, Wyman JF, Resnick B, Savik K. Yoga for managing knee osteoarthritis in older women: a pilot randomized controlled trial. BMC Complementary and Alternative Medicine. 2014;14:160. doi:10.1186/1472-6882-14-160.
11. Manchanda SC, Narang R, Reddy KS, Sachdeva U, Prabhakaran D, Dharmanand S, et al. Retardation of coronary atherosclerosis with yoga lifestyle intervention. J Assoc Physicians India. 2000;48:687–94.
12. Tran M.D., Holly R.G., Lashbrook J., Amsterdam E.A.(2001) Effects of Hatha Yoga Practice on the Health-Related Aspects of Physical Fitness. Preventive Cardiology 4, 165-170.
13. Tiedemann A, O'Rourke S, Sesto R, Sherrington C. A 12-week Iyengar yoga program improved balance and mobility in older community-dwelling people: a pilot randomized controlled trial. J Gerontol A Biol Sci Med Sci. 2013 Sep;68(9):1068-75. doi: 10.1093/gerona/glt087. Epub 13 Jul 2.
14. Yurtkuran M, Alp A, Yurtkuran M, Dilek K. A modified yoga-based exercise program in hemodialysis patients: a randomized controlled study. Complement Ther Med. 2007 Sep;15(3):164-71. Epub 2006 Aug 22.
15. Chohan IS, Nayar HS, Thomas P, Geetha NS. Influence of yoga on blood coagulation. Thromb Haemost. 1984 Apr 30;51(2):196-7.
16. Paula Chu, Rinske A Gotink, Gloria Y Yeh et al. The effectiveness of yoga in modifying risk factors for cardiovascular disease and metabolic syndrome: A systematic review and meta-analysis of randomized controlled trials. European J of Preventive Cardiology. Vol 23, Issue 3, 2016.
17. Cui J, Yan J, Yan L, Pan L, Le J, Guo Y. Effects of yoga in adults with type 2 diabetes mellitus: A meta-analysis. Journal of Diabetes Investigation. 2017;8(2):201-209. doi:10.1111/jdi.12548.
18. Lu Y-H, Rosner B, Chang G, Fishman LM. Twelve-Minute Daily Yoga Regimen Reverses Osteoporotic Bone Loss. Topics in Geriatric Rehabilitation. 2016;32(2):81-87. doi:10.1097/TGR.0000000000000085.

19. Schumann D, Anheyer D, Lauche R, Dobos G, Langhorst J, Cramer H. Effect of Yoga in the Therapy of Irritable Bowel Syndrome: A Systematic Review. Clin Gastroenterol Hepatol. 2016 Dec;14(12):1720-1731. doi: 10.1016/j.cgh.2016.04.026. Epub 2016 Apr 22.
20. Wang DJJ, Rao HY, Korczykowski M, Wintering N, Pluta J, Khalsa DS, et al. Cerebral blood flow changes associated with different meditation practices and perceived depth of meditation. Psychiatry Res Neuroimaging (2011) 191(1):60–710.1016/j.pscychresns.2010.09.011.
21. Jim Lagopoulos, Jian Xu, Inge Rasmussen, Alexandra Vik, Gin S. Malhi, Carl F. Eliassen, Ingrid E. Arntsen, Jardar G. Sæther, Stig Hollup, Are Holen, Svend Davanger, and Øyvind Ellingsen. Increased theta and alpha EEG activity during nondirective meditation. The Journal of Alternative and Complementary Medicine. November 2009, 15(11): 1187-1192. https://doi.org/10.1089/acm.2009.0113.
22. Dinesh T, Gaur G, Sharma V, Madanmohan T, Harichandra Kumar K, Bhavanani A. Comparative effect of 12 weeks of slow and fast pranayama training on pulmonary function in young, healthy volunteers: A randomized controlled trial. International Journal of Yoga. 2015;8(1):22-26. doi:10.4103/0973-6131.146051.
23. Paula Chu, Rinske A Gotink, Gloria Y Yeh et al. The effectiveness of yoga in modifying risk factors for cardiovascular disease and metabolic syndrome: A systematic review and meta-analysis of randomized controlled trials. European J of Preventive Cardiology. Vol 23, Issue 3, 2016.
24. Parshad O, Richards A, Asnani M. Impact of yoga on haemodynamic function in healthy medical students. West Indian Med J. 2011 Mar;60(2):148-52.
25. Aggithaya MG, Narahari SR, Ryan TJ. Yoga for correction of lymphedema's impairment of gait as an adjunct to lymphatic drainage: A pilot observational study. International Journal of Yoga. 2015;8(1):54-61. doi:10.4103/0973-6131.146063.
26. Singh SN, Jaiswal V, Maurya SP. 'Shankha Prakshalyana' (Gastrointestinal Lavage) in health and disease. Ancient Science of Life. 1988;7(3-4):157-163.
27. Brunner D, Abramovitch A, Etherton J. A yoga program for cognitive enhancement. Lidzba K, ed. PLoS ONE. 2017;12(8):e0182366. doi:10.1371/journal.pone.0182366.
28. Davidson RJ, Kabat-Zinn J, Schumacher J, Rosenkranz M, Muller D, Santorelli SF, Urbanowski F, Harrington A, Bonus K, Sheridan JF. Alterations in brain and immune function produced by mindfulness meditation. Psychosom Med. 2003 Jul-Aug;65(4):564-70.
29. Lutz A, Slagter HA, Dunne JD, Davidson RJ. Attention regulation and monitoring in meditation. Trends Cogn Sci. 2008;12:163–169.
30. Tran MD, Holly RG, Lashbrook J, Amsterdam EA. Effects of Hatha Yoga Practice on the Health-Related Aspects of Physical Fitness. Prev Cardiol. 2001 Autumn;4(4):165-170.
31. Rathore M, Trivedi S, Abraham J, Sinha MB. Anatomical Correlation of Core Muscle Activation in Different Yogic Postures. International Journal of Yoga. 2017;10(2):59-66. doi:10.4103/0973-6131.205515.
32. Jitatmananda S. Ch. Consciousness: Evolution of Life through Higher Mind. In Life, Mind and Consciousness. Papers read at a seminar on 16, 17 and 18 Jan 2004 at Ramakrishna Mission Institute of Culture Gol Park.
33. Mishra SK, Singh P, Bunch SJ, Zhang R. The therapeutic value of yoga in neurological disorders. Annals of Indian Academy of Neurology. 2012;15(4):247-254. doi:10.4103/0972-2327.104328.
34. Katuri KK, Dasari AB, Kurapati S, Vinnakota NR, Bollepalli AC, Dhulipalla R. Association of yoga practice and serum cortisol levels in chronic periodontitis patients with stress-related anxiety and depression. J Int Soc Prev Community Dent. 2016 Jan-Feb;6(1):7-14. doi: 10.4103/2231-0762.175404.
35. Uebelacker LA, Broughton MK. Yoga for Depression and Anxiety: A Review of Published Research and Implications for Healthcare Providers. R I Med J (2013). 2016 Mar 1;99(3):20-2.
36. Hewett ZL, Cheema BS, Pumpa KL, Smith CA. The Effects of Bikram Yoga on Health: Critical Review and Clinical Trial Recommendations. Evidence-based Complementary and Alternative Medicine : eCAM. 2015;2015:428427. doi:10.1155/2015/428427.

37. Telles S, Singh N, Balkrishna A. Finger dexterity and visual discrimination following two yoga breathing practices. International Journal of Yoga. 2012;5(1):37-41. doi:10.4103/0973-6131.91710.
38. McIver S., McGartland M., O'Halloran P. 'Overeating is not about the food': women describe their experience of a yoga treatment program for binge eating. Qualitative Health Research. 2009;19(9):1234–1245. doi: 10.1177/1049732309343954.
39. Akhtar P, Yardi S, Akhtar M. Effects of yoga on functional capacity and well being. International Journal of Yoga. 2013;6(1):76-79. doi:10.4103/0973-6131.105952.
40. Bhutkar MV, Bhutkar PM, Taware GB, Surdi AD. How Effective Is Sun Salutation in Improving Muscle Strength, General Body Endurance and Body Composition? Asian Journal of Sports Medicine. 2011;2(4):259-266.
41. Ross A, Friedmann E, Bevans M, Thomas S. National Survey of Yoga Practitioners: Mental and Physical Health Benefits. Complementary therapies in medicine. 2013;21(4):313-323. doi:10.1016/j.ctim.2013.04.001.
42. Oken BS, Zajdel D, Kishiyama S, et al. Randomized, controlled, six-month trial of yoga in healthy seniors: Effects on cognition and quality of life. Altern Ther Health Med 2006; 12:40–47.
43. Nekavand M, Mobini N, Sheikhi A, Roshandel S, Sheikhi A. A survey on the impact of relaxation on anexiety and the result of IVF in patients with infertility that have been referd to the infertility centers of Tehran university of medical sciences during 2012–2013. J Urmia Nurs Midwifery Fac. 2015;13(7):605–12.
44. Gaurav V. Effects of hatha yoga training on the health related physical fitness. International Journal of Sports Science and Engineering. 2011;5:169–173.
45. Farinatti PT, Rubini EC, Silva EB, Vanfraechem JH. Flexibility of the elderly after one-year practice of yoga and calisthenics. Int J Yoga Therap. 2014;24:71-7.
46. Kaswala D, Shah S, Mishra A, et al. Can yoga be used to treat gastroesophageal reflux disease? International Journal of Yoga. 2013;6(2):131-133. doi:10.4103/0973-6131.113416.
47. Saatcioglu F. Regulation of gene expression by yoga, meditation and related practices: a review of recent studies. Asian J Psychiatr. 2013 Feb;6(1):74-7. doi: 10.1016/j.ajp.2012.10.002. Epub 2012 Nov 27.
48. Huberty J, Leiferman JA, Gold KJ, Rowedder L, Cacciatore J, McClain DB. Physical activity and depressive symptoms after stillbirth: informing future interventions. BMC Pregnancy and Childbirth. 2014;14:391. doi:10.1186/s12884-014-0391-1.
49. Afonso RF, Balardin JB, Lazar S, et al. Greater Cortical Thickness in Elderly Female Yoga Practitioners—A Cross-Sectional Study. Frontiers in Aging Neuroscience. 2017;9:201. doi:10.3389/fnagi.2017.00201.
50. Monk-Turner E, Turner C. Does yoga shape body, mind and spiritual health and happiness: Differences between yoga practitioners and college students. Int J Yoga. 2010 Jul;3(2):48-54. doi: 10.4103/0973-6131.72630.
51. John PJ, Sharma N, Sharma CM, Kankane A. Effectiveness of yoga therapy in the treatment of migraine without aura: a randomized controlled trial. Headache. 2007 May;47(5):654-61.
52. Rao RM, Nagendra HR, Raghuram N, et al. Influence of yoga on postoperative outcomes and wound healing in early operable breast cancer patients undergoing surgery. International Journal of Yoga. 2008;1(1):33-41. doi:10.4103/0973-6131.36795.
53. Yogendra J, Yogendra H, Ambardekar S, et al. Beneficial effects of yoga lifestyle on reversibility of ischaemic heart disease: Caring Heart Project of International Board of Yoga. JAPI. 2004; 52:283.
54. Miles SC, Chun-Chung C, Hsin-Fu L, Hunter SD, Dhindsa M, Nualnim N, Tanaka H. Arterial blood pressure and cardiovascular responses to yoga practice. Altern Ther Health Med. 2013 Jan-Feb;19(1):38-45.
55. Paula Chu, Rinske A Gotink, Gloria Y Yeh et al. The effectiveness of yoga in modifying risk factors for cardiovascular disease and metabolic syndrome: A systematic review and meta-analysis of randomized controlled trials. European J of Preventive Cardiology. Vol 23, Issue 3, 2016.

56. Morgan N, Irwin MR, Chung M, Wang C. The effects of mind-body therapies on the immune system: meta-analysis. PLoS One. 2014 Jul 2;9(7): e100903. doi: 10.1371/journal.pone.0100903. eCollection 2014.
57. Huang AJ, Jenny HE, Chesney MA, Schembri M, Subak LL. A Group-Based Yoga Therapy Intervention for Urinary Incontinence in Women: A Pilot Randomized Trial. Female pelvic medicine & reconstructive surgery. 2014;20(3):147-154.
58. Falkenberg RI, Eising C, Peters ML. Yoga and immune system functioning: a systematic review of randomized controlled trials. J Behav Med. 2018 Feb 10. doi: 10.1007/s10865-018-9914-y.
59. Kumar S, Prasad S, Balakrishnan B, Muthukumaraswamy K, Ganesan M. Effects of Isha Hatha Yoga on Core Stability and Standing Balance. Adv Mind Body Med. 2016 Spring;30(2):4-10.
60. Taylor MJ. Yoga therapeutics: an ancient, dynamic systems theory. Tech Orthop. 2003;18:115–125.
61. Ross A, Friedmann E, Bevans M, Thomas S. National Survey of Yoga Practitioners: Mental and Physical Health Benefits. Complementary therapies in medicine. 2013;21(4):313-323. doi:10.1016/j.ctim.2013.04.001.
62. Ross A, Bevans M, Friedmann E, Williams L, Thomas S. "I Am a Nice Person When I Do Yoga!!!": A Qualitative Analysis of How Yoga Affects Relationships. Journal of holistic nursing: official journal of the American Holistic Nurses' Association. 2014;32(2):67-77. doi:10.1177/0898010113508466.
63. Jacobs TL, Epel ES, Lin J, Blackburn EH, Wolkowitz OM, Bridwell DA, Zanesco AP, Aichele SR, Sahdra BK, MacLean KA, King BG, Shaver PR, Rosenberg EL, Ferrer E, Wallace BA, Saron CD. Intensive meditation training, immune cell telomerase activity, and psychological mediators. Psychoneuroendocrinology. 2011 Jun;36(5):664-81. doi: 10.1016/j.psyneuen.2010.09.010. Epub 2010 Oct 29.
64. Karthik PS, Chandrasekhar M, Ambareesha K, Nikhil C. Effect of Pranayama and Suryanamaskar on Pulmonary Functions in Medical Students. Journal of Clinical and Diagnostic Research: JCDR. 2014;8(12): BC04-BC06. doi:10.7860/JCDR/2014/10281.5344.
65. Gothe NP, Kramer AF, McAuley E. The Effects of an 8-Week Hatha Yoga Intervention on Executive Function in Older Adults. The Journals of Gerontology Series A: Biological Sciences and Medical Sciences. 2014;69(9):1109-1116. doi:10.1093/gerona/glu095.
66. Vaze N, Joshi S. Yoga and menopausal transition. Indian Menopause Society. J Midlife Health. 2010;1:56–58.
67. Premenstrual symptoms: Effect of Yoga Exercise on Premenstrual Symptoms among Female Employees in Taiwan. Su-Ying Tsai. Int J Environ Res Public Health. 2016 Jul; 13(7): 721. Published online 2016 Jul 16. doi: 10.3390/ijerph13070721.
68. Siu PM, Yu AP, Benzie IF, Woo J. Effects of 1-year yoga on cardiovascular risk factors in middle-aged and older adults with metabolic syndrome: a randomized trial. Diabetol Metab Syndr. 2015;7:40.
69. Lau C, Yu R, Woo J. Effects of a 12-Week Hatha Yoga Intervention on Cardiorespiratory Endurance, Muscular Strength and Endurance, and Flexibility in Hong Kong Chinese Adults: A Controlled Clinical Trial. Evidence-based Complementary and Alternative Medicine : eCAM. 2015;2015:958727. doi:10.1155/2015/958727.
70. Davidson RJ, Lutz A. Buddha's Brain: Neuroplasticity and Meditation. IEEE signal processing magazine. 2008;25(1):176-174.
71. Jain N, Srivastava RD, Singhal A. The effects of right and left nostril breathing on cardiorespiratory and autonomic parameters. Indian J Physiol Pharmacol. 2005;49:469–74.
72. Büssing A, Ostermann T, Lüdtke R, et al. Effects of yoga interventions on pain and pain-associated disability: a meta-analysis. J Pain, 2012, 13: 1–9.
73. Jerath R., Edry J. W., Barnes V. et al. Iyengar Yoga Increases Cardiac Parasympathetic Nervous Modulation Among Healthy Yoga Practitioners. Evidence-based Complementary and Alternative Medicine: eCAM. 2007;4(4):511-517. doi:10.1093/ecam/nem087.
74. Strijk JE, Proper KI, van Mechelen W, van der Beek AJ. Effectiveness of a worksite lifestyle intervention on vitality, work engagement, productivity, and sick leave: results of a

75. Deshpande S, Nagendra HR, Nagarathna R. A randomized control trial of the effect of yoga on Gunas (personality) and Self esteem in normal healthy volunteers. Int J Yoga 2009;2:13-21.
76. Amaranath B, Nagendra HR, Deshpande S. Effect of integrated Yoga module on positive and negative emotions in Home Guards in Bengaluru: A wait list randomized control trial. International Journal of Yoga. 2016;9(1):35-43. doi:10.4103/0973-6131.171719.
77. Kelley KK, Aaron D, Hynds K, Machado E, Wolff M. The Effects of a Therapeutic Yoga Program on Postural Control, Mobility, and Gait Speed in Community-Dwelling Older Adults. Journal of Alternative and Complementary Medicine. 2014;20(12):949-954. doi:10.1089/acm.2014.0156.
78. Curtis K, Weinrib A, Katz J. Systematic Review of Yoga for Pregnant Women: Current Status and Future Directions. Evidence-based Complementary and Alternative Medicin : eCAM. 2012;2012:715942. doi:10.1155/2012/715942.
79. McCall MC, Ward A, Roberts NW, Heneghan C. Overview of systematic reviews: Yoga as a therapeutic intervention for adults with acute and chronic health conditions. Evid Based Complement Alternat Med 2013. 2013:945895.
80. Oken BS, Zajdel D, Kishiyama S, et al. Randominzed, controlled, six-month trial of yoga in healthy seniors: effects on cognition and quality of life. Altern Ther Health Med 2006;12:40–47.
81. Ross A, Bevans M, Friedmann E, Williams L, Thomas S. "I Am a Nice Person When I Do Yoga!!!": A Qualitative Analysis of How Yoga Affects Relationships. Journal of holistic nursing: official journal of the American Holistic Nurses' Association. 2014;32(2):67-77.
82. Manjunath NK, Telles S. Influence of Yoga and Ayurveda on self rated sleep in a geriatric population. Indian J Med Res. 2005;121:683–690.
83. Madanmohan, Mahadevan SK, Balakrishnan S, Gopalakrishnan M, Prakash ES. Effect of six weeks yoga training for weight loss following step test, respiratory pressures, handgrip strength and handgrip endurance in young healthy subjects. Indian J Physiol Pharmacol. 2008;52:164–70.
84. Birdee GS, Sohl SJ, Wallston K. Development and Psychometric Properties of the Yoga Self-Efficacy Scale (YSES). BMC Complementary and Alternative Medicine. 2016;16:3. doi:10.1186/s12906-015-0981-0.
85. Alexander CN, Rainforth MV, Gelderloos P. Trancendental meditation, self-actualization, and psychological health: A Conceptual overview and statistical meta-analysis. J Soc Behav Pers. 1991;6:189.
86. Prasad L, Varrey A, Sisti G. Medical Students' Stress Levels and Sense of Well Being after Six Weeks of Yoga and Meditation. Evid Based Complement Alternat Med. 2016;2016:9251849. doi: 10.1155/2016/9251849.
87. Kim HN, Ryu J, Kim KS, Song SW. Effects of yoga on sexual function in women with metabolic syndrome: a randomized controlled trial. J Sex Med. 2013 Nov;10(11):2741-51. doi: 10.1111/jsm.12283. Epub 2013 Jul 30.
88. Achilles N, Mösges R. Nasal saline irrigations for the symptoms of acute and chronic rhinosinusitis. Curr Allergy Asthma Rep. 2013 Apr;13(2):229-35. doi: 10.1007/s11882-013-0339-y.
89. Taibi DM, Vitiello MV. A pilot study of gentle yoga for sleep disturbance in women with osteoarthritis. Sleep medicine. 2011;12(5):512-517. doi:10.1016/j.sleep.2010.09.016.
90. Oikonomou MT, Arvanitis M, Sokolove RL. Mindfulness training for smoking cessation: a meta-analysis of randomized-controlled trials. J Health Psychol. 2016. April 4. pii: 1359105316637667.
91. Ross A, Friedmann E, Bevans M, Thomas S. National Survey of Yoga Practitioners: Mental and Physical Health Benefits. Complementary therapies in medicine. 2013;21(4):313-323. doi:10.1016/j.ctim.2013.04.001.
92. Chou R, Huffman LH. Nonpharmacologic therapies for acute and chronic low back pain: a review of the evidence for an American Pain Society/American College of Physicians clinical

practice guideline. Ann Intern Med. 2007;147:492–504. doi: 10.7326/0003-4819-147-7-200710020-00007.
93. Büssing A, Hedtstück A, Khalsa SBS, Ostermann T, Heusser P. Development of Specific Aspects of Spirituality during a 6-Month Intensive Yoga Practice. Evidence-based Complementary and Alternative Medicine: eCAM. 2012;2012:981523.
94. Hewett ZL, Pumpa KL, Smith CA, Fahey PP, Cheema BS. Effect of a 16-week Bikram yoga program on perceived stress, self-efficacy and health-related quality of life in stressed and sedentary adults: A randomised controlled trial. J Sci Med Sport. 2017 Aug 24. pii: S1440-2440(17)30994-5. doi: 10.1016/j.jsams.2017.08.006
95. Schmid AA, Miller KK, Van Puymbroeck M, DeBaun-Sprague E. Yoga leads to multiple physical improvements after stroke, a pilot study. Complement Ther Med. 2014 Dec;22(6):994-1000. doi: 10.1016/j.ctim.2014.09.005. Epub 2014 Oct 7.
96. Vempati RP, Telles S. Yoga-based guided relaxation reduces sympathetic activity judged from baseline levels. Psychol Rep. 2002;90:487–94.
97. Patil SG, Aithala MR, Das KK. Effect of yoga on arterial stiffness in elderly subjects with increased pulse pressure: A randomized controlled study. Complement Ther Med. 2015 Aug;23(4):562-9. doi: 10.1016/j.ctim.2015.06.002.
98. Daley WJ, Krum Holz RA, Ross JC. The venous pump in the legs as a determinant of pulmonary filling capacity. J Clin Invest. 1965;44:271.
99. Telles S, Naveen K, Dash M, Deginal R, Manjunath N. Effect of yoga on self-rated visual discomfort in computer users. Head & Face Medicine. 2006;2:46. doi:10.1186/1746-160X-2-46.
100. Paula Chu, Rinske A Gotink, Gloria Y Yeh et al. The effectiveness of yoga in modifying risk factors for cardiovascular disease and metabolic syndrome: A systematic review and meta-analysis of randomized controlled trials. European J of Preventive Cardiology. Vol 23, Issue 3, 2016.

Medical Benefits of Yoga

1. Agarwal SK. Therapeutic benefits of yoga. (Book) 2018.
2. Mishra SK, Singh P, Bunch SJ, Zhang R. The therapeutic value of yoga in neurological disorders. Annals of Indian Academy of Neurology. 2012;15(4):247-254. doi:10.4103/0972-2327.104328.
3. Kirkwood G, Rampes H, Tuffrey V, Richardson J, Pilkington K, Ramaratnam S. Yoga for anxiety: a systematic review of the research evidence. British Journal of Sports Medicine. 2005;39(12):884-891. doi:10.1136/bjsm.2005.018069.
4. Cramer H, Posadzki P, Dobos G, et al. Yoga for asthma: a systematic review and meta-analysis. Ann Allergy Asthma Immunol. 2014 Jun;112(6):503-510.
5. Peck H.L., Kehle T.J., Bray M.A., Theodore L.A. Yoga as an intervention for children with attention problems. Sch. Psychol. Rev. 2005;34:415–424.
6. Koenig K. P., Buckley-Reen A., Garg S. Efficacy of the get ready to learn yoga program among children with autism spectrum disorders: a pretest-posttest control group design. American Journal of Occupational Therapy. 2012;66(5):538–546. doi: 10.5014/ajot.2012.004390.
7. Cramer H, Lauche R, Haller H, Dobos G. A systematic review and meta-analysis of yoga for low back pain. Clin J Pain. 2013;29(5):450–460. doi: 10.1097/AJP.0b013e31825e1492.
8. Singh P, Chaturvedi A. Complementary and Alternative Medicine in Cancer Pain Management: A Systematic Review. Indian Journal of Palliative Care. 2015;21(1):105-115.
9. Gomes-Neto M, Rodrigues-Jr ES, Silva-Jr WM, Carvalho VO. Effects of Yoga in Patients with Chronic Heart Failure: A Meta-Analysis. Arquivos Brasileiros de Cardiologia. 2014;103(5):433-439. doi:10.5935/abc.20140149.
10. Garfinkel MS, Singhal A, Katz WA, Allan DA, Reshetar R, Schumacher HR., Jr Yoga-based intervention for carpal tunnel syndrome: a randomized trial. JAMA. 1998;280:1601–3.
11. Catherine Mak, Koa Whittingham, Ross Cunnington, Roslyn N Boyd. MiYoga: a randomised controlled trial of a mindfulness movement programme based on hatha yoga principles for

children with cerebral palsy: a study protocol. BMJ Open. 2017; 7(7): e015191. Published online 2017 Jul 10. doi: 10.1136/bmjopen-2016-015191.
12. Oka T, Tanahashi T, Chijiwa T, Lkhagvasuren B, Sudo N, Oka K. Isometric yoga improves the fatigue and pain of patients with chronic fatigue syndrome who are resistant to conventional therapy: a randomized, controlled trial. Biopsychosocial Medicine. 2014;8:27. doi:10.1186/s13030-014-0027-8.
13. Rajendra Kumar Pandey, Tung Vir Singh Arya, Amit Kumar, Ashish Yadav. Effects of 6 months yoga program on renal functions and quality of life in patients suffering from chronic kidney disease. Int J Yoga. 2017 Jan-Apr; 10(1): 3–8. doi: 10.4103/0973-6131.186158.
14. (COPD)Pomidori L, Campigotto F, Amatya TM, et al. Efficacy and tolerability of yoga breathing in patients with chronic obstructive pulmonary disease: a pilot study. J Cardiopulm Rehabil Prev. 2009 Mar-Apr;29(2):133-7.
15. Yogendra J, Yogendra H, Ambardekar S, et al. Beneficial effects of yoga lifestyle on reversibility of ischaemic heart disease: Caring Heart Project of International Board of Yoga. JAPI. 2004; 52:283.
16. Krishna BH, et al. Effect of yoga therapy on heart rate, blood pressure and cardiac autonomic function in heart failure. J Clin Diagn Res. 2014 Jan;8(1):14-6. doi: 10.7860/JCDR/2014/7844.3983. Epub 2014 Jan 12.
17. Kinser PA, Bourguignon C, Whaley D, Hauenstein E, Taylor AG. Feasibility, acceptability, and effects of gentle Hatha yoga for women with major depression: Findings from a randomized controlled mixed-methods study. Archives of psychiatric nursing. 2013;27(3):137-147. doi:10.1016/j.apnu.2013.01.003.
18. Innes KE, Selfe TK. Yoga for Adults with Type 2 Diabetes: A Systematic Review of Controlled Trials. Journal of Diabetes Research. 2016;2016:6979370. doi:10.1155/2016/6979370.
19. Khalsa, S.B.S., Khalsa, G.S., Khalsa, H.K., and Khalsa, M.K. Evaluation of a residential Kundalini yoga lifestyle pilot program for addiction in India. J. Ethn. Subst. Abuse. 2008; 7: 67–79.DOI: dx.doi.org/10.1080/15332640802081968.
20. McIver S, O'Halloran P, McGartland M. Yoga as a treatment for binge eating disorder: a preliminary study. Complement Ther Med. 2009 Aug;17(4):196-202. doi: 10.1016/j.ctim.2009.05.002. Epub 2009 Jun 13.
21. Panebianco M, Sridharan K, Ramaratnam S. Yoga for epilepsy. Cochrane Database Syst Rev. 2017 Oct 5;10:CD001524.
22. Curtis K, Osadchuk A, Katz J. An eight-week yoga intervention is associated with improvements in pain, psychological functioning and mindfulness, and changes in cortisol levels in women with fibromyalgia. Journal of Pain Research. 2011;4:189-201. doi:10.2147/JPR.S22761.
23. Hagins M, States R, Selfe T, et al. Effectiveness of Yoga for Hypertension: Systematic Review and Meta-Analysis Evidence-Based Complementary and Alternative Medicine. Volume 2013 (2013), Article ID 649836.
24. Duncan LG, Moskowitz JT, Neilands TB, Dilworth SE, Hecht FM, Johnson MO. Mindfulness-Based Stress Reduction for HIV Treatment Side Effects: A Randomized Wait-List Controlled Trial. Journal of Pain and Symptom Management. 2012;43(2):161-171. doi:10.1016/j.jpainsymman.2011.04.007.
25. Sengupta P, Chaudhuri P, Bhattacharya K. Male reproductive health and yoga. International Journal of Yoga. 2013;6(2):87-95. doi:10.4103/0973-6131.113391.
26. Mustian KM, Sprod LK, Janelsins M, et al. Multicenter, Randomized Controlled Trial of Yoga for Sleep Quality Among Cancer Survivors. Journal of Clinical Oncology. 2013;31(26):3233-3241. doi:10.1200/JCO.2012.43.7707.
27. Evans S, Lung KC, Seidman LC, Sternlieb B, Zeltzer LK, Tsao JCI. Iyengar Yoga for Adolescents and Young Adults With Irritable Bowel Syndrome. Journal of pediatric gastroenterology and nutrition. 2014;59(2):244-253.
28. Vaze N, Joshi S. Yoga and menopausal transition. Indian Menopause Society. J Midlife Health. 2010;1:56–58.

29. Premenstrual symptoms: Effect of Yoga Exercise on Premenstrual Symptoms among Female Employees in Taiwan. Su-Ying Tsai. Int J Environ Res Public Health. 2016 Jul; 13(7): 721. Published online 2016 Jul 16. doi: 10.3390/ijerph13070721.
30. Stephanie J. Sohl, Kenneth A. Wallston, Keiana Watkins, Gurjeet S. Birdee. Yoga for Risk Reduction of Metabolic Syndrome: Patient-Reported Outcomes from a Randomized Controlled Pilot Study. Evid Based Complement Alternat Med. 2016; 2016: 3094589.
31. Kisan R, Sujan M, Adoor M, et al. Effect of Yoga on migraine: A comprehensive study using clinical profile and cardiac autonomic functions. International Journal of Yoga. 2014;7(2):126-132. doi:10.4103/0973-6131.133891.
32. Guner S, Inanici F. Yoga therapy and ambulatory multiple sclerosis assessment of gait analysis parameters, fatigue, and balance. J Body Move Ther 2015;19:72–81.
33. Charlene Marie Muhammad, Steffany Haaz Moonaz. Yoga as Therapy for Neurodegenerative Disorders: A Case Report of Therapeutic Yoga for Adrenomyeloneuropathy. Integr Med (Encinitas) 2014 Jun; 13(3): 33–39.
34. Grover P, Varma VK, Pershad D, Verma SK. Role Of Yoga In The Treatment Of Neurotic Disorders: Current Status And Future Directions. Indian Journal of Psychiatry. 1994;36(4):153-162.
35. Rioux JG, Ritenbaugh C. Narrative review of yoga intervention clinical trials including weight-related outcomes. Altern Ther Health Med. 2013 May-Jun;19(3):32-46.
36. Shannahoff-Khalsa DS, Ray LE, Levine S, Gallen CC, Schwartz BJ, Sidorowich JJ. Randomized controlled trial of yogic meditation techniques for patients with obsessive-compulsive disorder. CNS Spectr. 1999 Dec;4(12):34-47.
37. Moonaz S, Bingham CO, Wissow L, Bartlett SJ. Yoga in sedentary adults with arthritis: effcts of a randomized controlled pragmatic trial. The Journal of rheumatology. 2015;42(7):1194-1202. doi:10.3899/jrheum.141129.
38. Lu Y-H, Rosner B, Chang G, Fishman LM. Twelve-Minute Daily Yoga Regimen Reverses Osteoporotic Bone Loss. Topics in Geriatric Rehabilitation. 2016;32(2):81-87. doi:10.1097/TGR.0000000000000085.
39. Surinder Sareen, Vinita Kumari, Karaminder Singh Gajebasia, Nimanpreet Kaur Gajebasia. Yoga: A tool for improving the quality of life in chronic pancreatitis. World J Gastroenterol. 2007 Jan 21; 13(3): 391–397.
40. Neena K Sharma, Kristin Robbins, Kathleen Wagner, Yvonne M Colgrove. A randomized controlled pilot study of the therapeutic effects of yoga in people with Parkinson's disease. Int J Yoga. 2015 Jan-Jun; 8(1): 74–79. doi: 10.4103/0973-6131.146070.
41. Kishore Kumar Katuri, Ankineedu Babu Dasari, Sruthi Kurapati, Narayana Rao Vinnakota, Appaiah Chowdary Bollepalli, Ravindranath Dhulipalla. Association of yoga practice and serum cortisol levels in chronic periodontitis patients with stress-related anxiety and depression. J Int Soc Prev Community Dent. 2016 Jan-Feb; 6(1): 7–14. doi: 10.4103/2231-0762.175404.
42. Prakasamma M, Bhaduri A. A study of yoga as a nursing intervention in the care of patients with pleural effusion. J Adv. Nurs. 1984 Mar;9(2):127-33.
43. Ram Nidhi, Venkatram Padmalatha, Raghuram Nagarathna, Ram Amritanshu. Effect of holistic yoga program on anxiety symptoms in adolescent girls with polycystic ovarian syndrome: A randomized control trial. Int J Yoga. 2012 Jul-Dec; 5(2): 112–117. doi: 10.4103/0973-6131.98223.
44. Tyagi I; Sharma UD; Bajaj P; Husain T; Gupta S; Lamba PS; Khan A. Evaluation of pink city lung exerciser for prevention of pulmonary complications following upper abdominal surgery. Indian Journal of Anaesthesia. 1991 Dec; 39(6): 198-203.
45. Bastille JV, Gill-Body KM. A yoga-based exercise program for people with chronic poststroke hemiparesis. Phys Ther. 2004; 84:33–48.
46. Chuntharapat S, Petpichetchian W, Hatthakit U. Yoga during pregnancy: effects on maternal comfort, labor pain and birth outcomes. Complement Ther Clin Pract. 2008;14(2):105–15.

47. Bernhard, J., Kristeller, J. and Kabat-Zinn, J. Effectiveness of relaxation and visualization techniques as a adjunct to phototherapy and photochemotherapy of psoriasis. J. Am. Acad. Dermatol. (1988) 19:572-73.
48. Jingxia Lin, Sherry KW Chan, Edwin HM Lee, Wing Chung Chang, Michael Tse, Wayne Weizhong Su, Pak Sham, Christy LM Hui, Glen Joe, Cecilia LW Chan, P L Khong, Kwok Fai So, William G Honer, Eric YH Chen. Aerobic exercise and yoga improve neurocognitive function in women with early psychosis. NPJ Schizophr. 2015; 1(0): 15047.
49. van der Kolk BA, Stone L, West J, et al. Yoga as an adjunctive treatment for posttraumatic stress disorder: a randomized controlled trial. J Clin Psychiatry. 2014;75:e559–e565. doi: 10.4088/JCP.13m08561.
50. Innes KE, Selfe TK, Agarwal P, Williams K, Flack KL. Efficacy of an Eight-Week Yoga Intervention on Symptoms of Restless Legs Syndrome (RLS): A Pilot Study. Journal of Alternative and Complementary Medicine. 2013;19(6):527-535. doi:10.1089/acm.2012.0330.
51. Evans S, Moieni M, Lung K, et al. Impact of Iyengar yoga on quality of life in young women with rheumatoid arthritis. The Clinical journal of pain. 2013;29(11):988-997. doi:10.1097/AJP.0b013e31827da381.
52. Adappa ND, Wei CC, Palmer JN. Nasal irrigation with or without drugs: the evidence. Curr Opin Otolaryngol Head Neck Surg. 2012 Feb;20(1):53-7. doi: 10.1097/MOO.0b013e32834dfa80.
53. Vancampfort D, Vansteelandt K, Scheewe T, Probst M, Knapen J, De Herdt A, De Hert M. Yoga in schizophrenia: a systematic review of randomised controlled trials. Acta Psychiatr Scand. 2012 Jul;126(1):12-20. doi: 10.1111/j.1600-0447.2012.01865.x. Epub 2012 Apr 6.
54. Loren M. Fishman, Erik J. Groessl, Karen J. Sherman. Serial Case Reporting Yoga for Idiopathic and Degenerative Scoliosis. Glob Adv Health Med. 2014 Sep; 3(5): 16–21.
55. Thind H, Jennings E, Fava JL, et al. Differences between Men and Women Enrolling in Smoking Cessation Programs Using Yoga as a Complementary Therapy. Journal of yoga & physical therapy. 2016;6(3):245. doi:10.4172/2157-7595.1000245.
56. Visweswaraiah NK, Telles S. Randomized trial of yoga as a complementary therapy for pulmonary tuberculosis. Respirology. 2004 Mar;9(1):96-101.
57. Huang AJ, Jenny HE, Chesney MA, Schembri M, Subak LL. A Group-Based Yoga Therapy Intervention for Urinary Incontinence in Women: A Pilot Randomized Trial. Female pelvic medicine & reconstructive surgery. 2014;20(3):147-154. doi:10.1097/SPV.0000000000000072.

RESOURCES

Yoga Books

- The Yoga Bible. Christina Brown. Walking Stick Press
- The Women's Health Big Book of Yoga: The Essential Guide to Complete Mind/Body Fitness. Kathryn Budig. Rodale Books
- Light on Yoga. B.K.S. Iyengar. Harper Collins Publishers
- Yoga as Medicine: The Yogic Prescription for Health and Healing. Timothy Mccall. Bantam.
- Evidence Based Health Benefits of Yoga. Shashi K. Agarwal, MD. CreateSpace Independent Publishing (Amazon)
- The Yoga Sutras of Patanjali. Integral Yoga Publications
- Evidence Based Therapeutic Effects of Yoga. Shashi K. Agarwal, MD. CreateSpace Independent Publishing (Amazon) Books
- Principles and Practice of Yoga in Health Care. Sat Bir Khalsa, Lorenzo Cohen, Timothy McCall, Shirley Telles. Handspring Publishing.
- Medical Therapeutic Yoga. Ginger Garner. Handspring Publishing.

Yoga Music

- https://open.spotify.com/album/3QBpwvP9jwNdVlksVogs9f
- https://www.doyouyoga.com/yoga-music/
- https://www.yogajournal.com/lifestyle/10-best-yoga-tunes-year
- Despierta by Mirabai Ceiba (www.mirabaiceiba.com)
- Sunshine by Matisyahu (www.matisyahuworld.com)
- Sleep meditations by Nirinjan Kaur (www.spiritvoyage.com)
- Bhakti without borders by Madi Das (https://kirtanshakti.bandcamp.com/album/bhakti-without-borders)
- Jai-jagdeesh (soundcloud.com/jai-jagdeesh)
- Ritual Mystical by M.C.Yogi (www.mcyogi.com)
- Kundalini Chillout: Liquid Mantra Remixes by Krishan (https://www.allmusic.com/album/kundalini-chillout-liquid-mantra-remixes-by-krishan-mw0002705460)
- Trevor Hall (www.trevorhallmusic.com)
- Illumine nation by Bachan Kaur (www.huemanbeing.com)
- Yoga Nidra by Max Gandossi (https://www.amazon.com/Yoga-Nidra-Original-Mix/dp/B00UEGC7EW)
- Papillion by Peter Samuels
- Beloved by Snatam Kaur (www.snatamkaur.com)

Yoga Teachers

- Check Yoga Journal for listing (1-800-600-9642)
- Write or call Yoga Alliance
  1560 Wilson Blvd #700, Arlington, VA 22209 (888) 921-9642

Yoga props

- http://www.yogaprops.com/
- https://www.yogaaccessories.com
- https://www.yogadirect.com
- https://www.yogaoutlet.com
- https://www.gaiam.com
- https://www.manduka.com

Professional Yoga Associations

- iayt.org (International Association of Yoga Therapists)
- yogaalliance.org (Yoga Alliance)

Non-professional Yoga Magazines

- Australian Yoga Life
- Integral Yoga Magazine
- LA Yoga
- OM Yoga & Lifestyle Magazine
- Yoga Journal

Professional Associations

- American Academy of Neurology (ana.org)
- American Association of Clinical Endocrinologists (aace.org)
- American Association of Cardiovascular and Pulmonary Rehabilitation (aacvpr.org)
- American College of Cardiology (acc.org)
- American College of Chest Physicians (chestnet.org)
- American College of Sports Medicine (acsm.org)
- American Diabetes Association (diabetes.org)
- American Heart Association (heart.org)
- American Lung Association (lung.org)
- American Neurological Association (myana.org)
- American Psychiatric Association (psychiatry.org)
- American Sexual Health Association (ashasexualhealth.org)
- American Society of Echocardiography (asecho.org)
- American Society of Nuclear Cardiology (asnc.org)
- American Stroke Association (strokeassociation.org)
- American Thoracic Society (thoracic.org)
- American Urological Association (urologyhealth.org)
- Endocrine Society (endo.org)
- Heart Failure Society of America (hfsa.org)
- International Society of Hypertension (ishworld.com)
- National Lipid Association (lipid.org)
- National Stroke Association (stroke.org)
- Obesity Society (obesity.org)

ABOUT THE AUTHOR

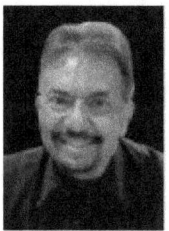

Shashi K. Agarwal, MD obtained his Internal Medicine Board Certification in 1979 and his Cardiovascular Board Certification in 1981. He completed his Cardiovascular Fellowship at the University of New Mexico, Albuquerque. He has been a Fellow of the American College of Cardiology and the American College of Physicians and many other professional associations in the past. He has presented research data both nationally and internationally and has published extensively in scientific journals all over the world. He is a reviewer for several medical journals. He is also a certified yoga teacher.

Dr. Agarwal may be reached at usacardiologist@gmail.com

Also by the author

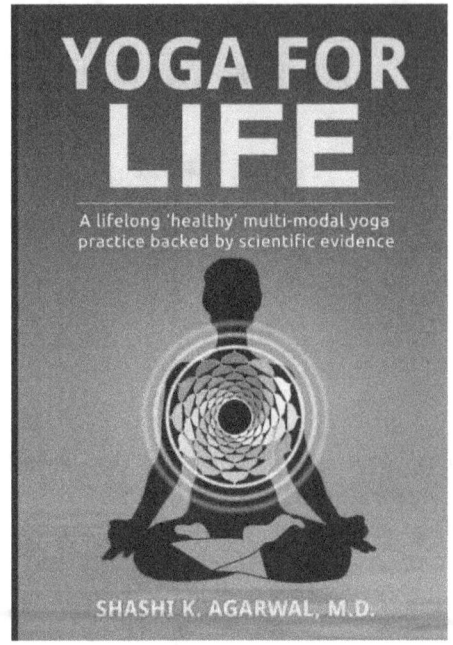

454 pages $18.99

AVAILABLE AT AMAZON.COM

AND OTHER RETAILERS

www.ingramcontent.com/pod-product-compliance
Lightning Source LLC
Chambersburg PA
CBHW081343280526
45788CB00009B/2756